The Health of Adult Britain
1841-1994

Volume 2

Chapters 15-27

Editors: John Charlton
Mike Murphy

Decennial Supplement No. 13

London: The Stationery Office

ISBN 0 11 691696 6

0116209097

Other reports in this series

Occupational Health - decennial supplement
ISBN 0 11 691618 4 price £29

The Health of our Children
ISBN 0 11 691643 5 price £21

The views expressed in this report are not necessarily those of the Office for National Statistics.

Contents

Tables and figures

Page

Page

22 Digestive diseases

23 Musculoskeletal diseases

Page

24   Accidents: trends in mortality and morbidity

Tables

Figures

25   Are we healthier?

Tables

Figures

26   The health and health care of older adults in England and Wales, 1841-1994

Tables

27   Trends and prospects at very high ages

Foreword

These two volumes bring together a wide range of information about the health of adults, covering a period of over 150 years. More than forty expert authors have generously donated their time to this comprehensive review, and our thanks are due to them for the result. The first volume presents general material on morbidity, mortality, and trends in behavioural and environmental factors known to be associated with health. The second considers specific major categories of diseases, the elderly, and changes in health generally in the most recent ten years.

The Health of Adult Britain is the third in a new series of decennial supplements, the previous two supplements being *Occupational Health* and *The Health of our Children*. A further volume, on socio-economic differences in health, is planned for publication in late 1997.

KAREN DUNNELL
Director of Health and Demographic Statistics
Office for National Statistics

Acknowledgements

The Editors are extremely grateful to the many colleagues in the ONS who have helped in one way or the other in producing these volumes, especially Anita Brock and John Waterman who laboured over proofs and graphs.

About the authors

Michael Adler is Professor of Sexually Transmitted Diseases at University College London Medical School. His main interests are in the epidemiology of HIV and sexually transmitted diseases, and the setting up of control programmes for these in both developed and developing countries.

Peter Burney is a Professor of Public Health Medicine at the United Medical and Dental School of Guy's and St Thomas's hospital in the University of London.

John Charlton is an epidemiologist and principal methodologist at the Office for National Statistics. His research interests include health outcomes, suicides and demographic trends.

Pat Coleman is a research associate in the Medical Care Research Unit with a long-standing research interest in sports injuries and more recently, accidents in adolescents and young adults.

Karen Dunnell is the Director of Demography and Health Division in the Office for National Statistics. Prior to that she worked in the Social Survey Division of the office, in a department of Public Health in a medical school and an independent health care research unit.

George Davey Smith is a professor in the Department of Social Medicine at the University of Bristol.

Richard Doll is an epidemiologist, Emeritus Professor of Medicine at Oxford University and an honorary consultant to the Imperial Cancer Research Fund in the Nuffield Department of Clinical Medicine in Oxford.

Shah Ebrahim is Professor of Clinical Epidemiology at the Royal Free Hospital School of Medicine, University of London. He is co-director of the British Regional Heart Study which is concerned with the aetiology of cardiovascular diseases. His research interests are in stroke aetiology and prevention, and the evaluation of health services for stroke.

Spence Galbraith is a retired medical epidemiologist, former Director of the Communicable Diseases Surveillance Centre.

Emily Grundy is a demographer working at the Age Concern Institute of Gerontology, King's College, University of London.

Anne Johnson is Professor of Epidemiology in the Department of Sexually Transmitted Diseases at the University College of London Medical School and honorary consultant in public health medicine. Her research interests are in epidemiology and the prevention of HIV and sexually transmitted diseases.

Kay-Tee Khaw is Professor of Clinical Gerontology in the University of Cambridge. She is an epidemiologist researching in prevention of chronic disease.

Richard Logan is a reader in clinical epidemiology at the University of Nottingham Medical School, UK. As a practising gastroenterologist he has developed a special interest in the epidemiology of digestive diseases.

Guy Marks is an epidemiologist and physician. Currently in practice as a consultant respiratory physician at Liverpool Hospital, and a research associate at the Institute of Respiratory Medicine, both in Sydney, NSW, Australia. This work was conducted whilst he was a visiting research fellow at the Department of Public Health Medicine, UMDS.

Christopher Martyn is a neurologist at the Wessex Neurological Centre, Southampton General Hospital and a clinical scientist with the Medical Research Council's Environmental Epidemiology Unit where he runs a research programme into the causes of cerebrovascular disease and other diseases of the nervous system.

Anna McCormick is a senior medical statistician for the Office for National Statistics, with particular interests in infectious diseases.

Mike Murphy is a medical epidemiologist who worked for the Office for National Statistics. He now works for the Imperial Cancer Research Fund at the University of Oxford in General Practitioner Research. His main interests are cancer and health care epidemiology.

Professor Jon Nicholl is the Director of the Medical Care Research Unit at the University of Sheffield. His early background was in road traffic accident research. His current research interests are accident and emergency services, including provision for major trauma and pre-hospital ambulatory care.

Andrew Phillips is a reader in epidemiology and biostatistics at the Royal Free Hospital School of Medicine. His interest is in the natural history of HIV infection and his recent work focuses on attempts to learn from mathematical models of viral and lymphocyte dynamics in HIV infection.

Paul Roderick is a public health physician working at the Wessex Institute for Health Research and Development at Southampton University.

Isabel dos Santos Silva is Senior Lecturer in Epidemiology in the Epidemiological Monitoring Unit at the London School of Hygiene and Tropical Medicine, working on cancer epidemiology.

Anthony Swerdlow is Professor of Epidemiology and head of the Epidemiological Monitoring Unit at the London School of Hygiene and Tropical Medicine.

Robert Swingler is a consultant of neurology at the Dundee teaching Hospital. His interests include multiple sclerosis and motor neurone disease.

Deborah Symmons is a senior lecturer in rheumatic disease epidemiology at the University of Manchester and Honorary Consultant Rheumatologist at East Cheshire NHS Trust.

Roger Thatcher was the Registrar General and Director of the Office of Population Censuses and Surveys from 1978 until he retired in 1986. His interests include mortality rates at high ages

Jonathan Van-Tam is a lecturer in public health medicine and epidemiology at the University of Nottingham Medical School, UK. His research interests include emergency and acute hospital care.

Chapter 15

Infection in England and Wales, 1838–1993

By

Spence Galbraith and Anna McCormick

Summary

- This chapter describes the pattern of infection in England and Wales over the past century and a half and considers possible causes of some of the changes that took place.

- Improvements in the sanitation, hygiene, living conditions and nutrition of the population began in the middle of the nineteenth century but these did not begin to bring about a decline in mortality until the 1870s. In the 1850s, 1 death in every 3 was attributed to infectious disease. At the turn of the century this had fallen to 1 in 5 and by the 1960s, infectious disease had become an insignificant cause of death.

- In the nineteenth century, mortality from tuberculosis in all forms exceeded that of all other epidemic infectious diseases combined. Tuberculosis declined slowly as nutrition and living conditions improved but remained a major cause of death until the introduction of specific chemotherapy in the 1950s.

- By the early twentieth century, gastrointestinal infections such as cholera, enteric fever and dysentery had been controlled by better hygiene and sanitation, particularly the purification of water supplies.

- Mortality from childhood infections fell as a consequence of the improving health of children, and morbidity declined rapidly after the introduction of immunisation. Poliomyelitis, diphtheria, tetanus, whooping cough, measles, mumps and rubella were virtually eliminated during the second half of the twentieth century.

- In the latter part of this century, there was a recrudescence of infection. Many apparently new infections appeared and some old infections returned. These were associated with greatly increased international travel and changes in social conditions and in life-style. Furthermore, some advances in medical practise have led to an increase in the number of persons highly susceptible to infection.

- In conclusion, the rate of change of human infection appears to be increasing as the speed of social, technical, environmental and population change accelerates. It is postulated that these changes increase the threat of the appearance of new diseases and the reappearance of some old diseases, and that it can be only a matter of time until the next microbial menace to our species emerges amongst us.

15.1 Introduction

The pattern of human infection in England and Wales changed radically between 1838 and 1990, a period that began soon after the arrival of Asiatic cholera in the country in 1831 and ended with the emergence of another new disease, the acquired immune deficiency syndrome (AIDS), in 1981.

The epidemics of cholera in 1831–32 and 1848–49 provided an important stimulus to the campaign to improve the appalling living and working conditions of the population, particularly the sanitation of the new urban industrial areas of the country (Pelling, 1978). The third major cholera epidemic occurred in 1853–54 and the last in Britain in 1866 (Underwood, 1947).

Mortality did not start to decline until the 1870s; the crude death rate then fell from over 20 per 1,000 to 16 per 1,000 in 1901–05 (OPCS, 1992). This fall mainly resulted from a decrease in deaths from infectious disease, principally tuberculosis, enteric fever, typhus, cholera, dysentery, smallpox and scarlet fever (see Figures 15.1 and 15.2). McKeown and Lowe (1974) attributed the fall in gastrointestinal infections to improvements in hygiene and sanitation, the fall in tuberculosis mainly to a rising standard of living, particularly improved nutrition, that of smallpox to widespread vaccination, and of scarlet fever to decreased virulence of the causative organism, the haemolytic streptococcus.

Infant mortality rates, however, remained virtually unchanged throughout the nineteenth century (see Chapter 3), a failure of the developing public health service, which was highlighted by the poor physical condition of recruits for the South African War at the turn of the century. A Government enquiry followed (Report, 1904), as a consequence of which maternity, child health and school health services were provided. In the present century, infant mortality fell rapidly, partly due to these services, from 156 per 1,000 live births in 1896–1900 to 36 in 1945–50. By then, the crude death rate was 11.8 per 1,000. Logan (1950) reviewed the achievements of the 100 years 1847–1947:

'Half a million persons died in England and Wales in 1947. If there had been no improvement in mortality over half a million more would have died. This is a measure of the progress that has been made in 100 years.'

Figure 15.1

Cholera, typhus, rabies, plague

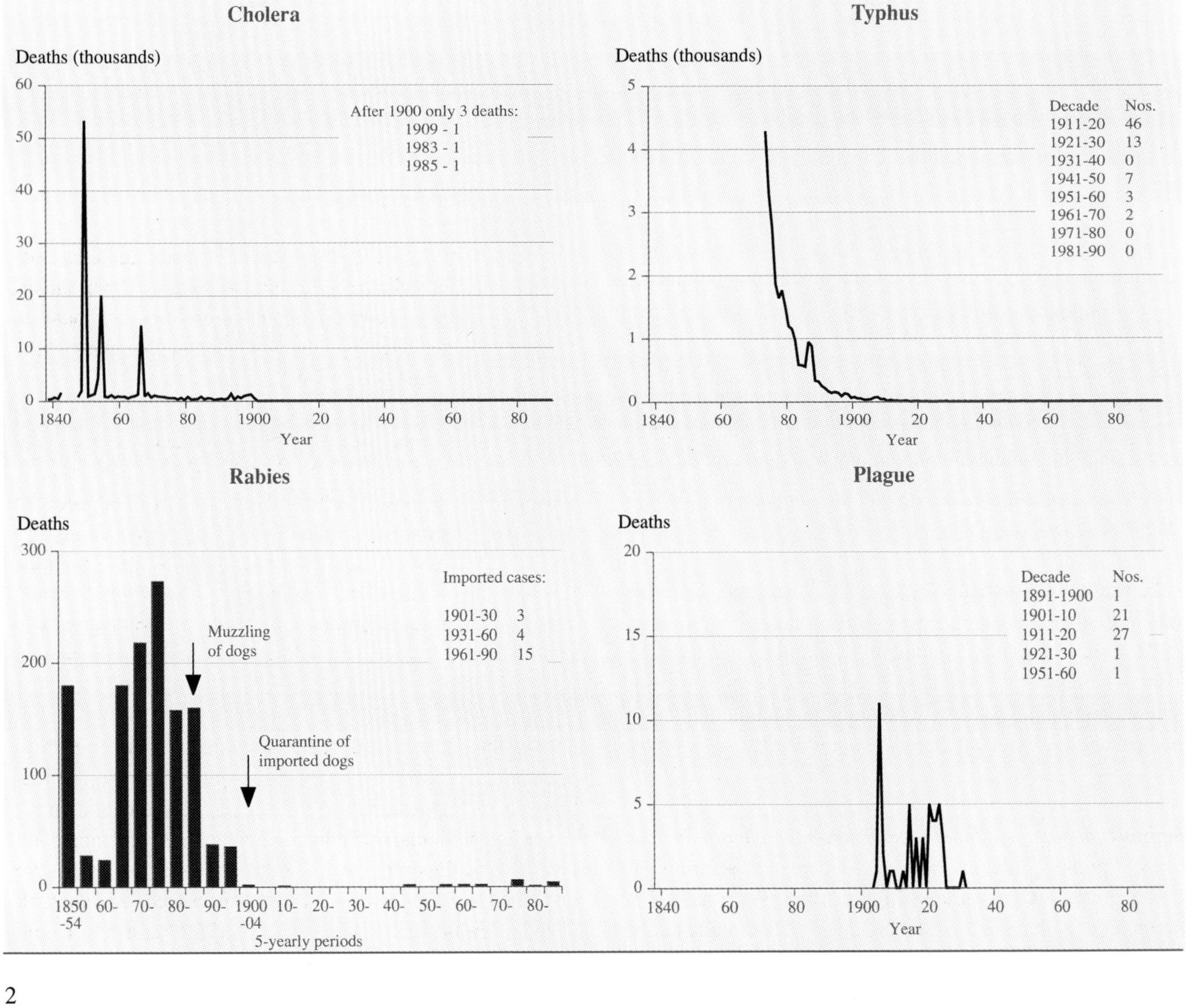

Figure 15.2

Smallpox, malaria, enteric fever and tuberculosis

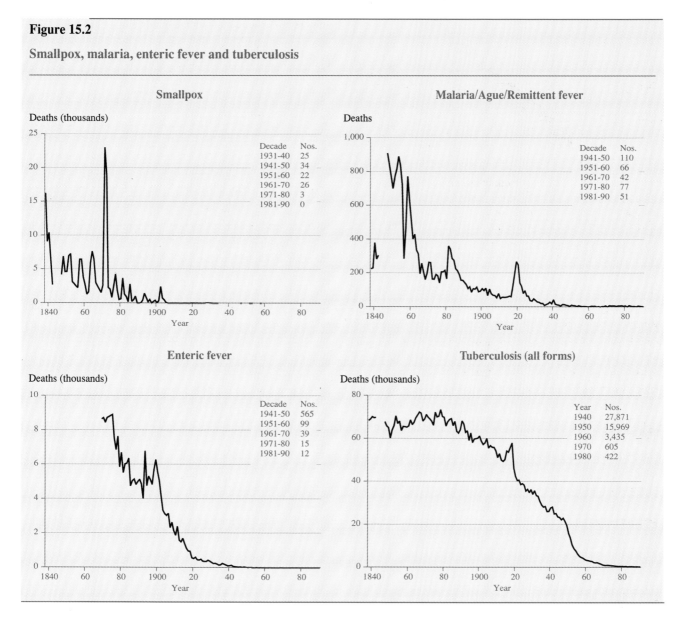

By the 1960s, deaths from most infectious diseases had declined sharply as a result of continuing improvements in hygiene and sanitation, rising standards of living, immunisation and, after the 1930s, also of specific therapeutic measures (McKeown and Lowe, 1974). In 1965 the standardised mortality ratio was 87 (1950 = 100), compared with 101 in 1945–50, 279 in 1901–05 and 344 in 1841–45; the crude death rate remained at 11.6 per 1,000 and did not reflect the downward trend in mortality because of the ageing population; infant mortality was 19 per 1,000 live births.

In the middle of the nineteenth century, one death in every three was attributed to infectious disease, about a third of which were caused by tuberculosis and a fifth by scarlet fever and diphtheria. By the turn of the century, infectious diseases accounted for one in five deaths and by the 1960s they had become an insignificant cause of death (see Chapter 4).

Morbidity as well as mortality declined, particularly after the 1930s; diphtheria, tetanus, whooping cough and poliomyelitis were controlled by immunisation, smallpox eradication was almost complete, bovine tuberculosis was virtually eliminated and brucellosis eradication was soon to begin. Many

other infections, such as streptococcal disease, meningococcal septicaemia and meningitis, and respiratory tuberculosis, were treatable by newly discovered antibiotics. The outlook for patients with infectious disease was transformed and the control of infection seemed almost complete.

Understandably, therefore, the belief arose and became widespread, that infection was no longer a significant threat to health. Such complacency, however, was short-lived, because in the 1970s a recrudescence of infection began. Many apparently new infections appeared and some old infections returned, associated with increasing international travel, changes in social conditions and lifestyle, and advances in medical practice. Infection once again became an important cause of morbidity and mortality.

This chapter considers the causes of variations in the pattern of human infection and reviews changes in some old infections and the appearance of some apparently new infections, and refers particularly to adults. The mortality and morbidity data used to illustrate the changing patterns of infection are described, and their uses and validity discussed, by Campbell (1965), Galbraith (1982), OPCS (1992) and Moro and McCormick (1988) and in Chapter 12.

3

15.2 Emerging causes of infection

Emerging infections may be the result of the appearance of a new infection, the discovery of a microbial cause of an existing disease or the recurrence of an old infectious disease. These may be a consequence of changes in micro-organisms, the human hosts, the environment or a combination of these.

15.2.1 The micro-organisms

The micro-organisms causing human infections may have arisen in several ways. Some pathogenic organisms possibly evolved in the remote past from the parasites of the ancestors of Homo sapiens. Other specifically human pathogens, which were able to persist for long periods in small nomadic groups of people, may have appeared later. Less speculative is the suggestion that some human pathogens probably emerged more recently after agriculture developed and larger populations formed in towns and cities. For example, small-pox and measles are both self-limiting, specifically human infections, and could not have been maintained without enough people to ensure a continuing group of susceptible subjects. These diseases possibly arose in the world's first civilisations, and may have evolved from similar organisms in the domestic animals with which human beings had become closely associated, the large populations then enabling indefinite transmission of organisms from person to person and the selection of strains best adapted to the human host (Cockburn, 1959).

New infections may be expected to arise in a similar way, now and in the future, because the greatly increased world population and movement of people in recent years has resulted in an unprecedented number of people being continuously in contact (Cockburn, 1967). Furthermore, changes in micro-organisms promoted by the widespread use of anti-microbial drugs in human beings and in animals and by large-scale immunisation programmes, may lead to the evolution of new pathogens. This is particularly likely to take place in hospitals because of intense use of anti-microbial drugs and the concentration of many highly susceptible people, some of whom may be suffering from infections.

15.2.2 The human host

Populations, when first exposed to a micro-organism, may be very susceptible to the infection, but develop non-specific resistance over time. Specific immunity follows infection or immunisation. Immunity is low in young and elderly people, and in those with defects of the immune system; it may be reduced by malnutrition, radiation, intercurrent disease, infection with the human immunodeficiency virus (HIV), and by drugs used in medical treatment.

Changes in behaviour may predispose to 'new' infections. For example, alteration in food habits of a population, such as eating raw fish, may result in infection with fish tapeworms new to that population. Changes in sexual behaviour may alter sexually transmissible diseases, such as the rise that took place during both World Wars and in the 1960s (Caterall, 1981), and the more recent appearance of rectal and oral infections as a consequence of homosexual practice; the use of injecting drugs will facilitate the spread of blood-borne micro-organisms, consequently infections with hepatitis B, C and D viruses and HIV may increase and become apparent.

Infections may emerge as a result of human penetration into remote areas of the world, where contact may occur with isolated groups of human beings and animals infected with micro-organisms not previously encountered. For example, some of the recently discovered viral haemorrhagic fevers probably arose in this way. Similar circumstances may occur in developed areas of the world by close contact with exotic animals kept in laboratories or as domestic pets, which may be infected with pathogens new to these areas. For example, Marburg virus disease first appeared in Marburg, Frankfurt and Belgrade, associated with infected monkeys imported from Uganda (Martini, 1973) and there have been many cases of human salmonellosis caused by unusual salmonella serotypes derived from imported pet terrapins (Orton and Henderson, 1972).

15.2.3 The environment

Pathogens may appear or reappear because of alterations in their modes of transmission. These may follow changes in climate, in agricultural methods, in industry and technology, and in the preparation of food and drink.

A rise in environmental temperatures may increase the global distribution of insect vectors of disease, such as mosquitoes carrying malarial parasites, and may bring insects into contact with a different range of micro-organisms to which they could become hosts and vectors (Cook, 1992).

Changes in the supply of food and water may lead to the appearance of 'new' diseases. For example, in the past, supplies of these commodities were obtained locally, but as towns and cities developed they were produced in bulk for distribution to the increased populations. Consequently, the risk of microbial contamination of larger quantities arose, such as sewage pollution of piped water supplies causing large outbreaks of cholera and typhoid fever. More recently, the same phenomenon has arisen as a result of the bulk production of animal feeding stuffs and the intensive rearing of food animals, particularly poultry, with consequent outbreaks of food-borne salmonellosis, sometimes with rare serotypes derived from their feed (Turnbull, 1979).

New food processes may provide new opportunities for the spread of pathogens. For example, after the introduction of canning of foods, outbreaks of staphylococcal food poisoning from canned peas took place. These arose because the cans developed minute transient leaks in the vulcanite seal during cooling, at a time when the cans were being handled; thus, organisms from the hands of workers, including toxigenic strains of *Staphylococcus aureus*, were occasionally sucked into the cans (Stersky *et al.*, 1980). In the same way, outbreaks of typhoid fever followed the cooling of cans of corned beef and other meat in raw river water polluted by sewage.

15.3 Recent variations in 'old' infections

15.3.1 Food-borne infections

Illness associated with the consumption of unwholesome food or drink must have occurred throughout human history, but until the second half of the nineteenth century it was usually attributed to chemical poisoning. The advent of microbiology, however, led to the discovery that food-borne illness most often had a microbial cause, caused either by an infection or by the toxic products of micro-organisms (Savage, 1913). Acute illness following the consumption of food, usually vomiting and/or diarrhoea, is commonly referred to as 'food poisoning' in the United Kingdom, irrespective of the cause.

Salmonellosis
Salmonellosis is the most common cause of food poisoning.

It is a zoonosis (i.e. a disease shared by humans and other vertebrates). It is usually transmitted by food, but person-to-person spread by the faecal-oral route may occur, especially in hospitals and institutions. Infection usually gives rise to an acute gastroenteritis, which may be severe in infants, elderly people and patients with intercurrent disease; sometimes the infection spreads beyond the gastrointestinal tract causing a septicaemic illness resembling typhoid fever. In animals infection is often symptomless.

Information about food poisoning was limited to outbreak reports until 1948, when statutory notification of food poisoning was introduced. These notifications comprised several types of bacterial, viral and toxic illnesses caused by food. Because salmonellosis was by far the most common, trends in notifications closely mirrored those of laboratory reports of salmonella infections. Laboratory reports, which began in 1941, were recorded as 'incidents' until 1980, that is, an outbreak and a single sporadic case each counting as one (Anonymous, 1950), and as numbers of laboratory reports from 1981. Both notifications and laboratory reports rose to a peak in the 1950s and then declined; another increase began around 1970 and was followed by a much greater rise in the late 1980s (see Figure 15.3).

Figure 15.3

Food poisoning and salmonellosis

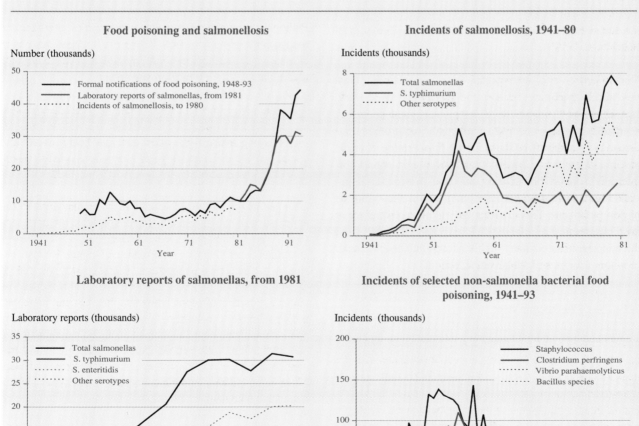

The first peak resulted from an increase in reports of *Salmonella typhimurium* and was attributed to infection in cattle and poultry, associated with changes in animal husbandry and in patterns of food consumption following the end of food rationing and the deregulation of abattoirs (McCoy, 1975). For example, in 1958 the development of phage typing of *S. typhimurium* led to the identification of an outbreak of 90 cases and one death caused by *S. typhimurium* phage type 20a in London and south-east England. This fine typing of the organism enabled the outbreak to be traced to symptomless intestinal infection in calves which had been purchased from a dealer who collected calves from many markets in the West Country (Anderson *et al.*, 1961). About 0.5 per cent of calves were infected with *S. typhimurium* phage type 20a at West Country markets, but after they had been kept together at the dealer's premises for several days before delivery to abattoirs at weekends, the infection rate rose to nearly 13 per cent. This greatly increased the chance of contamination of calf meat at slaughter and subsequent transfer of the organisms to shops and kitchens; indeed, all the cases in the outbreak were related to calf meat derived from the abattoirs in which calves were slaughtered on Sundays or Mondays.

The second rise, in the 1970s, resulted from an increase in reports of serotypes other than *S. typhimurium* (see Figure 15.3), and was associated with infection in poultry, usually a symptomless intestinal infection in the birds. Some of the serotypes, such as *S. hadar* and *S. agona*, were probably imported either in infected day-old chicks and hatching eggs, or in contaminated animal feeding stuffs. Infection then spread widely because of the intensive production of the poultry and the increased consumption of poultry meat (Palmer and Rowe, 1986).

The initial part of the third rise, in 1978–83, was due to an increase in reports of *S. typhimurium* and was probably related to bovine infection. The second part, beginning in 1985, was caused by an unprecedented increase in reports of *S. enteritidis* phage type 4, associated with infection in poultry. The mode of spread was different from that in poultry in the 1970s, because this organism not only infected the intestinal contents of the birds, but also the meat and eggs. Many outbreaks were associated with fresh eggs and poultry meat and in a case-control study, Cowden *et al.* (1989) showed that fresh shell eggs, egg products and precooked hot chicken were vehicles of infection in sporadic cases. Infection with *S. enteritidis* phage type 4 appeared in other countries of Europe at the same time as in England and Wales, suggesting that international supplies of hatching eggs and chicks from one or more hatcheries were probably infected. If this is so, then human infection is likely to continue until new salmonella-free breeding stocks are created, both for laying hens and for broiler birds.

Staphylococcal and clostridial infections

Staphylococcus aureus and *Clostridium perfringens* are less common causes of food poisoning, both of which are the result of poor food hygiene. *S. aureus* is usually derived from the skin of food handlers. Illness occurs only if food is contaminated with an enterotoxigenic strain of the organism, and then is kept at room temperature for at least 6 hours, enabling multiplication and production of toxin. *C. perfringens* is present in most meats. Illness occurs only if meat is cooked and then cooled very slowly, or kept at room temperature for a long time, or is reheated, thus allowing sufficient time and temperature for the organism to multiply profusely (Gilbert and Roberts, 1990).

Both these types of food poisoning were measured in incidents throughout the period under review (see Figure 15.3). They nearly always presented as outbreaks rather than single sporadic cases, and the number of lapses in food hygiene is better assessed by the number of incidents rather than by the number of reported cases that arose in consequence. Both these types of food poisoning increased at the same time as salmonellosis, reaching a peak in the 1950s, and then declined (see Figure 15.3). Subsequently, their incidence remained low, indicating a continuing improvement in standards of food hygiene.

This improvement in food hygiene, however, had no effect on the incidence of salmonellosis, which increased continuously, suggesting that other factors are probably more important in this disease. Indeed, human salmonellosis is probably more closely related to standards of hygiene of meat and poultry production than to hygiene in the kitchen. Consequently, human infection is likely to continue until the standards of hygiene of meat and poultry production approach those achieved in the water and dairy industries.

Botulism

Botulism is a rare and often fatal form of toxic food poisoning. The organism is ubiquitous, but toxin production occurs only in an anaerobic, alkaline, moist environment with a low salt concentration, providing that there is sufficient time for the organism to multiply. Only 10 outbreaks have ever been recorded in the United Kingdom, the last comprising 27 cases in 1989 in which the implicated food was hazelnut yoghurt. In this outbreak the disease was atypical and initially mistaken for a neurological syndrome, the Guillain-Barré syndrome, and was milder than in previous episodes, with only one death. The outbreak followed a change in the method of manufacture of hazelnut purée, included in the yoghurt, so as to reduce its sugar content. This inadvertently provided suitable conditions for the production of toxin (O'Mahony *et al.*, 1990). This outbreak suggested that the epidemiology and clinical presentation of botulism might be changing and that better methods of detection of acute neurological conditions, which are not notifiable in England and Wales, were required.

Other types of food poisoning

These include two new types of bacterial food-borne disease, which appeared in England and Wales in the 1970s as a result of changing food consumption. *Bacillus cereus* was often associated with reheated rice dishes and *Vibrio parahaemolyticus* with imported prawns; both were rare.

Listeriosis

Listeriosis is a zoonosis, first recognised in 1929. Initially it was reported as causing eye and skin infections in people in contact with infected animals. This clinical picture appeared to change, however, and by the 1960s the organism was recognised as an important cause of meningitis and septicaemia, particularly in infants, and in elderly and immunocompromised people, with a case fatality ratio of around 30 per cent (Neiman and Lorber, 1980). Food-borne transmission was first substantiated in the early 1980s in North America, where outbreaks were associated with coleslaw, milk and soft cheese.

In England and Wales, laboratory reports rose during the 1970s to nearly 100 per year, and then increased suddenly almost threefold in 1987–88 (see Figure 15.4). This rapid rise was the result of a widespread outbreak of food-borne infection caused by contaminated imported paté (Gilbert *et al.*, 1993). The causative organism, *Listeria monocytogenes*, grows slowly at temperatures between 1°C and 8°C, so that a small inoculum might outgrow competing organisms in foods refrigerated for long periods. The fall in incidence, which followed in 1989 and 1990, was associated with the introduction of control measures. These were the lower storage temperatures of food, and advice to susceptible people to avoid foods most likely to be contaminated, such as soft cheese and paté, as well as to improvements in the production methods of cheese and paté by the manufacturers.

Yersiniosis

Yersiniosis, caused by the organism *Yersinia enterocolitica*, is a zoonotic infection, often associated with infection in pigs, and is usually transmitted by food. It commonly presents with diarrhoea and abdominal pain (Cover and Aber, 1989). In England and Wales, laboratory reporting began in 1975 and by 1980 there had been just over 50 reports but, in the next decade, reports increased continuously reaching a peak in 1989, before falling sharply in 1989–91 (see Figure 15.4). The reason for the increase and the subsequent decline is unknown, but one possible explanation is that these changes may have resulted from changes in the refrigeration of foods.

The organism, like *L. monocytogenes*, grows slowly at refrigerator temperatures and the rise in reports may have been associated with increasing use of refrigeration. The sudden fall corresponded in time with that of listeriosis and may have been associated with the lower temperatures of food refrigeration (see Figure 15.4).

Dysentery

The two most common forms of dysentery are bacillary dysentery and amoebic dysentery. Both probably occurred frequently in the insanitary conditions of the nineteenth century, when they were likely to have been spread by water and food (Sandwith, 1914). Mortality data, first available as distinct from 'diarrhoea' in 1901, showed an average of 267 deaths per year in the first decade of this century. Deaths increased during the First World War, reaching a peak of 897 in 1917. In 1919, when notification began, there were 1,657 cases and 435 deaths, a fatality ratio of 26 per cent, and in 1925, 345 cases and 135 deaths, a fatality ratio of 39 per cent. Twenty years later, in 1945, the number of cases had increased to 16,278 with 165 deaths, a fatality ratio of 1 per cent. Glover (1947) alluded to a cause of this transformation:

> *Any enteritis or diarrhoea, however slight, which is found to be due to Shigella is now reported by the dreaded term "dysentery", which used to designate "one of the four great epidemic diseases of the world". "The scourge of armies" has become "the bane of residential nurseries".*

This transformation was probably also caused by a change in the causative organisms, as well as changing standards of hygiene and sanitation. *Shigella dysenteriae*, which causes severe disease, was common among soldiers returning from the Middle East during the First World War and may have been prevalent in the civilian population in earlier times. Some of the notifications may also have been relapses in amoebic dysentery in servicemen. In the 1920s, *S. flexneri* was often encountered in mental hospitals, where the illness was some-

Figure 15.4

Listeriosis and yersiniosis

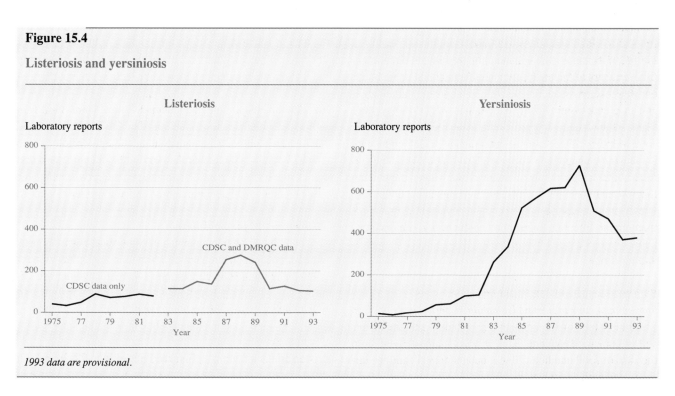

1993 data are provisional.

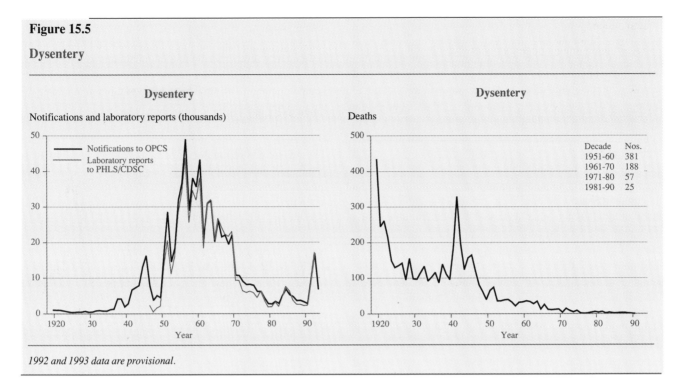

Figure 15.5

Dysentery

1992 and 1993 data are provisional.

times severe and accounted for more than half of the notifications and deaths. In the next two decades, *S. sonnei*, which usually gives rise to much milder diarrhoeal disease in young children, increased and notifications of dysentery reached a peak of over 16,000 in 1945 (see Figure 15.5). At the same time the seasonal distribution changed from late summer and autumn to winter and spring, and the mode of spread changed from food-borne and water-borne infection, which virtually ceased, to person-to-person spread by the faecal-oral route. The large rise in notifications between 1950 and 1970 probably resulted mainly from the increasing detection of many mild infections, as Glover (1947) suggested earlier.

The decline in notifications from the peak of over 49,000 in 1956 to less than 3,000 in 1979 and 1980 was probably caused by a decrease in the faecal-oral spread of *S. sonnei*. This was mainly brought about by improvements in sanitation in primary schools, many of which were rebuilt during this period. The communal, cold, damp, dark lavatories in the playground, which provided ideal conditions for the spread of the organism (Hutchinson, 1956), were replaced by warm, well-lit toilet facilities within the school building for smaller numbers of children. Another infection spread by the faecal-oral route, hepatitis A, also declined at the same time, but both diseases increased again in the late 1980s and early 1990s (see Figures 15.5 and 15.12) for reasons which are unknown.

15.3.2 Respiratory infections

Tuberculosis

Tuberculosis is caused by *Mycobacterium tuberculosis* and *M. bovis*. The former affects primarily the lungs and spreads by the air-borne route from an infected person with large numbers of living organisms in the sputum. *M. bovis* affects sites other than the lungs and usually spreads from infected cattle by the consumption of raw milk.

Tuberculosis probably reached a peak in incidence in England and Wales at the end of the eighteenth century (Gale, 1959). Deaths declined slowly as nutrition and living conditions improved, but the disease remained a major cause of death throughout the nineteenth and early twentieth centuries (see Figure 15.2). In the nineteenth century, mortality from tuberculosis in its many forms exceeded that from all the known epidemic infectious diseases combined. At that time, however, this was not apparent because the different forms of tuberculosis were regarded as different diseases. The disease was aptly described by the often quoted extract from John Bunyan's 'The life and death of Mr Badman' as: 'The captain of all these men of death.'

After the introduction of specific chemotherapy in the 1950s, deaths fell more steeply, because the new drugs quickly rendered patients non-infectious and thus rapidly controlled a potential source of infection for further cases. Mass miniature radiography to detect the disease and BCG (Bacille Calmette-Guérin) vaccine to prevent primary infection were introduced at the same time, but probably had a smaller impact on the control of the disease. Most of the decline in mortality, however, took place before these modern measures were introduced (see Figure 15.2).

Notifications of respiratory tuberculosis, which began in 1913, fell almost continuously except for an interruption during the Second World War (see Figure 15.6). The age distribution also changed, notifications declining more steeply in young adults, particularly young women, than in middle-aged and elderly people (Gale, 1959). This trend continued so that by the 1990s pulmonary tuberculosis in the indigenous white population had become a disease primarily of middle-aged and elderly men. In immigrant communities, who by then made up about half the total notifications, the picture was different, with a nearly equal sex distribution and with most notifications in young people.

Figure 15.6

Variations in some respiratory infections

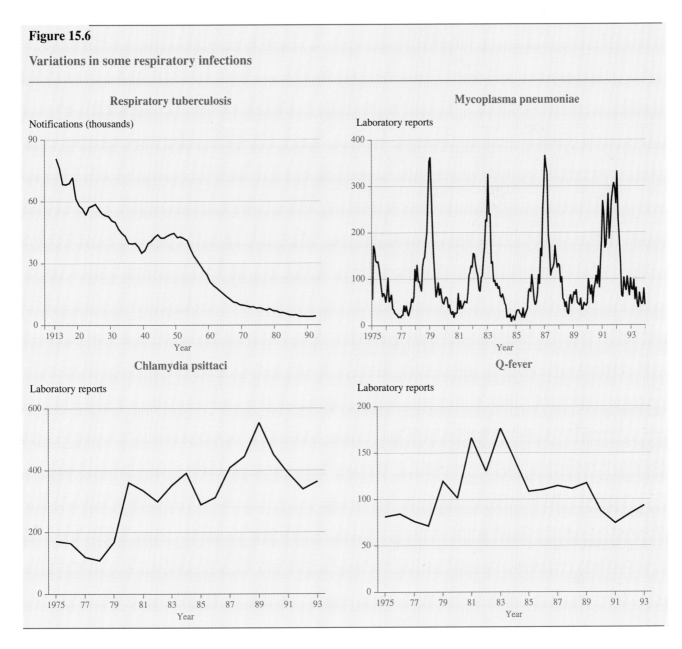

The decline in notifications ceased in 1987, when there were 4,010 recorded, and began to rise in 1988. By 1993, notifications had risen by 17.2 per cent, 49.5 per cent in non-respiratory tuberculosis and 8.5 per cent in respiratory notifications (Hayward and Watson, 1995). The rise in non-respiratory notifications was probably largely the result of improved notification, but the rise in respiratory tuberculosis was real and associated with poverty, homelessness and unemployment (Darbyshire, 1995). For example, in a radiological survey of homeless men in hostels in central London in 1984, 2 per cent were found to have tuberculosis, the highest prevalence ever recorded in the United Kingdom (Citron *et al.*, 1995). Ironically, it was the alleviation of these conditions that was mainly responsible for the fall in mortality in the last century.

Notifications increased in patients with HIV infection, which predisposes to tuberculosis, but the numbers remained small (Watson *et al.*, 1993). Antibiotic resistance of the strains of *M. tuberculosis* isolated from patients to one or more drugs also increased, but again remained low (Warburton *et al.*, 1993). It is likely, however, that tuberculosis will increase and spread further in HIV-infected people and others who

are highly susceptible to infection, and it is possible that multiple-resistant strains will appear, as has occurred in the United States of America, and some infections may become untreatable with existing anti-tuberculous drugs (Bloom and Murray, 1992).

The current methods of tuberculosis control by contact tracing, normally limited to people sharing the household of cases (Report, 1994), may prove inadequate to contain this new threat. For example, in 1979, an outbreak of tuberculosis in children, with 16 clinical cases, 11 of them symptomless, and a further 92 with strongly positive skin tests for tuberculosis, escaped detection by routine contact tracing. It was discovered by the extensive investigation of children who used a swimming pool where one of the pool attendants developed tuberculosis and was sputum smear positive (Rao *et al.*, 1980). Indeed, in a recent study in San Francisco using DNA fingerprinting of *M. tuberculosis*, only 10 per cent of new infections were detected by conventional contact tracing (Small *et al.*, 1994). Tuberculosis, like most other infectious diseases, is no longer transmitted only locally. A national surveillance scheme to detect common source outbreaks of primary tuberculosis, similar to that used for Legionnaires' disease (see below), is now needed to find highly infectious cases which are not within the households or otherwise close contacts of the index cases.

Influenza

Influenza has a long history, but it was not until the pandemic of 1847–48 that detailed mortality data were first available in England and Wales, when it was shown that influenza deaths alone greatly underestimated the extent of the disease (Farr, 1885). There was little influenza in England and Wales until the next pandemic of 1889–92 and then the pandemic of 1918–19 of unprecedented scale, which particularly affected healthy young adults. A pandemic occurred in 1947 and the last one in 1968, with the most recent serious epidemic in 1975–76 (Beveridge, 1977). The next pandemic is now overdue (Webster, 1994).

Further epidemics of influenza A virus infection will occur as the virus changes slowly (antigenic drift) and another pandemic when a sudden major antigenic change takes place in the virus (antigenic shift). The source of new pandemic strains is probably animal influenza viruses which become adapted to human beings or antigens from animal viruses, which become incorporated into human viruses and change them. These animal viruses are probably derived from pigs or ducks living in close association with people and often appear to arise in the densely populated areas of southern China (Shortridge and Stuart-Harris, 1982).

Influenza B virus does not have the same epidemic potential as influenza A virus, and outbreaks have usually been confined to children and young adults in schools and other closed communities.

Psittacosis

Psittacosis is an uncommon zoonosis giving rise to respiratory illness, often pneumonia, which is caused by *Chlamydia psittaci*; it is usually derived from birds. Laboratory reports increased from under 200 per year between 1975 and 1979 to a peak of 553 in 1989 and then fell to between 350 and 400 per year between 1990 and 1993 (see Figure 15.6). There was no apparent increase in cases associated with captive birds, nor was the rise accounted for by illness in poultry workers first identified during this period. Enzootic abortion in ewes, another chlamydial disease, received wide publicity at this time, but associated human infections did not increase.

The rise was probably due to the appearance of a new chlamydia, the TWAR agent, now known as *C. pneumoniae,* which causes respiratory infections and is transmissible from person to person. This agent was first isolated from the eye of a Taiwanese child (TW strain) and later from a student with acute respiratory illness in the United States of America (AR strain) (Bourke, 1993). Infections have been detected in Britain, but the organism is not yet distinguishable from *C. psittaci* by routine laboratory methods, so that the extent of the infection remains to be determined.

Q fever

Q fever is another uncommon zoonotic pneumonic illness, caused by *Coxiella burnetti*, which is usually reported in men exposed to infected animals, most often sheep. Laboratory reports more than doubled in the early 1980s, associated with several outbreaks reported during this period (Winner *et al.*, 1987) and then declined to below 100 per year, similar to the previous decade (see Figure 15.6).

Other respiratory infections

Other respiratory infections include the parainfluenza viruses, which cause croup, bronchitis and pneumonia, especially in children, and epiglottitis in elderly people. These viruses are much more predictable than the influenza viruses; types 1 and 2 are usually epidemic in the late autumn and type 2 in the summer. *M. pneumoniae* is another cause of pneumonia, often in young adults, and fluctuates regularly with epidemics recurring every 4 years (see Figure 15.6). Respiratory syncytial virus causes outbreaks of bronchiolitis and pneumonia in young children recurring regularly every winter, as well as outbreaks of respiratory infection in old people's homes.

15.3.3 Sexually transmitted diseases

Trends in sexually transmitted diseases are covered in detail in Chapter 16.

15.3.4 Streptococcal and meningococcal disease

Streptococcal disease

Scarlet fever is a childhood streptococcal infection, which has varied in incidence and severity; it was a mild disease at the beginning of the nineteenth century, but increased in severity to a peak in 1860–70 (Gale, 1959). Between 1840 and 1884, the number of deaths from scarlet fever ranged from just over 9,000 to 32,500 each year, with a peak of 32,543 in 1870. Deaths then fell gradually to less than 4,000 per year at the end of the century, to under 400 in 1930 and to nil in 1960. Statutory notification of the disease began in 1936, and numbers fell from around 80,000 per year in the 1940s to less than a tenth of this in the 1990s (see Figure 15.7). Deaths from erysipelas and puerperal fever, both caused by the streptococcus, also fell (see Figure 15.7). There were only 22 deaths from erysipelas and nine from puerperal fever in the decade 1981–90. Streptococcal pneumonia also declined (Loudon, 1987). Rheumatic fever and acute nephritis, both manifestations of streptococcal infection, declined as did rheumatic heart disease and chronic nephritis, the late effects of these diseases.

The use of antibiotics reduced mortality from streptococcal disease, but it remains uncertain whether they influenced the decline in incidence. The history of scarlet fever suggests that a more important factor may have been changing virulence of the streptococcus. It is possible, therefore, that reversion in severity may occur again in the future. Penicillin-resistant organisms have already arisen and multiple-resistant organisms may appear later, rendering specific chemotherapy increasingly difficult. Generalised streptococcal infections continue to be reported (Ispahani *et al.*, 1988), although only

Figure 15.7

Streptococcal disease

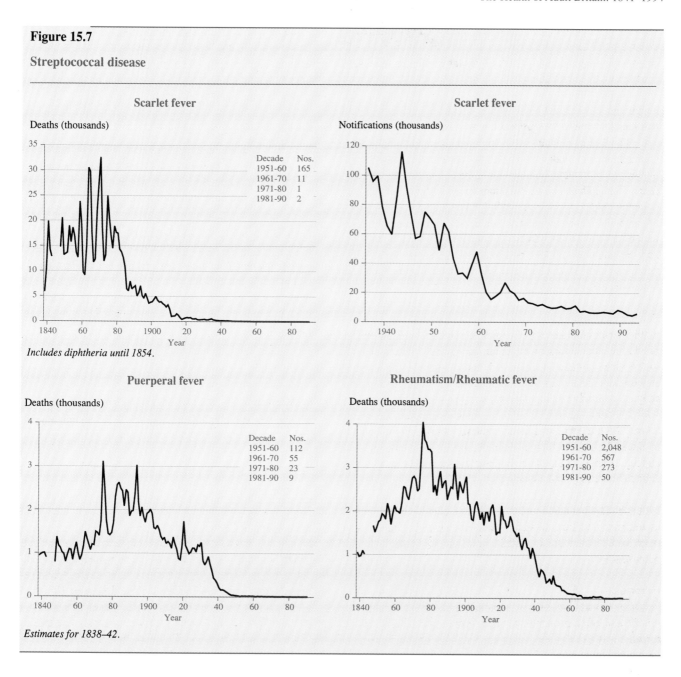

Scarlet fever

Deaths (thousands)

Decade	Nos.
1951-60	165
1961-70	11
1971-80	1
1981-90	2

Includes diphtheria until 1854.

Scarlet fever

Notifications (thousands)

Puerperal fever

Deaths (thousands)

Decade	Nos.
1951-60	112
1961-70	55
1971-80	23
1981-90	9

Estimates for 1838–42.

Rheumatism/Rheumatic fever

Deaths (thousands)

Decade	Nos.
1951-60	2,048
1961-70	567
1971-80	273
1981-90	50

a few cases occur each year and no increase has taken place. In the last decade, however, several cases of nephritis occurred in young men in closed communities following streptococcal skin infections and in 1993, necrotising fasciitis received wide publicity in Britain, although no rise in incidence occurred. In the United States of America, localised outbreaks of rheumatic fever have been reported (Bisno, 1991), but this has not occurred in Britain.

Meningococcal disease

Meningitis or cerebrospinal fever appears to have been uncommon in England and Wales until the twentieth century (Gale, 1959). The first major outbreak took place during the First World War. This was probably a consequence of mixing young people from communities who had not previously been exposed to particular strains of *Neisseria meningitidis*, and who were therefore non-immune, with groups in whom the strains were circulating. Overcrowding was also an important factor. For example, in barrack rooms, cases of meningococcal meningitis appeared when the bed spacing had to be reduced to less than 3 feet, but new cases disap-

peared again when the bed spacing was increased (Glover, 1920).

In 1930–32, another smaller outbreak occurred and a larger outbreak followed during the Second World War, in 1940–41, when notifications greatly exceeded those in the 1915–18 epidemic. The fatality rate, however, was lower because of the introduction of specific treatment with sulphonamides in the 1930s (Abbott *et al.*, 1985). There were smaller outbreaks in the mid-1970s and again beginning 10 years later, which is continuing (see Figure 15.8). In this present outbreak, there have been about 1,000 notified cases of meningococcal meningitis and septicaemia, with about 100 deaths each year, most of them in previously healthy young adults. The outbreak has been caused mainly by a serogroup B strain of the organism new to this country, which had previously been prevalent in northern Europe (Poolman *et al.*, 1986). An unusual feature of this infection has been its persistence in small localities for several years; indeed, the outbreak is persisting longer than the previous outbreak in the 1970s.

Figure 15.8

Meningococcal disease

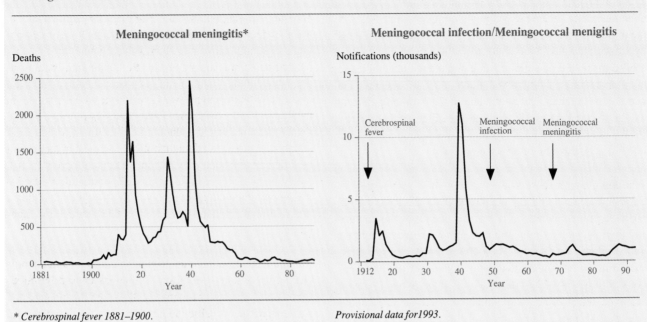

* Cerebrospinal fever 1881–1900.

Provisional data for1993.

Figure 15.9

Diphtheria, tetanus, whooping cough and poliomyelitis

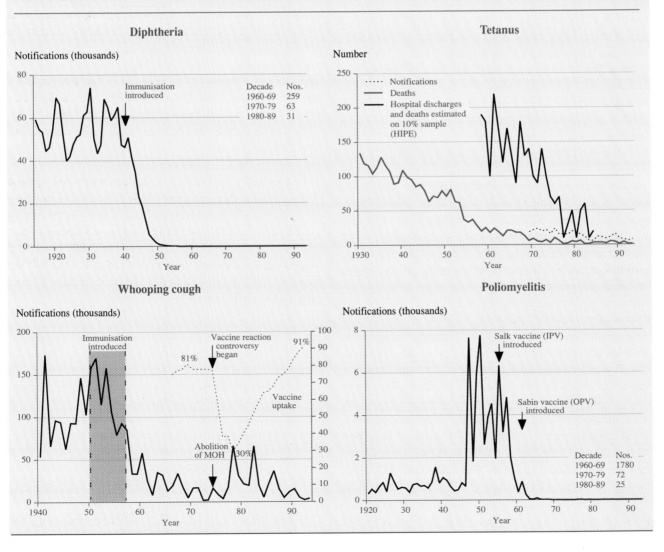

15.3.5 Diseases controlled by immunisation

Diphtheria, pertussis, tetanus and poliomyelitis

Diphtheria first became widespread in England and Wales in the middle of the nineteenth century, but was overshadowed by scarlet fever. In 1886–90 deaths from diphtheria first exceeded those of scarlet fever and it remained a leading cause of death in children until 1941 (Gale, 1959). Immunisation was then introduced and by the end of the following decade the disease had almost disappeared (see Figure 15.9). In the 1980s, only 30 cases were reported, many of them imported infections or contacts of imported cases.

Whooping cough (pertussis) has a much longer history in England and Wales than diphtheria. Deaths remained at around 10,000 a year from 1847 until the first decade of this century and then declined steeply as the health and care of children improved, and reached less than 400 by 1950. Immunisation started in the 1950s, deaths continued to fall and notifications fell sharply. This decline was interrupted in 1974, however, following a study which suggested that encephalopathy and brain damage might be a rare complication of immunisation. At the same time, by an unfortunate coincidence, the post of the doctor responsible for the management of immunisation programmes, the medical officer of health, was abolished in the NHS reorganisation of 1974 (see Figure 15.9). By 1978, only 30 per cent of children under 2 years were immunised and large outbreaks of whooping cough followed in 1978 and 1982. Immunisation co-ordinators were appointed in 1985, replacing the function of the medical officer of health (Begg and Nicoll, 1994) and new evidence showed that the association between immunisation and encephalopathy was not causative. Vaccine uptake rates increased and the decline in the disease recommenced. By 1994, uptake rates had reached 93 per cent and the expected 4-yearly outbreak failed to occur for the first time; whooping cough had at last been controlled in England and Wales.

Tetanus immunisation began around 1960. The disease declined; by the 1990s there were less than 10 notifications per year, none of them in children and most in elderly women who had not been immunised as adults in the services. This near elimination of the disease was brought about by the improved surgical care of wounds and by routine immunisation in childhood (see Figure 15.9).

Poliomyelitis changed in the early twentieth century from an endemic disease in young children, 'infantile paralysis', to an epidemic disease of young adults, 'paralytic poliomyelitis'. This change was associated with improvements in hygiene and sanitation, which tended to limit the faecal-oral spread of the virus in infants and young children, in whom the infection was usually symptomless. As a consequence, fewer children grew up with naturally acquired immunity, and a pool of susceptible young adults accumulated. Immunisation was introduced in the 1960s, first with Salk killed virus vaccine given by injection (IPV) and then with Sabin live attenuated vaccine given orally (OPV). Notifications then declined rapidly and the infection virtually disappeared (see Figure 15.9). About one third of 25 cases reported during the

1980s acquired the infection abroad, many of which were in adults who had not been immunised in childhood.

Measles, rubella, mumps and Haemophilus influenzae

Measles deaths followed a similar pattern to those of whooping cough and fell to less than 100 each year by the time immunisation was introduced in 1968. Although immunisation was slow to gain general acceptance, notifications fell by about two thirds to an average of about 90,000 per year in the early 1980s. When in 1988, measles/mumps/rubella (MMR) vaccine was introduced, a higher uptake of immunisation was achieved and notifications then fell to the lowest recorded annual total of 9,599 in 1993 (see Figure 15.10). Although numbers of notifications fell, notification rates increased in teenage children and young adults, necessitating a programme to immunise children in these susceptible age-groups.

Rubella immunisation was originally introduced in schoolgirls to prevent congenital malformations caused by infection during subsequent pregnancy. Although this programme was successful in subsequently reducing the incidence of malformed children, it proved impossible to eliminate congenital infection. To achieve this, routine immunisation of all children was started with MMR vaccine in 1988. General practice consultation rates for rubella, derived from data collected by the Royal College of General Practitioners (RCGP), then fell sharply (see Figure 15.10). Notifications of rubella began only in 1989, when there were 24,570, and this fell to 9,719 in 1993. Information is not yet available to assess the affect of MMR on congenital rubella.

Mumps immunisation, included in MMR vaccine, began for the first time in 1988. General practice consultation rates (RCGP) and laboratory reports fell sharply (see Figure 15.10). Notifications started in 1989 and fell from 20,713 to 2,147 by 1993.

More recently, in October 1992, immunisation against *Haemophilus influenzae* group B (HIB) meningitis and invasive disease was introduced. HIB meningitis occurs mainly in children under 5 years of age and is less common than meningococcal meningitis but, during the 1980s, laboratory reports of the infection more than doubled to over 500 per year. By 1993 these had fallen to 140, about half the level of the 1970s (see Figure 15.10).

15.3.6 Imported infections

> This fortress built by nature for herself
> Against infection and the hand of war
> This happy breed of men, this little world,
> This precious stone set in the silver sea,
> Which serves in the office of a wall,
> Or as a moat defensive to a house...
> Shakespeare, *King Richard II* (Act 2, Scene 1)

The seas around England no longer afford protection against infection and Shakespeare's 'little world' has gone; many old

Figure 15.10

Measles, rubella, mumps and bacterial meningitis

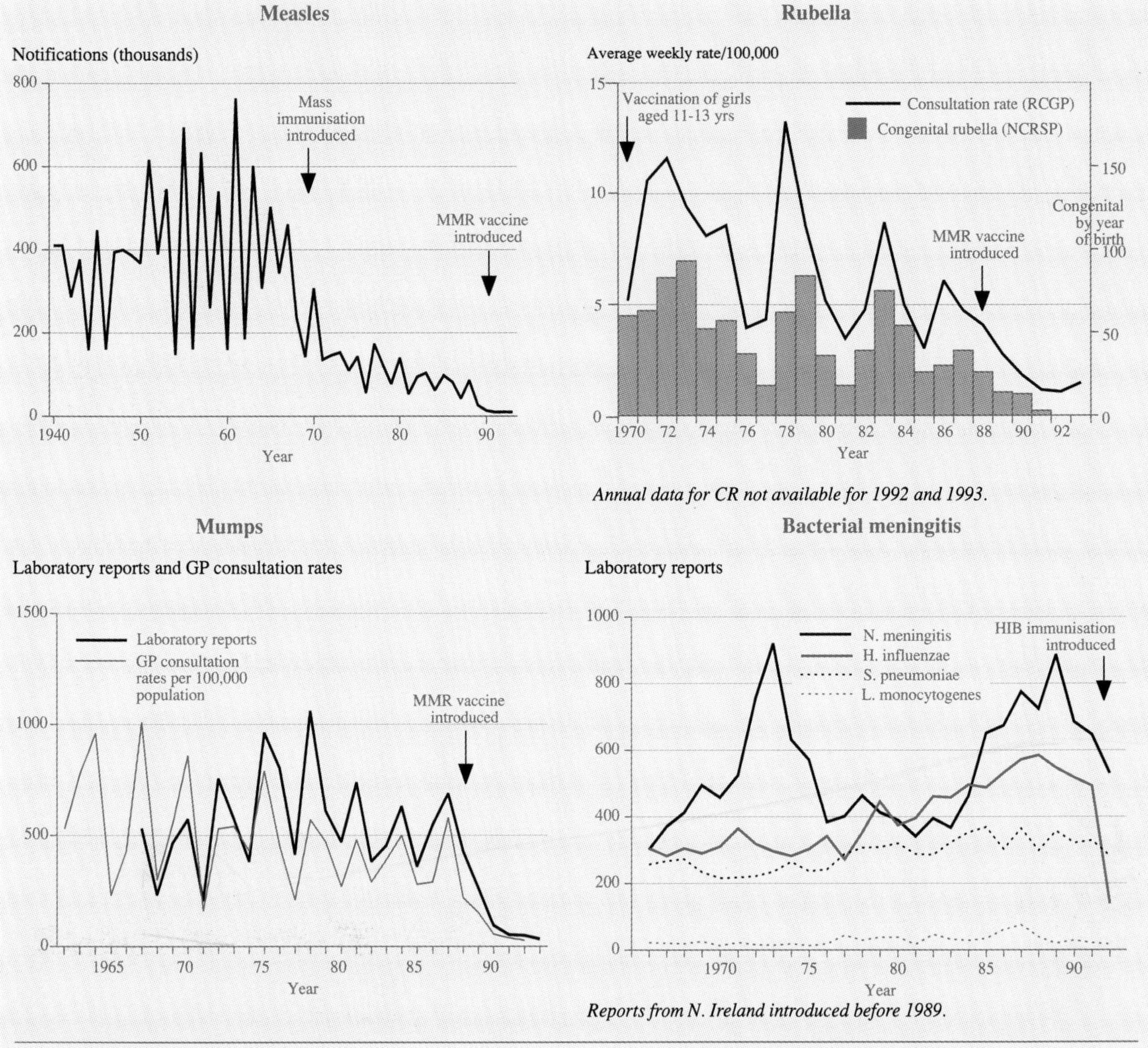
Measles
Notifications (thousands)
800
600
400
200
0
1940
50
60
70
80
90
Year
Mass immunisation introduced
MMR vaccine introduced
Rubella
Average weekly rate/100,000
15
10
5
0
Vaccination of girls aged 11-13 yrs
Consultation rate (RCGP)
Congenital rubella (NCRSP)
150
100
50
0
Congenital by year of birth
MMR vaccine introduced
1970
72
74
76
78
80
82
84
86
88
90
92
Year
Annual data for CR not available for 1992 and 1993.
Mumps
Laboratory reports and GP consultation rates
1500
1000
500
0
Laboratory reports
GP consultation rates per 100,000 population
MMR vaccine introduced
1965
70
75
80
85
90
Year
Bacterial meningitis
Laboratory reports
1000
800
600
400
200
0
N. meningitis
H. influenzae
S. pneumoniae
L. monocytogenes
HIB immunisation introduced
1970
75
80
85
90
Year
Reports from N. Ireland introduced before 1989.

Source. CSF isolates reported to CDSC provisional figures for 1993

diseases have returned and some new infections have appeared in the wake of a phenomenal increase in human travel (Bruce-Chwatt, 1977). Diarrhoeal illness of varying severity and aetiology, 'traveller's diarrhoea', is the most common infection, but many other sometimes life-threatening and highly infectious diseases have been imported in recent years (Bannister, 1990).

Imported malaria increased 20-fold from less than 100 annual notifications in the 1960s to around 2,000 per year in the 1990s (see Figure 15.11), mostly as a result of a rise in imported malignant tertian malaria, caused by the parasite *Plasmodium falciparum*, from Africa. The re-emergence of malignant tertian malaria, both in Africa and in India, was responsible for the increase in malaria notifications in the last two decades (see Figure 15.11). Although of obvious clinical importance, imported malaria has little public health significance because it is unlikely to spread in England and Wales. Another less common imported insect-borne infection was typhus; notifications rose from 3 in 1961–70 to 28 in 1971–80 and 43 in 1981–90, mostly caused by tick-borne typhus acquired in the Mediterranean, also known as boutenneuse fever. Dengue fever, also an insect-borne imported infection, increased; laboratory reports rose to a peak of 34 in 1990 following outbreaks in the Caribbean.

Classical cholera disappeared from Britain early in the present century. Cholera caused by a different type of the organism, *Vibrio cholerae* El tor, which was confined to Indonesia for several decades, began to spread to neighbouring countries in 1961 and reached Britain in 1970. Since then there have been nearly 100 imported infections with two deaths (see Figure 15.11). No spread of infection occurred, apart from a symptomless infection in the wife of a case, who nursed her husband at home. Indeed, spread is very unlikely, so long as present standards of hygiene and sanitation are maintained.

Figure 15.11

Some imported infections

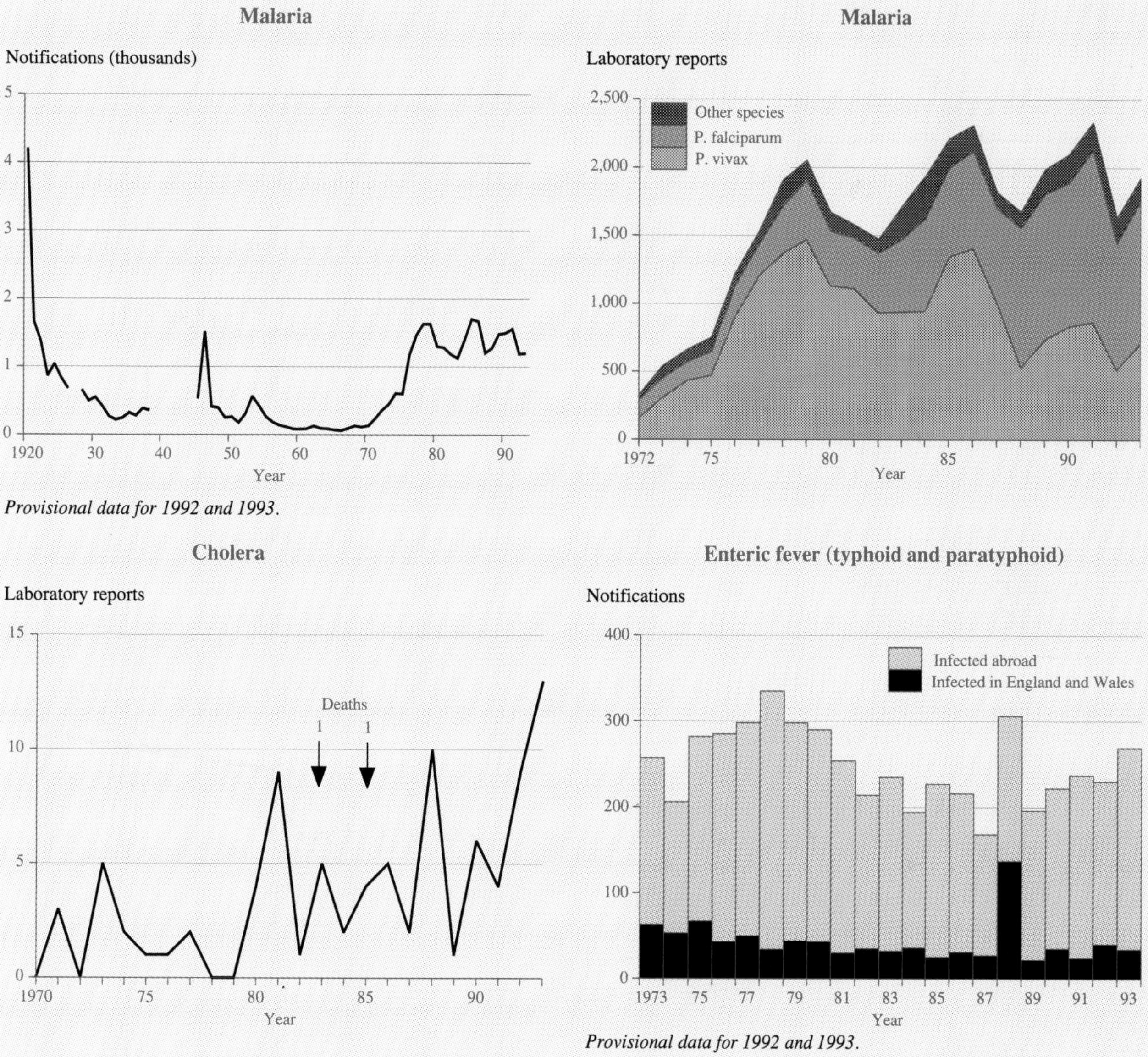

Malaria

Notifications (thousands)

Provisional data for 1992 and 1993.

Malaria

Laboratory reports

Cholera

Laboratory reports

Enteric fever (typhoid and paratyphoid)

Notifications

Provisional data for 1992 and 1993.

In 1992 another strain, designated *V. cholerae* 0139, previously thought not to cause epidemic cholera, caused large epidemics in India and Bangladesh. By 1993 global spread had begun, with imported cases reported in Europe, including Britain (Cheasty and Rowe, 1994).

Enteric fever (typhoid and paratyphoid) became almost exclusively an imported disease, with less than 400 notifications annually since 1973 (see Figure 15.11), over 85 per cent of them in people infected abroad. In about one third of the cases infected in England and Wales, the source was found to be a case or carrier from abroad, living in the household. Many other bacterial, viral and parasitic gastrointestinal infections have been imported (Bannister, 1990).

Sexually transmitted diseases, including AIDS, were often acquired abroad. For example, for new cases of syphilis between 1964 and 1981, about 15 per cent of those in men and 5 per cent of those in women acquired the infection abroad, but the corresponding proportions for cases of gonorrhoea

were 5 per cent and 1 per cent. When penicillin-resistant strains of *Neisseria gonorrhoea* were first reported in the 1970s, most infections were acquired abroad, but the proportion of cases infected in the United Kingdom gradually increased and by 1982 most infections were contracted at home (Galbraith, 1985).

15.4 Newly described and emerging diseases

15.4.1 'New' gastrointestinal infections

Campylobacter enteritis

This infection was recognised as a common cause of acute self-limiting diarrhoeal disease in the 1970s, soon after laboratory techniques were developed to detect the organism (see Figure 15.12). Since 1981, it has been the most common known bacterial cause of acute diarrhoea in Britain

(Cowden, 1992). The causative organisms are found in the aqueous environment, farm animals, domestic pets and birds. Milk, water and poultry are the most common reported sources of outbreaks. In some parts of the country there is a spring peak in incidence associated with milk delivered to the door and then pecked by birds. About 10 per cent of reported cases are in travellers. Direct spread from animals is not common and person-to-person spread is very unusual. Most cases are sporadic and the spread and source remain unknown.

It seems likely that most infections are food-borne and associated with infection in poultry. Very high rates of infection have been found both in birds in broiler units and in poultry meat. Indeed, the recent detection of *Campylobacter enteritis* may have been the result of a substantial increase of human infection related to changes in poultry rearing. The introduction of intensive broiler production could have led to the amplification of the infection in the birds before slaughter. Studies have shown that birds in broiler units may become infected from contaminated water supplies to these units, and that the infection is usually symptomless and confined to the intestinal tract. The infection rate increases to reach a maximum at about 8 weeks of age, that is, about the time of slaughter, when around 70 per cent of birds may be infected. Spread of the organism then takes place by faecal contamination of the broiler carcases during slaughter and later to other foods during food preparation in the kitchen (Healing *et al.*, 1992).

Cryptosporidiosis

This was established as an important cause of diarrhoea in farm animals, particularly calves and lambs, in the 1970s. Human infection was first recorded in 1976, mainly in immuno-compromised patients. It commonly occurred in association with HIV infection, causing severe life-threatening diarrhoea. It was not until the 1980s, when reliable laboratory tests for crytosporidium oocysts in faeces became available, that it was found to be a common cause of mild diarrhoeal illness in previously healthy people. Direct spread from animals and from person-to-person by the faecal-oral route appear to be common. Food-borne spread is unusual, but several water-borne outbreaks have been reported, raising the possibility that contaminated drinking water may be a source of infection in immuno-compromised people (Casemore, 1990).

The appearance of water-borne cryptosporidiosis may have been associated with increased recognition of the infection. It may also have been associated with an increase in incidence which could have arisen because of the more intensive agricultural and recreational use of water catchment areas, increasing the risk of contamination of the water by animals. At the same time, there was a change of flocculants used in water purification, because of concern about the use of aluminium compounds previously in common use. The organism is resistant to chlorine and inexperience with the new treatment processes may have allowed the organisms to pass into the water supply. The number of laboratory reports increased to a peak in 1989, and the annual number then became stable at around 5,000.

Giardiasis

Giardiasis was found to be a cause of outbreaks of water-borne illness in travellers in the 1960s, but only two water-borne outbreaks have been detected in England and Wales. Person-to-person spread by the faecal-oral route is probably most common. Direct spread from pets and other animals occurs and may account for some of the infections. Food-borne infection appears to be very unusual. Laboratory reports rose continuously to reach about 6,000 per year in the late 1980s and then remained steady at around this number each year.

Haemorrhagic colitis and haemolytic uraemic syndrome (HUS)

Haemorrhagic colitis and haemolytic uraemic syndrome (HUS) caused by verocyto-toxin producing *Escherichia coli* (VTEC) type 0157, were recognised in the 1980s. It was first described in the United States of America as the cause of an outbreak of severe bloody diarrhoea. The vehicle of infection was inadequately cooked hamburgers and the origin was traced to infection in cattle. Although the incidence of VTEC-related disease in England and Wales is low, infection can lead to HUS, which in children is a common cause of renal failure.

The infection is usually derived from cattle and is usually transmitted by meat, meat products or milk. Several outbreaks occurred in Britain and laboratory reports increased to over 500 per year (see Figure 15.12) (Thomas *et al.*, 1993). A further rise in reports is likely as case ascertainment improves, and this may continue until more information is acquired about the source and mode of spread of the infection, enabling control measures to be introduced.

Viral causes of gastroenteritis

These began to be detected when electron microscopy became widely available in the 1970s, and the increase in laboratory reports which followed resulted mainly from increased recognition (see Figure 15.12) (Blacklow and Greenberg, 1991).

The following are the three most commonly reported viruses:

*   Rotaviruses, an important cause of winter epidemic diarrhoea in children; a different strain of the same virus causes illness in adults and elderly people. Spread is by the faecal-oral route. Laboratory reports increased to about 15,000 per year.

*   Adenoviruses, group F, types 40 and 41, cause diarrhoea particularly in infants. Again, spread is by the faecal-oral route but, unlike rotavirus infection, there is no seasonal variation. About 1,500 cases have been reported each year.

*   Small round structured viruses (SRSVs), which cause epidemic diarrhoea in adults that is sometimes food-borne; this is associated with shellfish harvested from sewage-polluted water or with other foods contaminated by infected food handlers. The infection also spreads from person-to-person by the faecal-oral route. Over 100 outbreaks and 1,000 cases were reported in 1993 (see Figure 15.12).

Figure 15.12

Some new infections

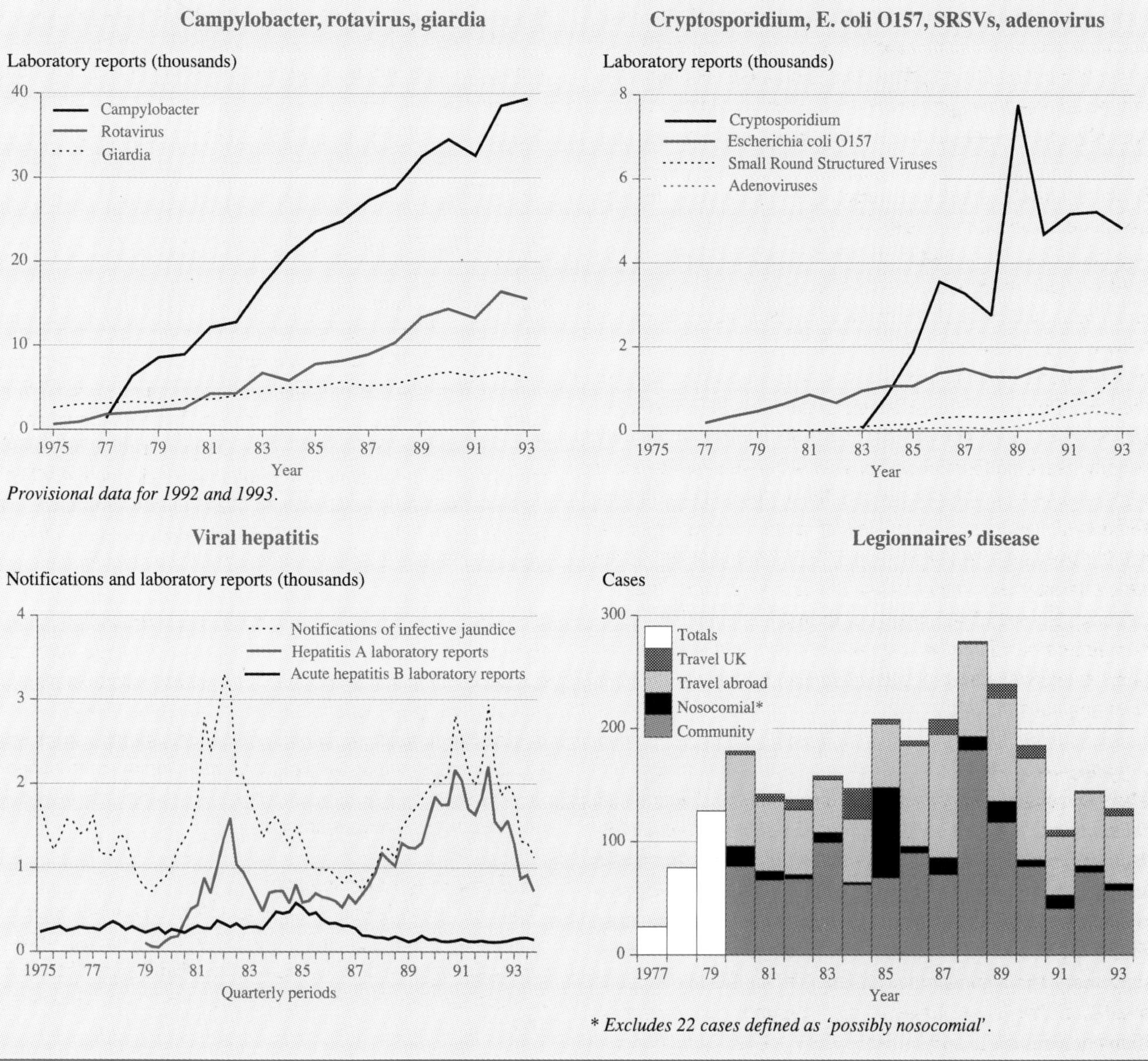
Campylobacter, rotavirus, giardia
Laboratory reports (thousands)
40
30
20
10
0
Campylobacter
Rotavirus
Giardia
1975
77
79
81
83
85
87
89
91
93
Year
Provisional data for 1992 and 1993.
Cryptosporidium, E. coli O157, SRSVs, adenovirus
Laboratory reports (thousands)
8
6
4
2
0
Cryptosporidium
Escherichia coli O157
Small Round Structured Viruses
Adenoviruses
1975
77
79
81
83
85
87
89
91
93
Year
Viral hepatitis
Notifications and laboratory reports (thousands)
4
3
2
1
0
Notifications of infective jaundice
Hepatitis A laboratory reports
Acute hepatitis B laboratory reports
1975
77
79
81
83
85
87
89
91
93
Quarterly periods
Legionnaires' disease
Cases
300
200
100
0
Totals
Travel UK
Travel abroad
Nosocomial*
Community
1977
79
81
83
85
87
89
91
93
Year
* Excludes 22 cases defined as 'possibly nosocomial'.

15.4.2 'New' zoonoses

Marburg and Ebola virus diseases and Lassa fever

Marburg and Ebola virus diseases, Lassa fever and other similar haemorrhagic fevers became prominent in the 1960s and 1970s when several outbreaks occurred in Africa and one in Europe, with very high mortality rates. These infections may have arisen recently because of human encroachment into hitherto remote areas of the world. Very few cases have been imported into Britain, and the infections do not appear to pose a threat of community spread in Britain at present, because transmission in this country is from person-to-person by direct contact with blood or tissue fluids. Nevertheless, they are an important hazard in hospitals and laboratories in Britain, which care for patients recently arrived from Africa. In a recent outbreak of Ebola-like virus infection among imported monkeys from the Philippines in the United States of America, spread is thought to have taken place by the airborne route. Although there was a high mortality rate among the monkeys and human infection occurred, this strain did not cause human disease (Brown, 1993). This episode raised the possibility, however, that a similar human pathogen with a high mortality, spreading by the airborne route, might arise in the future.

Haemorrhagic fever with renal syndrome

This is caused by hanta virus and was first recognised in an outbreak of haemorrhagic disease in the Korean War in the 1950s. Other manifestations were subsequently encountered in northern Europe, where a milder disease, nephnopathia epidemica, caused by viruses similar to that identified in Korea, was reported, and most recently in the United States of America where the pulmonary syndrome was identified. Rodents are the usual hosts. The infection is spreading in parts of North America and continental Europe and, although less than 10 infections have been detected in Britain, the disease is likely to be detected with increasing frequency in the future (Bremner, 1994).

Lyme disease

Lyme disease is a newly recognised manifestation of erythema chronicum migrans, which had long been endemic in forest areas of Scandinavia and central Europe. The cause is a tick-borne spirochaete, the definitive host of which is the deer. The appearance of the disease in Lyme, Connecticut, United States of America in 1977 was associated with reforestation and residential development in the vicinity (O'Connell, 1993). Less than 200 cases have been detected in England and Wales in the last 7 years, but this may increase, particularly in places where reforestation has taken place in and around residential areas.

15.4.3 'New' environmental infections

Legionnaires' disease

This was first recognised in an outbreak of acute respiratory disease in the United States of America in 1976. The causal bacterium is widespread in the aqueous environment. The appearance of the disease was probably associated with the increasing use of systems capable of generating aerosols which convey the organism to humans, such as water cooling systems of air-conditioning plants and whirlpool spas. About 200 cases per year were reported in the 1980s in England and Wales, and many outbreaks were detected by active surveillance. About half the cases reported were shown to have acquired the infection abroad and about 15 per cent of the indigenous infections were hospital-associated. The national active surveillance scheme comprised recording the likely buildings and places of infection of all cases diagnosed by laboratories, and then the appropriate investigation of any site common to two or more cases. In the last 5 years the numbers of reported cases have almost halved (see Figure 15.12), a success probably attributable to control measures which followed this successful surveillance scheme (PHLS Communicable Disease Surveillance Centre, 1993).

Primary amoebic meningoencephalitis (PAM)

PAM was detected by a careful epidemiological and laboratory study of a cluster of 10 deaths from purulent bacteriologically-negative meningitis in Port Augusta, South Australia, between 1961 and 1972. The organism thrives in natural warm springs and warm static fresh water and gains access to the brain through the nose during energetic swimming or immersion in contaminated water (Ma *et al.*, 1990). Only one recent case occurred in England, in 1978, after swimming in a pool filled partially with water from a natural warm spring. Further cases are unlikely to arise with continuing high standards of maintenance of swimming pools.

Acanthamoeba keratitis

This is an uncommon eye infection, first reported in 1974, caused by a free-living environmental amoeba which is widespread in the watery environment. Most reported cases have been in people who wear contact lenses. The recent appearance of the infection was associated with the development and common use of contact lenses, particularly soft lenses worn for long periods, and inadequate contact lens hygiene, such as cleaning them in tap water (Ma *et al.*, 1990).

15.4.4 'New' microbes for old diseases

Viral hepatitis

Five causal viruses have been identified in the last 20 years. Hepatitis A and E viruses are enteric viruses, and hepatitis B, C and D viruses are often blood-borne; B and C viruses may also be sexually transmitted (Teo, 1992).

Hepatitis A virus (HAV) is the most common cause of viral hepatitis in Britain, formerly known as infective jaundice or catarrhal jaundice. The infection spreads mainly by the faecal-oral route in young children, but may also spread by food, often shellfish grown in sewage-polluted estuaries, and sometimes by food contaminated by an infected food handler. The infection is usually mild and often symptomless in young children, but may cause severe illness in adults. Notifications which reflect the trend in HAV infection declined from over 23,500 in 1969 to just over 3,000 in 1979 probably associated with improved hygiene and sanitation in schools. After this, the disease increased in two epidemics in 1981–83 and 1990–92, during which several food-borne outbreaks were reported (see Figure 15.12). Shellfish-associated disease declined following the improved heat treatment of cockles, but outbreaks are likely to continue from time to time because oysters are usually eaten raw and may harbour HAV, and other foods may be contaminated by infected food handlers.

Hepatitis E virus was only recently identified. It has caused water-borne outbreaks of severe jaundice in Asia and Central America but has not yet been reported in Britain.

Hepatitis B virus (HBV) was first identified in the 1970s. The infection was previously known as serum jaundice, because, in the 1940s, it followed the use of contaminated serum. In retrospect, it was also the main cause of arsphenamine jaundice, early in this century. Arsphenamine was an arsenical preparation given by intravenous injection in the treatment of syphilis, and it was the inadequate sterilisation of the syringes which led to outbreaks of jaundice (Mortimer, 1995). Laboratory reports began in the early 1970s and remained at about 1,000 per year from 1975 until the mid 1980s, when an outbreak took place among intravenous drug users. Reports have since declined to nearly half the original number (see Figure 15.12), possibly associated with control measures in drug users and to changes in sexual behaviour consequent upon the AIDS epidemic.

Hepatitis D virus (Delta virus) is a co-infection with HBV, which has been reported in intravenous drug users giving rise to a severe fulminating hepatitis. Hepatitis C is a recently recognised cause of blood-borne hepatitis. Screening of donor blood is now carried out, so that the infection is likely to decline.

Childhood exanthemata

Parvovirus B19 was found to be the cause of erythema infectiosum, a common, usually mild, frequently symptomless, rubella-like infection in childhood. In adults, however, the illness may be severe and prolonged and may be associated with arthritis. The infection has two other serious consequences. First, in patients with chronic haemolytic anaemia, infection induces aplastic crises. Second, in pregnancy, infection in the second trimester may cause spontaneous abortion and in the second and third trimesters may damage the foetal blood-forming tissues giving rise to hydropsfetalis, sometimes with a fatal outcome (Pattison, 1994). The cause of another childhood infection, roseola infantum, was also discovered recently, human herpesvirus-6. This infection presents with a rash which is often misdiagnosed as measles, so that newly available specific tests for this virus will be valuable, excluding these misdiagnosed cases in assessing the efficacy of measles vaccine.

Pet-associated zoonoses

Rochalimaea henselae was found to be the cause of cat-scratch disease, an uncommon zoonosis manifested by enlarged glands in the area of a cat or dog bite or scratch. The organism was discovered following the identification of another similar organism, Rochalimaea quintana, as the cause of a rare disease, bacillary angiomatosis, which had appeared in AIDS patients (PHLS Communicable Disease Surveillance Centre, 1991).

Two other rare zoonoses appeared. Nearly 30 cases of cowpox, often associated with cats, have been reported in the last 20 years. It is usually a mild viral skin infection, but it poses a serious risk in immuno-compromised people (Anonymous, 1994). The definitive host of the virus is not known, but it is likely to be small field rodents from which cats and cows acquire the infection. Human infection has probably appeared because of declining immunity following the cessation of vaccination against smallpox with vaccinia virus, a closely related virus to cowpox. Another apparently new illness was septicaemia caused by Capnocytophaga canimorus, an organism of the normal flora of the mouth of dogs and cats. The disease may occur in previously healthy people but is usually seen in those who are highly susceptible to infection, particularly those who have undergone splenectomy (PHLS Communicable Disease Surveillance Centre, 1991). It has probably come to notice because of the increasing numbers of susceptible people in the population.

15.4.5 Hospital acquired and opportunistic infections

In the middle of the nineteenth century, hospital acquired infection was common after childbirth, and was almost inevitable after surgical operations. Simpson (1871) commented:

'A man laid on the operating table in one of our surgical hospitals is exposed to more chances of death than the English soldier on the field of Waterloo.'

By the end of the century, antiseptic surgery had been followed by aseptic surgery, hospital design and practice had improved and, with the development of bacteriology, surgical practice was revolutionised. It seemed that hospital infection was a thing of the past. Early in this century, however, it was realised that in fever hospitals cross-infection was common, particularly streptococcal infection. The so-called 'return cases' of scarlet fever were shown to be the result of reinfection in hospital with a different strain of S. pyogenes (Selwyn, 1991). This was confirmed in the 1920s, when methods of typing the organism were developed. The introduction of typing of S. pyogenes subsequently enabled the identification of cross-infection in other circumstances, for example in maternity and burns units and in general wards in the 1930s. Indeed, streptococcal cross-infection dominated the hospital scene until the arrival of penicillin in the 1940s.

Hospital infection with Staphylococcus aureus began to re-emerge at this time and became increasingly important when penicillinase-producing staphylococci appeared, resistant to this antibiotic. There followed, in the 1950s and 1960s, many and widespread outbreaks of sepsis in hospitals caused by virulent strains of penicillinase-producing S. aureus, one of which, phage type 80/81, spread worldwide (Williams et al., 1960). In the next decade, the staphylococcus declined and was replaced by gram-negative bacteria, often resistant to many antibiotics, such as Pseudomonas aeruginosa, Klebsiella spp. and Enterobacter spp. More recently, the staphylococcus reappeared (epidemic methicillin-resistant S. aureus (EMRSA)) and, although less virulent than the strains of the 1950s, it has caused clinical infections in many hospitals.

Many new hospital infections have also appeared caused by bacteria, viruses, fungi and parasites, often organisms previously unrecognised or regarded as non-pathogenic. These followed in the wake of major developments in hospital practice. For example, the increasingly widespread use of antibiotics and chemotherapy, immuno-suppression following transplants and in the treatment of disease, and the introduction of many new prostheses and new surgical techniques. Furthermore, the survival of increasing numbers of highly susceptible patients and elderly people increased the numbers at special risk of infection in hospitals. This pool of susceptible people has been added to since the 1980s by the spread of the acquired immune deficiency syndrome (AIDS). Infections which are usually mild in healthy people may spread to hospitals where highly susceptible patients may develop severe and sometimes fatal disease. For example, outbreaks of salmonellosis in maternity, premature baby and paediatric units may have a high case fatality rate. Similarly, outbreaks of enterovirus infections in special care baby units have occurred with high fatality rates. Chickenpox and herpes zoster are particularly dangerous in patients with leukaemia and lymphoma undergoing therapy. Legionnaires' disease has occurred in hospital outbreaks in which the case fatality rate was over 30 per cent, three times that of community acquired disease. Lastly, influenza in wards and homes for elderly people often has a high fatality rate.

Although such outbreaks in hospitals may be devastating, cause much disruption and receive great prominence, the number of cases involved is small compared with the total number of patients with infections in hospital. For example, the overall burden of hospital infection in England and Wales was estimated in 1980 by a prevalence survey involving 18,186 patients in 43 hospitals. This survey showed that 19.1

Figure 15.13

The acquired immune deficiency syndrome

AIDS

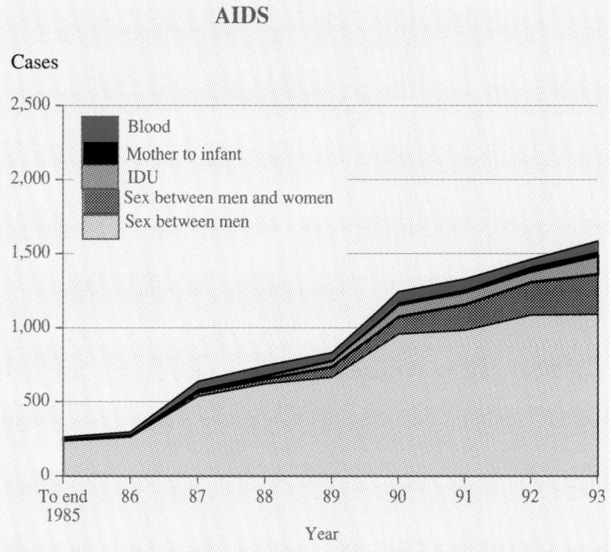

per cent of patients had an infection, in half of whom, 9.2 per cent of the total, it was acquired in hospital (Meers *et al.*, 1981), representing around 12,500 patients with a hospital-acquired infection in acute hospitals in England and Wales at any one time.

15.4.6 HIV infection and AIDS

Increasing clinical requests for a drug used to treat *Pneumocystis carinii* pneumonia led to the identification of clusters of cases of this unusual type of pneumonia and of Kaposi's sarcoma among homosexual men in New York and California in 1981. The acquired immune deficiency syndrome (AIDS) was defined, the viral cause of which was first established in France in 1983. This is a new human infection which probably arose in the recent past in Central Africa and then the particular social circumstances in the 1970s facilitated its dissemination.

The virus spreads by blood, body fluids and tissues, so that the most common methods of transmission have been: sexual contact, especially when mucous membranes are breached by previous disease or trauma, the sharing of syringes,

needles and other skin-piercing equipment, the use of contaminated blood and blood products, and mother to foetus. The first recognised case of AIDS occurred in Britain in December 1981, and by 1993 over 8,500 cases and more than 5,500 deaths had been reported.

Homosexual transmission has predominated and although the increase in this exposure category now appears to be slowing, it may rise again in young men who have not adopted safe sexual practices. Heterosexual transmission has been much lower than homosexual, but has shown a continuing increase, which is likely to continue in the future. Transmission by injecting drug use increased in the 1980s and appeared to be slowing in 1990–92, then increased again in 1993, but the overall downward trend may return if needle sharing does not increase. The epidemic among people with haemophilia and other people who received contaminated blood or blood products in the past has been controlled (see Figure 15.13).

15.5 Conclusions

....however secure and well-regulated civilized life may become, bacteria, Protozoa, viruses, infected fleas, lice, ticks, mosquitoes and bedbugs will always lurk in the shadows ready to pounce when neglect, poverty, famine, or war lets down the defences. And even in normal times they prey on the weak, the very young and the very old, living among us, in mysterious obscurity waiting their opportunities.

Hans Zinsser, *Rats, Lice and History*, 1935.

This review confirms the truth of these comments of Hans Zinsser in his well-known book, published 60 years ago. The pattern of infection in England and Wales, and indeed worldwide, has changed continually over the last 150 years and, moreover, the rate of change appears to be increasing as the speed of human social, technical, environmental and population changes accelerate. These changes increase the threat of the appearance of new diseases and the re-appearance of old diseases and have led to the appreciation that these emerging and re-emerging infections require global action to detect them quickly and to carry out rapid investigation to bring about their control (Lederberg *et al.*, 1992; Murphy, 1994). It is now recognised that it can only be a matter of time until the next microbial menace to our species emerges amongst us.

Chapter 16

Communicable diseases: sexually transmitted diseases, including AIDS

By
Michael Adler, Andrew Phillips and Anne Johnson

Summary

- Before the creation of a clinical service for sexually transmitted diseases, data collection was confined to mortality and serological surveys of syphilis in populations.

- The widespread use of penicillin since the Second World War has been effective in reducing the number of deaths and long-term complications due to syphilis.

- There was a marked increase in cases of gonorrhoea and all other sexually transmitted diseases in the 1960s and 1970s. This may be attributed partly to changes in sexual behaviour and contraceptive practice.

- Clinic-based morbidity data alone do not give a reliable estimate of the number of cases of sexually transmitted diseases in the population. A fuller picture requires information about people treated in other settings, and from those who are asymptomatic or symptomatic but not seeking treatment.

- There has been an increase in the number of reports of AIDS cases in Britain every year since 1982. Ninety three per cent of all AIDS cases reported by the end of 1991 had occurred in people aged under 50 and 60 per cent were within the 20–25 year age-band.

- The proportion of cases of both HIV and AIDS infection attributable to heterosexual transmission is increasing. In 1991 they comprised 23 per cent of all newly reported HIV infections and 13 per cent of AIDS cases.

- Although the number of cases remains relatively small, the incidence of AIDS in women is increasing. Injecting drug users also constitute a small but growing group in which the incidence of AIDS is increasing.

- The Public Health Laboratory Service report suggests that by the end of the century the number of new cases of AIDS in homosexual men will level off, but that those acquiring HIV from heterosexual sex and injecting drug users will continue to increase.

16.1 Sexually transmitted diseases (excluding AIDS)

16.1.1 Introduction

Sexually transmitted diseases (STDs) have always been a major public health problem and continue to be so. Before the creation of a clinical service for these diseases, following the Royal Commission on Venereal Diseases (1916), data were few and inadequate, being largely confined to mortality and serological surveys of syphilis in populations (Adler, 1980a).

During the nineteenth and early twentieth centuries legislation created a climate of stigma associated with the venereal diseases (syphilis, gonorrhoea and chancroid). The Contagious Disease Acts of 1864 and 1866 required the compulsory registration and police supervision of all prostitutes, plus regular examinations and hospital detention if thought necessary. The Royal Commission on Poor Laws of 1909 also recommended detention orders for patients with venereal diseases, and the Royal Commission on Divorce (1912) commented that the passing on of these diseases was an act of cruelty second to none as grounds for divorce. Such legislation implicitly recognised the magnitude of the problem, but created a climate of secrecy and shame rather than a programme of control of venereal diseases.

The Royal Commission on Venereal Diseases recommended the establishment of a free, open access, medical service for patients with such diseases funded by local and central government. The local authorities were given the responsibility for organising the service within county and general hospitals. The creation of the National Health Service in 1948 resulted in regional hospital boards and boards of governors taking on the running of the service for venereal disease. Since that time the numbers of clinics and consultants have increased. Currently there are 180 consultants working in 270 clinics in Britain. The setting up of clinics allowed the collection of routine data about the number of cases seen by diagnostic category for the first time.

16.1.2 Mortality

Deaths caused by syphilis were frequently seen before the widescale use of penicillin. These usually occurred many years after the initial infection and were related to involvement of the brain and heart. In 1910, 4,375 deaths caused by syphilis were reported (see Table 16.1). This was probably a considerable underestimate, because physicians often gave other diagnoses on the death certificate, such as locomotor ataxia, aneurysm, hemiplegia, apoplexy, etc., for fear of offending relations and as a result of the stigma attached to syphilis. William Osler (1917) estimated that total deaths were closer to 60,000 instead of the reported number of just over 4,000.

Serological surveys carried out at the same time suggested that 12 per cent of the adult male population of London and 7 per cent of the female population had acquired syphilis (Morris, 1917).

Table 16.1

Deaths from syphilis (neurosyphilis, tabes dorsalis, etc.)

Year	Number of deaths
1910	4,375
1920	4,150
1930	3,185
1940	3,198
1950	1,732
1960	1,567
1970	185
1980	59
1990	18

Source: ONS

The availability and use of penicillin after the Second World War resulted in a substantial reduction in the mortality and number of cases of syphilis diagnosed within clinics (see Table 16.1). Deaths from gonorrhoea were rare, even before the discovery of penicillin, but caused considerable morbidity (e.g. urethral stricture, epididymitis and salpingitis).

16.1.3 Morbidity data

There are a number of limitations to the data collected about STDs (see Table 16.2). The data collected from clinics relate to cases, not patients, and there is a lack of uniform criteria for diagnosing and reporting. These clinic-based data do not give a total picture of sexually transmitted diseases in the population. The total picture would require, in addition, the number of people (1) treated in the community or in other clinical settings and (2) who are asymptomatic or symptomatic, but not seeking care.

Clinic attendance
Consultants in charge of genitourinary medicine clinics are required to make annual returns to the Department of Health of the number of cases seen in their respective clinics. The original notification form to indicate cases seen in clinics (SBH 60) was limited to syphilis, gonorrhoea and chancroid. It has been recognised over the years that many other organisms can be spread by sexual contact and the diseases associated with them have been added to the SBH 60 over the years (see Table 16.3). In 1988 this form was redesigned as the KC 60 with clearer subcategories for various diseases and the addition of HIV infection and AIDS.

There have been considerable variations in the number of cases seen within clinics by diagnosis over the years. Latest data (1993) indicate that over 739,000 cases are seen within clinics in the United Kingdom (see Table 16.4). Unfortunately, these data are always a minimum of 2 years out of date.

Table 16.2

Drawbacks for current statistics for sexually transmitted disease, England and Wales

I Clinical statistics
   - (a) Lack of uniform criteria for diagnosis and reporting
   - (b) Figures relate to number of cases

II Community statistics
   - (a) Omission of certain categories of patients
     - Those treated in the community outside clinics
     - Symptomless
     - Symptomatic not seeking care

Table 16.3

Notification of sexually transmitted diseases

Year	Diseases reported
1916	Syphilis, gonorrhoea, chancroid
1951	+ Non-gonococcal urethritis
1967	+ Trichomoniasis
1971	+ Candidiasis Scabies Pediculosis pubis Herpes simplex Molluscum contagiosum Non-specific genital infection
1988	SBH60 → KC60

Table 16.4

Sexually transmitted disease United Kingdom, 1993

Disease	Number of cases
Non-specific genital infection	112,438
Genital warts	99,691
Candidiasis	66,291
Gonorrhoea	12,647
Genital herpes	27,627
Trichomonas	5,609
Syphilis	1,439
Scabies and lice	5,787
Chancroid/donovanosis/ lymphogranuloma venereum	55
Other conditions requiring treatment	128,217
Other conditions not requiring treatment	200,582
All other conditions and diagnosis	79,415
Total	739,798

Source: CDSC

There was a marked fall during the 1950s of cases of gonorrhoea, probably as a result of the widespread production and use of penicillin. The 1960s and 1970s saw this reversed with rapid increases in cases of gonorrhoea diagnosed and treated in clinics. It is not totally clear what caused the increase in gonorrhoea and all other STDs, but may be in part attributed to concurrent changes in sexual behaviour (see section 16.1.4). Other factors are the increasing use of the oral contraceptive pill and intrauterine devices, which has reduced the use of barrier techniques such as the condom and their associated protective effects. As a result of greatly improved services offered by clinics, their ability to trace sexual contacts and the reduction in the stigma associated with sexually acquired infections, more people are seeking treatment who may not have done so previously. In view of this it is not certain whether the increases seen for most STDs are real or apparent.

The increase in gonorrhoea in the 1960s and 1970s was followed by a fall in the 1980s, particularly in homosexual men in response to the emerging AIDS epidemic (see Figure 16.1). There is some evidence of a recent reversal of this trend (Evans *et al.*, 1993).

In the United Kingdom, a decline in syphilis has been witnessed and maintained (see Figure 16.2). Congenital syphilis has been almost eradicated, partly because of the decline of female syphilis, but mainly because of antenatal screenings and prompt treatment of those found to be infected. The numbers fell from about 1,500 per year in the 1940s to only a single case in 1992. There had been an increase in all types of syphilis among men during the 1970s, whereas the rate in women had continued to fall. This disparity was explained

Figure 16.1

Total annual cases of gonorrhoea seen in STD clinics, England and Wales

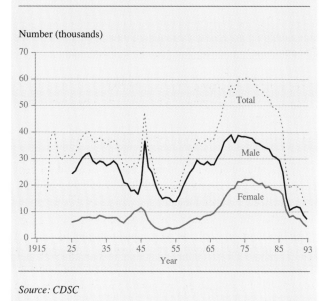

Number (thousands)

Source: CDSC

Figure 16.2

Total annual cases of syphilis seen in STD clinics, England and Wales

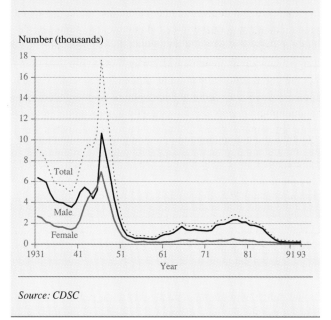

Number (thousands)

Source: CDSC

by the fact that most cases of primary and secondary syphilis (58 per cent) occurred among homosexual men. However, as with gonorrhoea, there has been a decline in cases of syphilis in homosexual men seen in STD clinics in theUnited Kingdom as a result of changing sexual practices with the advent of HIV infection and AIDS but, as indicated previously, this may reverse.

Genital herpes and warts are the two conditions that have shown the greatest increase in departments of genitourinary medicine in England in the last decade. In 1978, 89,406 cases of herpes and 24,136 of warts were seen in STD clinics, rising to 27,065 and 93,317 respectively by 1995. Again, it is difficult to interpret these trends with absolute certainty, because the rises could result from either a real increase or increased uptake of services following media interest and health education.

Pelvic inflammatory disease (PID) occurs as a complication of gonococcal and chlamydial infections and is, therefore, seen in departments of genitourinary medicine/STD clinics. Until the modification of the reporting form in 1988, PID was not recorded by aetiological agent and figures were, therefore, hard to obtain.

Hospital admissions

Usually, patients with STDs do not require hospitalisation. Patients with pelvic inflammatory disease may be admitted, particularly if seen by gynaecologists, but less frequently by a physician in genitourinary medicine as indicated above. Past studies show that approximately 90 per cent of cases of PID diagnosed within STD clinics or departments of genitourinary medicine are not hospitalised (Adler, 1980b). The Hospital In-Patient Enquiry (HIPE) and, from 1987, Hospital Episode Statistics (HES) give an indication of trends; it is not a representative picture of all women in whom a diagnosis of

pelvic inflammatory disease is made and the two sets of data are not strictly comparable. Admissions for patients with pelvic inflammatory disease have continued to increase each year and accounted for just over 21,000 in-patient episodes in 1990. Additional problems in terms of quantifying pelvic inflammatory disease lie in establishing a correct clinical diagnosis. Studies comparing the use of clinical and laparoscopic criteria indicate that the use of the former gives a correct diagnosis in only 65 per cent of cases with a false-positive diagnosis rate of 23 per cent. In the remaining 12 per cent of cases other conditions, such as ectopic pregnancy, appendicitis and endometriosis, are found (Jacobson and Westrom, 1969). In the United Kingdom, most patients diagnosed with pelvic inflammatory disease have their diagnosis based on clinical grounds alone.

Non-hospital data sources

A complete picture of the true prevalence and morbidity of the STDs would require data from non-hospital sources (see Table 16.1).

Patients diagnosed and treated outside STD clinics: Patients with an STD may be seen and treated in general or private practice, or in antenatal and gynaecology clinics. In the past, surveys have been performed in gynaecology, antenatal and family planning clinics to provide fairly crude estimates of the prevalence of certain STDs. These studies were limited to specific age-groups and those who had opted to seek medical care. To some extent the different rates reported in these types of studies reflect demographic and consulting differences and not 'true' differences in disease prevalence. As the women studied only represented one part of the total population at risk of contracting an STD, the findings cannot be related to a defined population at risk, and correct incidence or prevalence rates cannot be obtained.

'Patients' who are symptomless or symptomatic, but not seeking care: Patients who are symptomless may never be seen unless they are a named sexual contact and attend a clinic as a result of partner notification. Likewise, there will be a group of patients with symptoms of an STD who ignore these and never consult. A population-based study carried out in a defined population of women (209,100) in England was designed to identify patients with and without symptoms needing care or failing to seek care at all (Adler *et al.*, 1981). Those patients who ignored their symptoms were identified by screening carried out in general practice, antenatal and family planning clinics. Likewise, the symptomless women who are unaware of their disease and do not consult were picked up by screening in these three agencies. The difference between symptomatic and symptomless patients with regard to when they may seek care is arbitrary. Obviously, overlap does occur and the theoretical division was only created in an attempt to construct a way of identifying the different agencies that need to be sampled if a total picture of STDs is to be obtained.

As the study was carried out in a defined population sampling symptomatic, asymptomatic, consulters and non-consulters, it was possible to calculate prevalence rates. This study indicated that the proportion of women in the United Kingdom with gonococcal infections who are not receiving care is low, that the clinic service of STDs is effective in controlling disease, and that only small amounts of disease remain undetected.

Ad hoc surveys of trends

On occasion, the occurrence of gonorrhoea and syphilis has been used as a surrogate measure of sexual behaviour. For instance, numerous studies in the last 5 years have looked at rectal gonorrhoea in homosexual men following the advent of HIV infection and extensive health education. Within the United Kingdom such studies have indicated an original fall in rectal gonorrhoea followed by a recent increase, as such

men have been unable to sustain safer sex and younger homosexual men who were not touched by the early campaigns, joined the 'gay scene'.

16.1.4 Sexual behaviour

The epidemiology of STDs depends on three factors:

1. The pattern of behaviour in the population
2. The extent of undiagnosed and untreated infection in the community
3. The availability and effectiveness of treatment

It is frequently difficult to discern the relative contribution of these components to patterns of disease. There are very few historical data on sexual lifestyle in the general population. Early in the century, anecdotal evidence suggested that a substantial proportion of STDs were acquired through contact between clients and prostitutes, particularly associated with the armed forces. This may account for the high incidence of gonorrhoea and syphilis at the time of the First and Second World Wars.

In 1990 and 1991, a random sample survey of sexual lifestyle was undertaken among 18,896 men and women aged 16–59 years in Great Britain (Johnson *et al.*,1994). This indicated that there have been marked changes in sexual behaviour since the 1950s. The median age of first intercourse has fallen rapidly (see Table 16.5). The proportion of individuals having sex before marriage has risen such that less than 1 per cent of men and women aged 16–24 in 1990 were married at the time of first intercourse, as compared with 14 per cent of men and 38 per cent of women aged 45–59. There is some evidence that people whose first intercourse took place in the

Table 16.5

Median age at first intercourse by current age of respondent.

Age group	Men	Women
16-19	17	17
20-24	17	17
25-29	17	18
30-34	17	18
35-39	18	18
40-44	18	19
45-49	18	19
50-54	19	20
55-59	20	21

Source: Johnson et al. (1994)

Figure 16.3

Proportion of respondents reporting 10+ heterosexual partners ever by year of first sexual intercourse

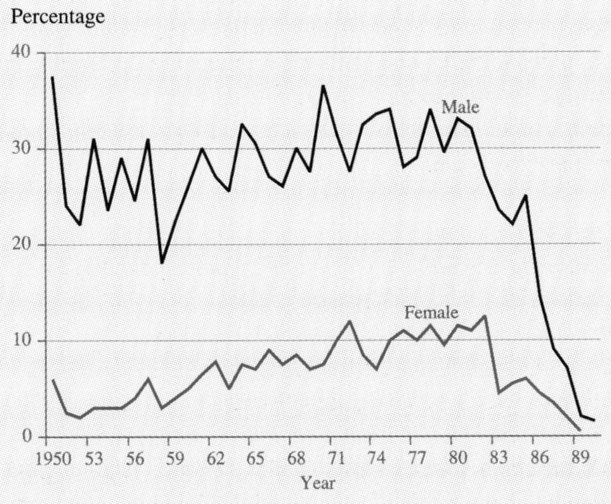

Source: Johnson et al. (1994)

1960s and 1970s have had more lifetime sexual partners than earlier cohorts. It is too early to tell what the trends are for those whose first intercourse occurred subsequently (see Figure 16.3). These trends started before the availability of oral contraception or legalisation of abortion. There appears to have been a general liberalisation of attitudes to sexual relationships, sex outside marriage and sex for pleasure, rather than procreation. These changes may, in part, account for the increased incidence of gonorrhoea in the 1970s. Following the 'safer sex' education campaigns of the late 1980s in response to the HIV epidemic, there have been substantial changes in male homosexual behaviour (Johnson and Gill, 1989). This includes the reduction in numbers of partners and unprotected anal intercourse. There is little evidence of substantial change in heterosexual behaviour, however, although condom use may have increased slightly.

16.2 The acquired immune deficiency syndrome

16.2.1 Introduction

The article describing five cases of *Pneumocystis carinii* pneumonia (PCP) in young homosexual men in Los Angeles did not even make the front page of *Morbidity and Mortality Weekly Report* (MMWR) for the US Centers for Disease Control (CDC) in June 1981 (CDC, 1981). It heralded, however, the development of a worldwide pandemic of diseases induced by infection with the human immunodeficiency virus type 1 (HIV) over the ensuing decade. The diseases include opportunistic infections such as PCP and cytomegalovirus retinitis, malignancies such as Kaposi's sarcoma and primary brain lymphoma, a wasting syndrome and a dementia complex. Infected people with any of the diseases are said to have the acquired immune deficiency syndrome (AIDS). Soon after that first report in the MMWR the first case of AIDS was identified in Britain.

By 1984 it was established that HIV infection is the cause of AIDS, but it was already clear that this could take some years. Now, 10 years later, the natural history of the infection and means of spread of the virus have been clarified further, although many details remain unclear. The time elapsing between infection with HIV and the development of AIDS has been found to be extremely variable. Some people develop AIDS within 1–2 years of infection whereas others remain healthy some 15 years after, the longest that such cases have yet been followed to date. About 50 per cent develop AIDS by 12 years after infection. It cannot be certain yet whether, given sufficient time, HIV infection will always lead to AIDS. A consistent finding of prospective studies of HIV-infected individuals is that older people tend to progress to AIDS more rapidly after HIV infection than younger people (Eyster *et al.*, 1987). No other demographic or behavioural factors have been shown to have a marked effect on the rate of progression of HIV infection.

More recently it has been discovered that a second human immunodeficiency virus exists. The two viruses have been designated HIV-1 and HIV-2. The former accounts for the vast majority of HIV infections worldwide, whereas HIV-2 appears to be mainly restricted to parts of West Africa. Although this virus is known to induce AIDS in at least some cases, it appears to do so more slowly on average than does HIV-1. There is also some suggestion that HIV-2 is less easily transmitted than HIV-1.

Once AIDS has developed, the death rate is very high, with a median survival time in developed countries of about 18 months (Lundgren *et al.*, 1994a). This value varies according to the extent of immunosuppression at the time of AIDS diagnosis, the age of the patient – older patients again do worse – and the particular AIDS-defining diseases present (Lundgren *et al.*, 1994a). The survival in those with a primary lymphoma of the brain as the AIDS diagnosis disease, for example, is usually less than 1 year whereas in those with only oesophageal candida it can often be as much as 3–4 years (Lundgren *et al.*, 1994a). Currently available treatments – prophylaxis to prevent PCP and antiviral therapy, principally with the nucleoside analogue zidovudine, introduced in the late 1980s - appear to have had only a marginally beneficial effect on prognosis, whether initiated before or after AIDS diagnosis (Concorde Co-ordinating Committee, 1994; Lundgren *et al.*, 1994b).

As of June 1995, 1,169,811 cumulative AIDS cases in adults and children have been reported to the World Health Organisation (WHO). In addition, as of June 1995, they have estimated there are around 18.5 million adults infected with HIV with an additional 1.5 million children.

16.2.2 HIV/AIDS in Britain

In Britain there is a voluntary confidential scheme for clinical doctors to report cases of AIDS. For England, Wales and Northern Ireland reports are sent to the Communicable Disease Surveillance Centre and for Scotland they are sent to the Communicable Diseases (Scotland) Unit (now called the Scottish Centre for Infectious and Environmental Health, SCIEH). It is estimated that the under-reporting rate for AIDS cases is no more than 15 per cent, and possibly lower than 10 per cent. Figure 16.4 shows the number of reports of AIDS cases, by year of report, for the United Kingdom. Every year since the first reports in 1982 has shown an increased number of reports from the previous year. Up to the end of 1991 there had been a total of 5,356 reports of AIDS cases. Ninety-three per cent of these AIDS cases occurred in people under the age of 50 and 60 per cent within the 20–35 year age-band. Also shown in Figure 16.4 are numbers of deaths in reported AIDS cases. The very poor survival associated with AIDS means that the number of deaths shadows the number of AIDS cases quite closely.

Newly identified HIV-infected people are also reported, by laboratories performing the tests, to the surveillance centres. As the infection is largely asymptomatic for many years in most individuals, the number of reports are clearly likely to

Figure 16.4

Number of AIDS cases and deaths with AIDS by year of first report, England and Wales

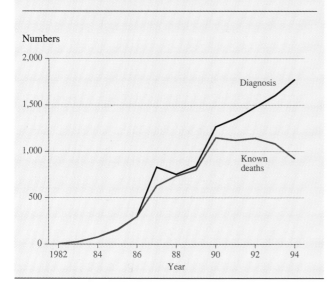

be an underestimate of the total number of infected persons, many of whom remain untested. Reports of 16,228 HIV-infected people were received by the end of 1991. Thus, by this date, for every AIDS case identified a further two people had been identified as infected with HIV, who did not have AIDS.

16.2.3 HIV exposure categories

The most common route of transmission of HIV worldwide is through sexual intercourse – mainly heterosexual sex. It can also be transmitted, however, through sharing drug injection needles and syringes, receipt of blood transfusions or blood products, and other blood contacts, such as needlestick injuries, and from mother to child in utero and through breast-feeding.

In most developed countries, including Britain, HIV infection attributed to intercourse between men has been much more widespread than that attributed to heterosexual sex. This is likely to be the result of the larger average number of sexual partners for homosexual men compared with heterosexual men and women, and of anal intercourse being a more efficient means of transmitting HIV than vaginal intercourse. Figure 16.5 shows the percentage of AIDS cases reported that are attributed to male homosexual transmission. This includes a small number of AIDS cases in homosexual men who also injected drugs, so the percentages could be slight overestimates. Overall, 78 per cent of cases were attributed to anal intercourse between men. However, this high figure is declining and was only 74 per cent in 1991.

Figure 16.5 also shows the corresponding percentages for other transmission categories. Numbers of AIDS cases attributable to injecting drug use and heterosexual sex are small, but have both gradually increased since 1985. The small percentage of AIDS cases attributable to injecting drug use contrasts sharply with the situation in other European countries, such as Italy and Spain, where this means of transmission is more common than transmission through male homosexual sex. The increasing proportion of cases attributed to heterosexual transmission is found for HIV infection as well as for AIDS itself. In 1991, 23 per cent of all newly reported HIV infections were ascribed to transmission through heterosexual intercourse, compared with 13 per cent of AIDS cases. This indicates the growing significance of heterosexual transmission in the British epidemic.

Figure 16.5

Proportion of AIDS cases in different exposure categories, England and Wales

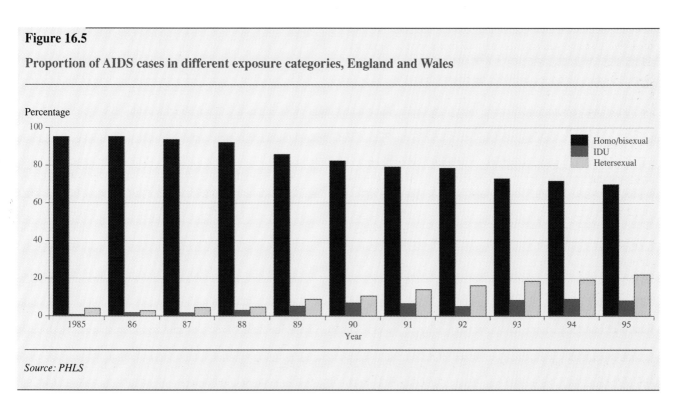

Source: PHLS

Figure 16.6

Number of AIDS cases by year of report for women, England and Wales

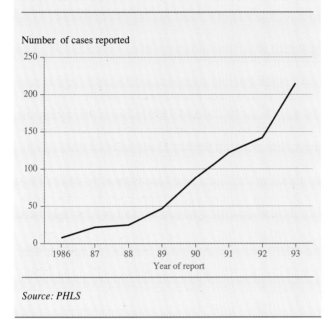

Source: PHLS

Figure 16.7

Distribution of AIDS cases up to the end of 1991 by region of diagnosis, England and Wales

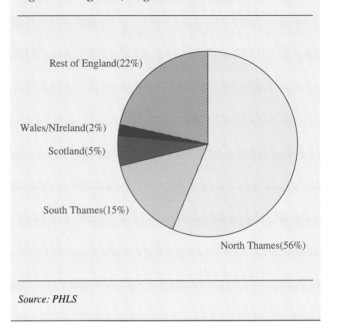

Source: PHLS

16.2.4 HIV/AIDS in women

Although the number of cases remains relatively small, the incidence of AIDS in women has increased markedly (see Figure 16.6). A total of 288 women were reported to have AIDS and a further 1,019 found to be HIV positive, but did not have AIDS, by the end of 1991. Fifty-nine per cent of the AIDS cases and 65 per cent of the total HIV infections were ascribed to infection with HIV, via heterosexual sex. Of these AIDS cases in women infected through heterosexual sex, the majority (64 per cent of a sample of 171) had a sexual partner from a country where the heterosexual spread of HIV is common. Only 27 women with heterosexually acquired AIDS, before the end of 1991, had no partner from such a country and no partner with other HIV risk factors (bisexual, blood/components recipient, injecting drug user).

16.2.5 Distribution of HIV infection in Britain

Figure 16.7 indicates the geographical distribution of AIDS case reports up to the end of 1991. It can be seen that the epidemic is heavily focused on the four Thames regions, especially the North Thames region; these four regions together account for over half of all reports nationally.

16.2.6 Future prospects

In 1993, the Chief Medical Officers commissioned reports for England and Wales (Report of a Working Group, 1993), and for Scotland (Communicable Diseases Unit, 1993), on the predicted number of AIDS cases up to 1997 (1995 for Scotland). To make these projections, the working groups used information on the number of AIDS cases reported to June

1992, the number of HIV infection reports, the distribution of time periods from HIV infection to the development of AIDS, HIV prevalence estimates from unlinked anonymous surveys and data from the National Survey of Sexual Attitudes and Lifestyles conducted in 1991.

The Unlinked Anonymous Surveys (1995) have been carried out among various groups, including attenders at genitourinary medicine clinics, injecting drug users and pregnant women. About one in six (17 per cent) of homo/bisexual men attending central London genitourinary medicine clinics since 1990 (and having syphilis tests performed) were infected with HIV-1. The figure for the rest of London was 3.1 per cent and 4.3 per cent for clinics outside London. The prevalence of HIV-1 infection among male heterosexual attenders at genitourinary medicine clinics, who were not known to have injected drugs, was 1.7 per cent in central London, 0.3 per cent in the rest of London and 0.1 per cent outside London. Women attending genitourinary medicine clinics in central London, who were not known to have injected drugs, had a prevalence of 0.7 per cent. In outer London the prevalence was 0.4 per cent and in the rest of England and Wales 0.1 per cent. The prevalence rate for HIV-1 infection in injecting drug users in London and the South East was 4.0 per cent in men and 2.8 per cent in women. The prevalence of HIV-1 infection among pregnant women receiving antenatal care was 0.18 per cent in inner London, 0.02 per cent elsewhere in the South East and 0.004 per cent (i.e. 6 of a sample of 160,735 women) outside the South East. These data provide further evidence that, so far, the risks have been concentrated among homo/bisexual males and injecting drug users, especially in the London area.

The National Survey of Sexual Attitudes and Lifestyles obtained information on sexual history and lifestyle on a random sample of about 20,000 British men and women (Johnson *et al.*, 1992). In the report commissioned by the Chief Medical Officer for England and Wales, this was used to estimate the size of the various exposure groups. The information was then combined with that from the unlinked anonymous surveys, to provide an estimate that the prevalence of HIV infection in adults in England and Wales at the end of 1991 was 27,180 (Johnson *et al.*, 1992; Report of a Working Group, 1993). Of these, 14,890 were thought to be homo/bisexual men, 4,450 injecting drug users or former users, 6,340 had had heterosexual exposure only and 1,500 were exposed to blood or blood products (Giesecke *et al.*, 1994).

The projections from the Chief Medical Officer's report suggested that there will be 2,025 new cases of AIDS in England and Wales in 1997 (compared with 1,340 reports of new AIDS cases in 1991) and 2,010 new cases in 1999 (Report of a Working Group, 1996). It is projected that the number of new cases in homosexual men will flatten off – and perhaps even decline slightly – after 1994, but that numbers of injecting drug users, and those acquiring HIV from heterosexual sex, will continue to increase rapidly.

HIV/AIDS is a new disease which has an almost 100 per cent case-fatality rate and, because it is communicable, and tends to affect young adults, has quickly taken up a position of major importance among causes of death in Britain (McCormick, 1994). Current research gives little grounds for optimism that a vaccine or, even more unlikely, a cure will be available for several years. Although the epidemic in Britain has not developed exponentially in the way that many first feared, we are, nevertheless, currently still experiencing a year-on-year increase in the number of reported cases. This, and the extent to which HIV is spreading throughout other countries of the world, mean that AIDS is likely to be a major threat to the public health in Britain for many years to come.

16.3 Conclusions

Over the last 150 years, morbidity and mortality from STDs have shown marked changes, largely as a result of effective treatment, but changes in incidence may also have been influenced by changing patterns of sexual behaviour.

Sexually transmitted diseases were responsible for considerable mortality and morbidity before both the setting up of specialist clinics and the advent of penicillin. In spite of a subsequent reduction in the sequelae of STDs, the number of cases diagnosed within clinics continues to increase (e.g. chlamydial infection, genital herpes and warts), even though there have been reductions in the number of patients with syphilis and gonorrhoea.

The network of clinics within the United Kingdom provides an effective platform for the control of all STDs and HIV infection. However, it is essential to promote the primary prevention of STDs through effective health education. This is particularly important with the advent of HIV infection, but also because of the increase in other viral STDs (particularly genital warts and herpes) for which there is as yet no cure.

Chapter 17

Time trends in cancer incidence and mortality in England and Wales

By
Anthony Swerdlow, Richard Doll
and Isobel dos Santos Silva

Summary

- Cancer is one of the main causes of morbidity and death in England and Wales – almost a quarter of a million cases are registered each year and over 140,000 people die of cancer, a quarter of all deaths.

- The chapter considers trends in mortality over the period 1970–91 and incidence over the period 1971–87, for those aged 15–84 in England and Wales.

- Mortality from cancer overall at ages 15–84 has decreased by 5 per cent in men and increased by 9 per cent in women. Trends varied by age. In men, decreases have occurred at all ages below 70; above this age there has been a small increase. In women, there have been decreases below age 50 and increases at ages 50 and above.

- Incidence rates of all cancers have increased by 8 per cent in men and 17 per cent in women. At each age-group, incidence rates either increased or remained little changed. The difference between the trends in mortality and incidence at young ages largely reflects improved survival for a few cancers, as a result of greatly improved treatment.

- Lung cancer is the most common fatal cancer in men. Lung cancer mortality has decreased at all ages in men and at ages under 50 in women, but has increased in women aged 50 and above. These trends largely reflect trends in cigarette smoking.

- The most common fatal cancer in women is breast cancer. Mortality rates from this tumour have decreased in women aged under 50, but at older ages rates increased until 1985–89, although not subsequently.

- Trends for cancer of the oesophagus, stomach, colon and rectum, cervix, ovary, prostate, testis and brain, and Hodgkin's disease, non-Hodgkin's lymphoma, myeloma and leukaemia, are also discussed. At older ages mortality from several of these malignancies has increased, but at younger ages there have been decreases for several malignancies, including large decreases for testicular cancer and Hodgkin's disease as a result of improved treatment. Rates of several cancers that are important in old age are decreasing at younger ages, and these decreases are expected to spread progressively to older ages in the future; the outlook is, therefore, moderately encouraging.

17.1 Introduction

Cancer is one of the main causes of morbidity and death in England and Wales. Almost a quarter of a million cases are registered annually, and over 140,000 deaths – a quarter of all deaths – are certified annually as due to cancer. This chapter presents data on cancer incidence trends in England and Wales from 1971 to 1987 and cancer mortality trends from 1970 to 1991. Because of limitations of space, cohort trends are not analysed and consideration is restricted to the most common cancer sites, plus certain other sites where recent trends have been of particular interest (see Table 17.1). Similar data are, of course, also available for Scotland. For reasons of space, these are not presented here, but are briefly considered elsewhere in the volume, in particular in the chapter on morbidity data from health service utilisation.

17.2 Materials and methods

17.2.1 Mortality

Data were extracted from ONS mortality files on all deaths occurring in England and Wales in 1970–91 in residents, for which the underlying cause of death on the death certificate had been coded to a malignant neoplasm (International Classification of Diseases Eighth Revision (ICD8) 140–209; ICD9 140–208, 238.4, 289.8) (WHO, 1967, 1978). In addition, we extracted data on death from nervous system tumours coded as benign or of uncertain or unspecified behaviour (ICD8 225.0–.4, 225.9, 238.1–.5; ICD9 225, 237.5–.6, 239.6). The deaths were categorised for analysis according to actual year of death, not year of registration of death as in previously published statistics. (The former is strictly correct for epidemiological investigation, although the difference is small since the great majority of deaths in any particular year are registered in the same year.) Deaths were coded to ICD8 for deaths registered in 1970–78 and ICD9 for deaths registered from 1979 onwards. Changes occurring from differences between the ICD8 and ICD9 codes were allowed for as in Swerdlow and dos Santos Silva (1993). Population data to give denominators for calculation of rates were taken from ONS annual population estimates.

Age-standardised mortality rates by site were calculated for the periods 1970–74, 1975–79, 1980–84, 1985–89 and 1990–91. These rates were calculated for the age-bands 15–34, 35–49, 50–69, 70–84 and 15–84, in each case after direct standardisation by single year of age; more detailed age-specific data will be published elsewhere. The 1981 population of England and Wales was used as the standard, since the purpose of the analyses was to compare rates in the country over time, not to compare rates between England and Wales and other countries. Age-standardised rates in each period are also presented as percentages of the 1970–74 age-standardised rate, to provide a simple measure of the magnitude of the changes over time. We did not calculate rates at ages 85 and above, because cause of death data at these ages are likely to be unreliable.

17.2.2 Incidence

Data were extracted from ONS cancer registration files on all cancers registered as incident in residents of England and Wales in 1971–87. The former year was the first after a reorganisation of national cancer registrations that improved the completeness of data collection; the latter was the most recent for which ONS held reasonably complete data at the time of data extraction for these analyses. Details of the national cancer registration scheme from which the data derive, and of interpretational issues when using these data, can be found in Swerdlow (1986). Bridge coding between ICD revisions and calculation of age-standardised rates were conducted as for the mortality analyses. Rates were calculated for the periods 1971–74, 1975–79, 1980–84 and 1985–87.

Comparison between the magnitude of the changes in incidence and mortality over time needs to take into account several factors, and to be conducted with judgment. As the incidence data presented are for a shorter period than the mortality data, equal rates of change will lead to a larger percentage change over the period for which data are available for mortality than for incidence. Mean percentage changes per annum would also not be entirely comparable, however. There is a lag between incidence and mortality from cancers, and the average duration of this lag varies by cancer site. The earlier years of mortality data in the present analyses, therefore, correspond to years of incidence before those for which data are presented here.

Since the mortality data are available for a longer period and to a more recent date than those for incidence, they are presented first.

17.3 Results

17.3.1 All cancers

Mortality
The trends in total certified cancer mortality have differed in men and women and at different ages. At 15–84 years, the mortality has decreased by 5 per cent in men but has increased by 9 per cent in women. In men, decreases have occurred at all ages under 70 years and have been most marked at young ages, with a decrease of over 30 per cent at ages 15–34. In contrast, there has been a small increase at ages 70–84 years. In women, the decrease has been less marked (about 20 per cent at ages under 50) and increases have occurred at all ages over 50, being greatest (almost 20 per cent) at ages 70–84 years (see Table 17.2 and Figure 17.1).

Some of the increase at old ages is an artefact, due partly to a change in the rules for choosing the underlying cause of death when more than one cause was mentioned on the death certificate, and partly to a change in the practice of doctors. The first occurred in 1984 when a change was made to ONS cause coding rules, such that when the underlying cause from Part I of the death certificate was a terminal or non-specific

Figure 17.1

Mortality from all cancer, by age and sex, England and Wales, 1970–91

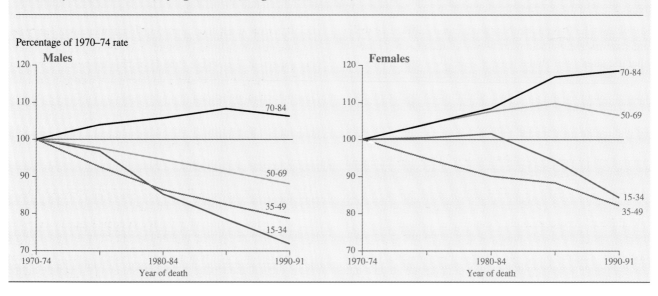

Percentage of 1970–74 rate

condition, such as bronchopneumonia or heart failure, and Part II gave a major cause such as cancer, then the major cause was to be taken as underlying. This resulted in an increase of 4.8 per cent in deaths attributed to cancer at ages 75 years and above, but only a 1.5 per cent increase for ages younger than this (Grulich *et al.*, in press). The second was shown by an increasing tendency for doctors to describe cancer (if known to be present) as the underlying cause of death rather than as an associated condition. Each of these artefacts was particularly marked for men with cancer of the prostate (Grulich *et al.*, in press).

Incidence

Registered all-site cancer incidence rates increased by 8 per cent in men and 17 per cent in women. In men, there were substantial increases at both ends of the age spectrum (15–34 and 70–84 years) and little change in between. In women,

rates have increased at all ages other than 35–49 years, at which the incidence remained fairly constant (see Table 17.2).

The difference between the trends in mortality and incidence at young ages largely reflects improvements in survival for a few cancers, as a result of greatly improved treatment. Differences at all ages may, in some instances, be artefactual, resulting from changes with time in the criteria for distinguishing between benign and malignant tumours or from the introduction of screening, which may have resulted in the registration of cases that would not have appeared clinically for many years, if at all. Changes in the completeness of registration could also have affected recorded trends in incidence, although the available evidence suggests that there has been little change in completeness for the country as a whole over the period considered (Swerdlow *et al.*, 1993). Part of the increase in both recorded incidence and mortality rates at older

Figure 17.2

Mortality from cancer of the oesophagus, by age and sex, England and Wales, 1970–91

Percentage of 1970–74 rate

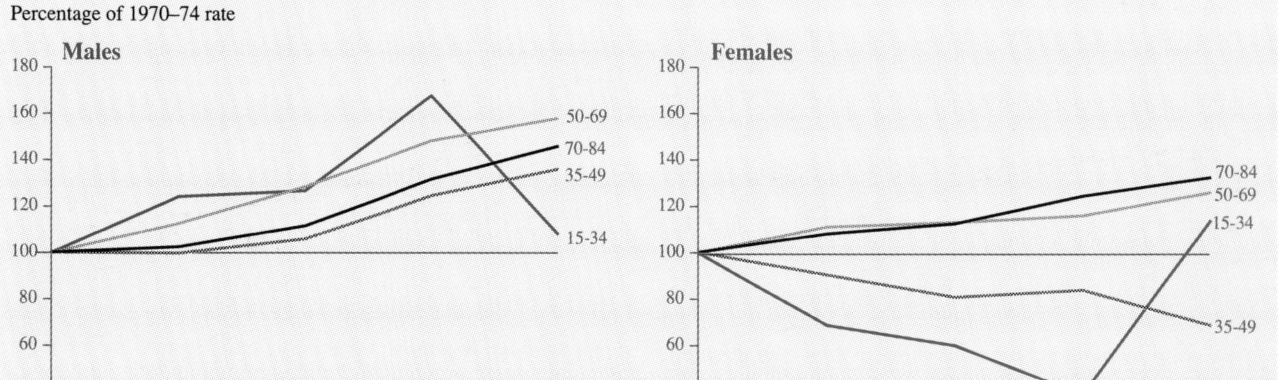

ages is likely to have been the result of improved diagnosis of solid cancers of some internal sites and haematological malignancies, mainly because of the introduction of more elaborate and reliable diagnostic technologies. The extent to which such factors have affected the trends differs for different cancers and is discussed below in relation to cancer of specific sites.

17.3.2 Cancer of the oesophagus

Mortality

The mortality rate from cancer of the oesophagus at ages 15–84 has increased by a half in men and by a quarter in women over the study period (see Table 17.3 and Figure 17.2). In men, increases have occurred at each age-group over age 34, although more at ages 50 and over than at 35–49. In women, there were also increases at ages 50 and above, but a decrease occurred at 35–49. At ages 15–34 years, the numbers in both sexes were small and the trends were irregular.

Incidence

Incidence rates of oesophageal cancer also increased over the study period, again more for men (27 per cent at ages 15–84) than women (14 per cent) (see Table 17.3). In men, there were increases at each age, but substantially the greatest was at ages 15–34. In women, there were increases at ages 50 and above, a decrease at ages 35–49, and erratic trends based on small numbers at ages 15–34. For men, there was some indication that recorded mortality rates may have risen more rapidly than recorded incidence over a comparable period, which might reflect changes in registration or death certification practice for tumours of the lower third of the oesophagus and cardia.

The increases in oesophageal cancer rates are likely to reflect increasing *per caput* alcohol consumption since the end of the Second World War (Spring and Buss, 1977; Brewers & Licensed Retailers Association, 1994). Smoking is also a risk factor for oesophageal cancer, but smoking has declined since 1960 in men and since the mid-1970s in women. Dietary deficiencies may also be involved in oesophageal cancer aetiology, and it is possible that the different trends in women and men may, to some extent, reflect sex-specific changes in diet and alcohol intake.

17.3.3 Cancer of the stomach

Mortality

Mortality rates from stomach cancer decreased steadily at each age-group in each sex, with decreases for ages 15–84 of 42 per cent in males and 50 per cent in females over the period (see Table 17.4 and Figure 17.3). In each sex, the percentage decrease was greater at younger ages, except that trends at ages 15–34 were irregular, based on smaller numbers.

Incidence

Incidence rates also decreased in each sex (see Table 17.4). Again, the decrease was greater at younger ages, except that at 15–34 years, particularly in females, there was a potentially worrying reversal of the downward trend in recent years.

The decreasing rates of stomach cancer form part of a pattern of decreases across the Western world, including Britain, over several decades. The reason is uncertain, but it seems likely that improved food storage, notably by refrigeration, and greater availability of fresh fruit and vegetables in the diet (MAFF, 1991) may be at least part of the reason. Improvement in social conditions early in life leading to decreased infection with *Helicobacter pylori* may also have played a part.

Figure 17.3

Mortality from cancer of the stomach, by age and sex, England and Wales, 1970–91

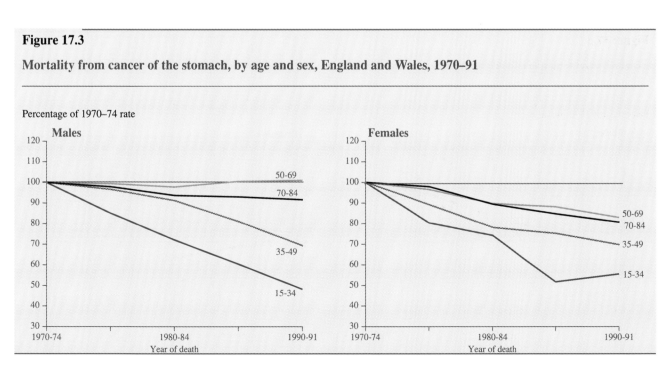

Figure 17.4

Mortality from cancer of the colon and rectum, by age and sex, England and Wales, 1970–91

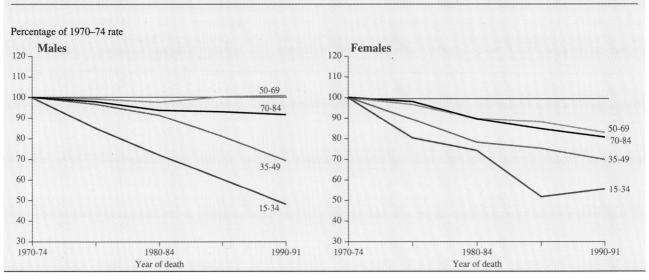

Percentage of 1970–74 rate

17.3.4 Cancers of the colon and rectum

Mortality

Mortality from cancers of the colon and rectum at ages 15–84 decreased slightly in men and by almost 20 per cent in women over the study period (see Figure 17.4). Trends diverged by age in men: at ages under 50, rates decreased markedly whereas at ages 50 and above, rates did not. In women, rates decreased in all age-groups, particularly the youngest.

Incidence

Incidence of cancers of the colon and rectum at ages 50 and above increased in men and was unchanged in women over the study period, whereas at younger ages there were decreases (see Table 17.5). The net result for ages 15–84 was a 6 per cent increase in men and no change in women.

The more downward trend in mortality than incidence rates for colon and rectal cancers corresponds with improvements in survival over the last 20 years. Some of the decrease in incidence at young ages could be due to better case finding and treatment of familial adenomatous polyposis, but the condition is not common enough (about 1/8,000) to account for all of the decrease. The decline in incidence at younger ages contrasts with rising incidence rates recorded in most European countries (Coleman *et al.*, 1993), although decreases have been seen in certain parts of Australasia and North America. Since dietary factors are probably the main cause of colorectal cancers, the decreasing incidence at younger ages in England and Wales is likely to be due to changes in diet – for instance, decreases in fat consumption and increases in intake of fresh fruit and vegetables (MAFF, 1991) – although the precise components are not known.

Figure 17.5

Mortality from cancer of the lung, by age and sex, England and Wales, 1970–91

Percentage of 1970–74 rate

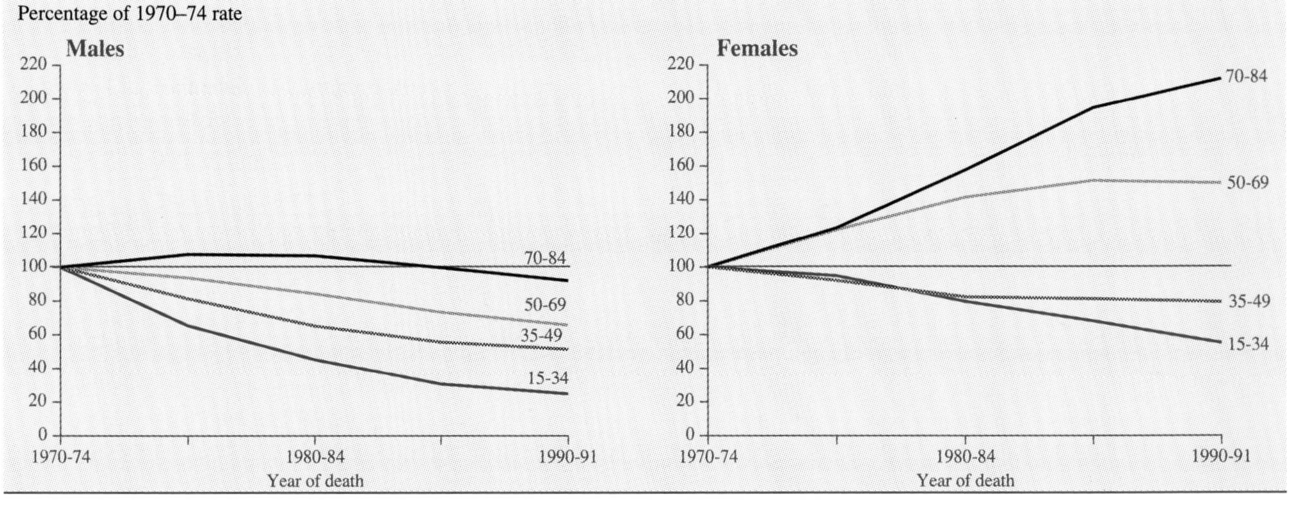

17.3.5 Cancer of the lung

Mortality

Lung cancer is the most common fatal cancer in men in England and Wales. Mortality rates decreased progressively throughout the study period at ages under 70, especially at young ages (see Figure 17.5). At ages 70–84, the rate increased until 1980–84 but decreased thereafter. In women, for whom rates were substantially lower than in men, the changes were less favourable. Rates rose markedly at ages 50 and over and declined at younger ages, but by much less than in men of similar ages. As a result of the differences in trend by sex, the female rate (0.18 per 100,000 per year) at ages 15–34 in 1990–91 was close to that for males (0.24 per 100,000) whereas 20 years earlier, the male rate had been three times that in females.

Incidence

Lung cancer incidence trends were fairly similar to those for mortality (see Table 17.6). There were large decreases in the rates for men under age 70 and an increase, followed by a decrease, at ages 70–84. In women, rates increased greatly at ages over 50, but declined at ages 35–49, and declined at ages 15–34 up to 1984, but then increased. In 1985–87, at ages 15–34, the incidence rate in women (0.68 per 100,000) was slightly greater than that in men (0.60 per 100,000), and in each sex the incidence rate was over twice the corresponding mortality rate. In contrast, at other age-groups and in earlier years, mortality rates were only slightly below incidence rates, reflecting the poor survival from this cancer. Judging from available national data on survival, which are somewhat out of date (OPCS, 1986), the high incidence to mortality ratio at young ages in recent years is not explicable by survival. It is based on modest numbers, may be due to chance, and needs re-examination as future data become available.

The trends in lung cancer rates in men and women essen-

tially reflect trends in smoking habits and tar contents of cigarettes over time. Consumption of cigarettes by men in England and Wales reached a peak in 1960 and has since diminished greatly, almost halving by 1985, whereas in women peak consumption was in the mid-1970s, with a lesser diminution since then. Tar yields of cigarettes have been dropping since the Second World War (Wald *et al.*, 1988). A small part of the decreasing rates may also be attributable to the massive reduction in air pollution in urban areas in England and Wales over the last 40 years (Doll, 1990). The chapter on trends in smoking-related diseases presents further discussion of these issues.

17.3.6 Malignant melanoma of the skin

Mortality

The mortality rate from cutaneous melanoma at ages 15–84 doubled in men and increased by 50 per cent in women from 1970–74 to 1990–91 (see Figure 17.6). The increase has been greater at older ages than at younger; indeed, at ages 15–34, rates have been steady (men) or slightly decreasing (women) and at 35–49 the increase has been substantial only in men.

Incidence

Incidence rates for cutaneous melanoma have increased in all age-groups over the study period (see Table 17.7). The increases were around twofold in each sex and age-group, generally slightly greater for men than women and greater for ages 35 and over than for ages 15–34. For the years for which both mortality and incidence data were available, the incidence rates of melanoma increased more steeply than the mortality rates.

Cutaneous melanoma incidence has been rising rapidly in white populations around the world for several decades. The likely reason in England and Wales, as in other countries, is

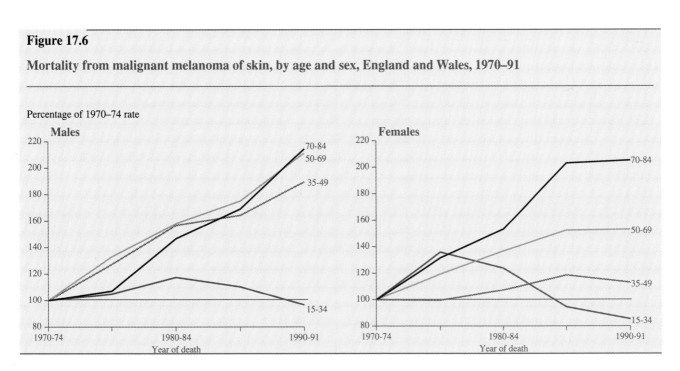

Figure 17.6

Mortality from malignant melanoma of skin, by age and sex, England and Wales, 1970–91

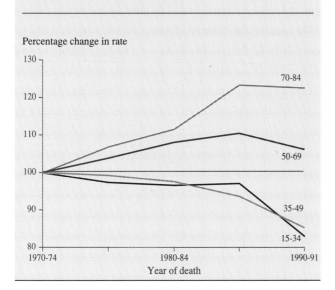

Figure 17.7

Mortality from cancer of female breast, by age, England and Wales, 1970–91

Percentage change in rate

Figure 17.8

Mortality from cancer of the cervix, by age, England and Wales, 1970–91

Percentage change in rate

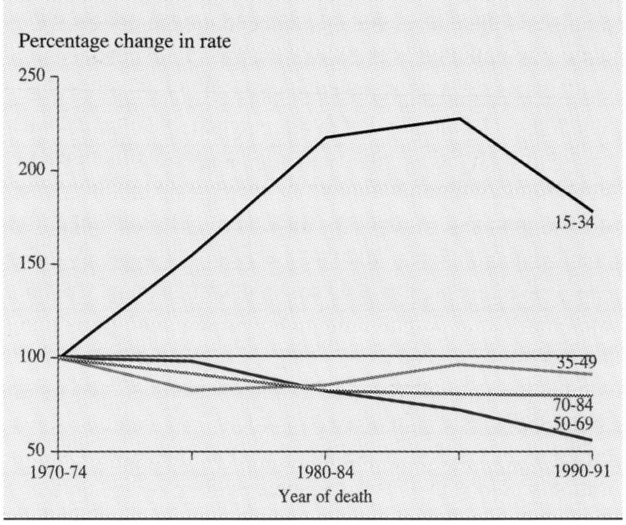

an increase in intermittent sun exposure of untanned skin, on beach holidays and in other leisure pursuits. The greater rate of increase for melanoma incidence than mortality in England and Wales is also seen in data for other white populations. It is partly a result of improved treatment and of earlier presentation of melanomas at a stage when they can be treated more successfully. Also, however, there has probably been an increase in the tendency to biopsy melanocytic lesions of borderline malignancy.

17.3.7 Breast cancer in women

Mortality
Breast cancer mortality in women decreased by about 15 per cent at ages under 50, with a greater rate of decrease after 1989 than previously (see Figure 17.7). At ages 50 and above, rates increased up to 1989, but since then they have declined at ages 50–69 and stabilised at ages 70–84, to give overall increases of 6 per cent at ages 50–69 and 23 per cent at 70–84 through the study period. Although small in percentage terms, these increases are numerically important because breast cancer is so common. Part, but not most, of the increase in the oldest age-group can be accounted for by changes in ONS rules for coding cause of death (see section 17.3.1).

Incidence
Breast cancer incidence in women has remained virtually unchanged at ages under 50, and increased by just over 10 per cent at ages 50 and above (see Table 17.8).

For the years for which both incidence and mortality data were available, the trends were similar for each, suggesting that survival has not changed substantially. Direct information on survival from cancer in England and Wales throughout the period are not available, but for selected registries survival data for cancers incident 1978–80 to 1983–85 have been published (Berrino *et al.*, 1995); these show only a slight

improvement in breast cancer survival between these years. For the most recent years, however, the downturn (or, at the oldest ages, stabilisation) of mortality rates gives more grounds for optimism. This might reflect the increasing use of tamoxifen and other treatments of proven efficacy (Early Breast Cancer Trialists' Collaborative Group, 1992). The reasons for the increasing incidence of breast cancer at older ages are unclear: earlier age at menarche (Dann and Roberts, 1993), perhaps consequent on better diet in childhood, and changes in childbearing patterns (dos Santos Silva and Swerdlow, 1995), will have contributed. The reduction in the most recent years is discussed further by Beral *et al.* (1995).

17.3.8 Cancer of the cervix uteri

Mortality
The mortality rate from cervical cancer at ages 15–84 diminished over the period by about a quarter, but this overall trend disguised differing trends by age (see Figure 17.8). At ages 15–34, the rate more than doubled from 1970–74 to 1985–89, although there was some diminution thereafter. In contrast, at ages 50–69, the rate decreased throughout the period, by over 40 per cent in total. At other age-groups the changes were comparatively small: there was a slight decrease at ages 35–49, and a 20 per cent decrease at ages 70–84.

Incidence
In incidence data, there was a fairly similar pattern (see Table 17.9). At ages 15–34, the rate in 1985–87 was twice that in 1971–74. At ages 35–49, there was an initial decrease but then an increase and at older ages, rates decreased moderately over the period.

Recorded rates of cervical cancer are potentially influenced by the proportion of uterine cancers for which the exact site is not specified. These tumours are coded to a different 3-digit ICD code from cervix. In the England and Wales data for the study period, however, the percentage of uterine cancers whose site was unspecified was not large (around 10 per cent of all uterine cancer deaths and 5 per cent of all uterine cancer registrations). The changes in rates of unspecified uterine cancers (e.g. 0.20 per 100,000 increase for mortality, 0.03 per 100,000 increase for incidence, for ages 15–84 for the period overall) were too small to explain the changes in recorded cervical cancer rates. The aetiology of cervical cancer relates mainly to a sexually transmitted infection, the evidence pointing to types of the human papilloma virus. Past time trends in cervical cancer mortality up to 1971, by birth cohort, have been shown by Beral (1974) to parallel closely changes in sexually transmitted disease incidence rates. The recent increase in cervical cancer rates in young women is likely also to be due to greater exposures to oncogenic sexually transmitted infection at young ages, following widespread use of the oral contraceptive pill (which may also have an independent effect in increasing risk). The fact that the increase occurred for mortality as well as incidence indicates that it was not the result of increased case-finding due to screening, or to changes in diagnostic criteria for malignancy in borderline malignant lesions. The increase in rates in young women in the United Kingdom is not unique in direction internationally, but is unusually large (Coleman *et al.*, 1993).

17.3.9 Cancer of the ovary

Mortality
At ages under 50 years, the ovarian cancer mortality rate decreased, reaching about 60 per cent of its 1970–74 value by 1990–91 (see Figure 17.9). At ages 50–69, there was no change in mortality over the period and at ages 70–84, the rate increased by over 20 per cent. The aggregate of these divergent trends left the rate for ages 15–84 little altered over time.

Incidence
In incidence data, the decreases at younger ages were less than in mortality data and the increases at ages 50 and over were greater (see Table 17.10).

The main known factors affecting risk of ovarian cancer are parity and oral contraceptive use. Past ovarian cancer mortality trends in England and Wales have been shown to correlate well with changes in mean parity (Beral *et al.*, 1978), and the recent decreases at younger ages are probably due to oral contraceptive use (dos Santos Silva and Swerdlow, 1995). The more favourable trends for mortality than for incidence at ages under 70 are probably a result of better survival, with the introduction of chemotherapy for ovarian cancers. The limited data available on survival in England and Wales show modest improvements between cases diagnosed 1978–80 and those diagnosed 1983–85 (Berrino *et al.*, 1995).

17.3.10 Cancer of the prostate

Mortality
Very few deaths occurred from cancer of the prostate at ages under 35 (see Figure 17.10). At older ages the mortality rate increased by about 40–50 per cent over the period overall, after an initial decrease at ages 35–49 only.

Incidence
Incidence rates of cancer of the prostate also increased, by 30 per cent for ages 15–84 and by fairly similar amounts at each age group except 15–34 (see Table 17.11). At this latter age rates were erratic, based on small numbers, with a particularly high rate in 1985–87.

Asymptomatic carcinoma of the prostate is common and can often be found at prostatectomy or autopsy in older men. There is, therefore, considerable scope for artefactual increases in recorded prostatic cancer incidence and mortality rates from the increasing use of transurethral resection of the prostate to treat benign hypertrophy (Potosky *et al.*, 1990). The impact of diagnostic artefact on the mortality trends is likely to have been much smaller, however. Part of the increase in mortality, especially at older ages, is due to a change in ONS coding procedures and, probably, a part is due also to change in certification practice (see section 17.3.1). Much of the mortality increase, however, is likely to have been real.

17.3.11 Cancer of the testis

Mortality
Mortality rates from testicular cancer decreased steeply in each age-group, especially at the youngest ages, during the study period (see Figure 17.11). The rate for ages 15–84 in 1990–91 was 40 per cent of that in 1970–74. The trends in incidence for this malignancy, however, were different. At ages under 50, rates increased by over 40 per cent, at 50–69 by almost 20 per cent and only at 70–84 was there a decrease, of almost 10 per cent (see Table 17.12).

Incidence
The increasing incidence of testicular cancer at younger ages

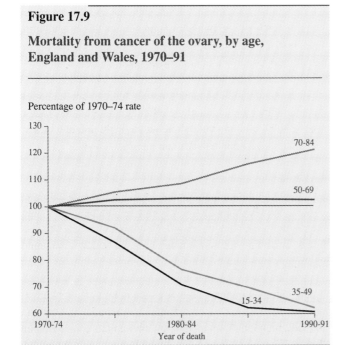

Figure 17.9

Mortality from cancer of the ovary, by age, England and Wales, 1970–91

Percentage of 1970–74 rate

70-84

50-69

35-49

15-34

1970-74   1980-84   1990-91

Year of death

Figure 17.10

Mortality from cancer of the prostate, by age, England and Wales, 1970–91

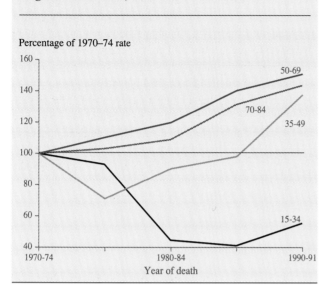

Percentage of 1970–74 rate

Year of death

Figure 17.11

Mortality from cancer of the testis, by age, England and Wales, 1970–91

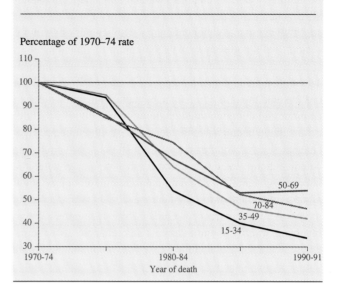

Percentage of 1970–74 rate

Year of death

is part of a long-term increase which has taken place for at least 80 years (Davies, 1981), the reasons for which are not known. Recent evidence has suggested that prenatal exposure to high levels of maternal oestrogens (Henderson *et al.*, 1983) or early puberty and lack of exercise (Forman *et al.*, 1994) might be partly responsible. The decreasing mortality, despite increasing incidence, reflects the great successes of radiotherapy and chemotherapy for this tumour.

17.3.12 Cancer of the brain and other nervous system

Mortality

Mortality from malignancy of the nervous system showed a similar pattern in each sex: rates at ages under 50 showed no change or a small decline, whereas rates at ages 50–69 increased by about a quarter and at 70–84 by almost 200 per cent (see Figure 17.12). Since clinical differentiation between malignant and benign nervous system tumours can be difficult, we also analysed trends for deaths from all neoplasms of the nervous system, whether reported as benign, malignant, or of uncertain or unknown behaviour (not shown in Figure 17.12 and Table 17.12). The increases for this category were generally slightly less and the decreases slightly greater, than in the analysis for malignancies of the nervous system. The same general pattern by age was, however, present: large increases in rates occurred at ages 70–84, there were small increases at ages 50–69 and, at ages under 50, there were decreases of 15 per cent to 30 per cent over the study period.

Figure 17.12

Mortality from cancer of the nervous system, by age and sex, England and Wales, 1970–91

Percentage of 1970–74 rate

Males

Females

Year of death

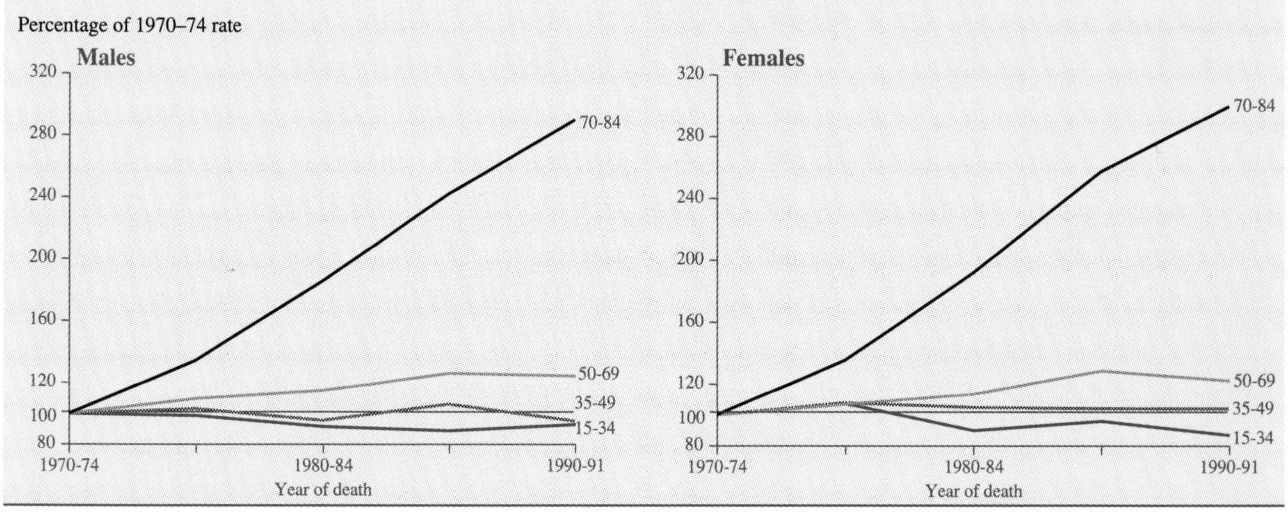

Incidence

The trends for incidence were similar. Rates of nervous system malignancy doubled at ages 70–84 and changed by 10 per cent or less at younger ages (see Table 17.13). Rates of all neoplasms of the nervous system generally showed a slightly more upward trend than malignancies of the nervous system, but not greatly so.

The increases in recorded incidence and mortality from nervous system tumours at older ages have been seen in many countries and appear to be, at least in part, a reflection of more complete diagnosis, especially with the introduction of computerised axial tomography (CAT) scans. It is uncertain whether there is also a real component to the increase. The decreasing mortality at young ages, greater for all nervous system tumours than for those coded to malignancy, is likely to be due to better treatment of benign tumours plus, possibly, some improvement in diagnostic precision.

17.3.13 Hodgkin's disease

Mortality

The mortality rate from Hodgkin's disease in males decreased by 60 per cent at ages 15–84 over the study period, with almost identical decreases at each age-group within this (see Figure 17.13). In females, there was a similar decrease for ages 15–84, again with no clear variation by age. The improvement in mortality in females aged 15–34 ceased for the most recent period (1990–91), but this was based on smaller numbers than for the other periods in the analysis.

Incidence

There were also substantial decreases in incidence of Hodgkin's disease, although less marked than those for mortality (see Table 17.14). For ages 15–84, incidence decreased by 27 per cent in men and 19 per cent in women from 1971–87, with decreases of around 40 per cent in each sex at ages 50

and above, a smaller decrease in each sex at ages 35–49 and in men aged 15–34, and an increase in women aged 15–34.

The large decreases in mortality from Hodgkin's disease without comparable decreases in incidence, reflect the great improvements in survival that have been brought about by intensive chemotherapy and radiotherapy over the last 25 years. Part of the reason for the decrease in incidence rates is a tendency for certain histological types of lymphoma (notably lymphocyte depleted malignancies), which used to be classified to Hodgkin's disease, to be categorised instead as non-Hodgkin's lymphoma (G Vaughan Hudson, personal communication). This does not explain most of the decrease in incidence rates, however, the reason for which remains unknown.

17.3.14 Non-Hodgkin's lymphoma

Mortality

The mortality rate from non-Hodgkin's lymphoma (NHL) has almost doubled for ages 15–84 in each sex over the period, but within this there has been a clear variation in secular trend by age (see Figure 17.14). At ages 70–84, there were increases of 130 per cent in each sex, at ages 35–69 there were smaller increases and at ages 15–34 there were decreases of 13 per cent in males and 27 per cent in females.

Incidence

In incidence data too there was an almost doubling of rates in each sex over the study period, with the largest increases at older ages (see Table 17.15). Unlike the mortality data, however, there were increases (of 10–20 per cent) even at ages 15–34. A small part of the increase in NHL incidence can be explained by the advent of AIDS-associated NHL and by NHL occurring after immunosuppression for organ transplantation. Lymphomas due to these causes are much too rare, however, to explain more than a small proportion of the rise

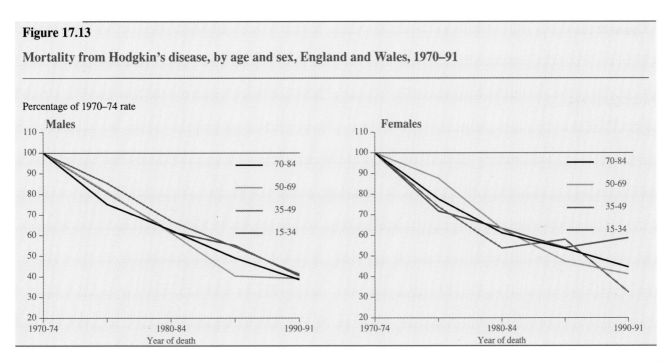

Figure 17.13

Mortality from Hodgkin's disease, by age and sex, England and Wales, 1970–91

Figure 17.14

Mortality from non–Hodgkin's lymphoma, by age and sex, England and Wales, 1970–91

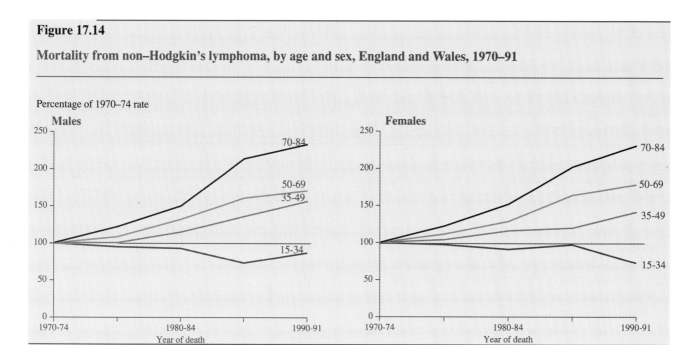

Percentage of 1970–74 rate

and they mainly affect trends at younger ages, which are not those at which the largest increases in incidence rates have occurred. Several other factors, including pesticides and phenoxyherbicides, have been suggested as possible causes of NHL and of its increasing incidence, but their aetiological roles remain uncertain. A minor part of the increase is the result of transfer of cases in recent years that would previously have been categorised as Hodgkin's disease (see above). A part of the increase in rates might also have occurred through improved coding of lymphomas of sites other than lymph nodes (e.g. of stomach, brain and testis) which, according to the ICD should be coded to NHL, but if the histology was not stated or the ICD was not followed correctly, would be coded to the ICD code of the extra-nodal site. This could not account for the full magnitude of the increases, however, since lymphomas of extra-nodal sites account for only about 20 per cent of the total (Coleman *et al.*, 1993). A pathology review in Yorkshire of cases over a 20-year period, concluded that the large increase in NHL rates that had occurred was not an artefact of changed pathological criteria or changes in registration completeness or coding (Barnes *et al.*, 1986).

Improved diagnostic investigation might have been involved in the rising rates, but it seems unlikely that artefacts can fully account for the increase. There may well have been a large real increase in incidence.

The divergent trends for incidence and mortality from NHL at young ages are due to the introduction and then improvement in intensive chemotherapy. This treatment cannot be used aggressively at older ages, which may explain the lesser divergence between incidence and mortality trends at these ages.

Figure 17.15

Mortality from multiple myeloma, by age and sex, England and Wales, 1970–91

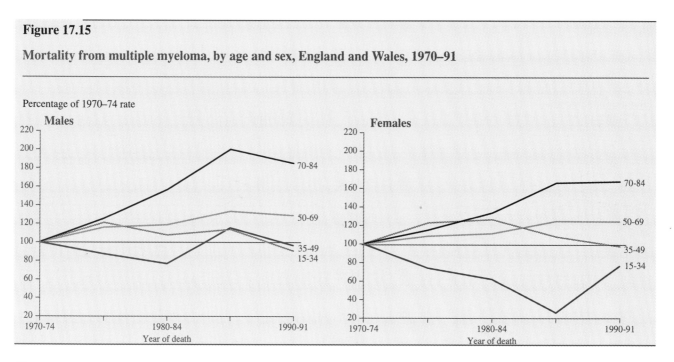

Percentage of 1970–74 rate

17.3.15 Multiple myeloma

Mortality

Mortality rates from myeloma at ages 15–84 increased by about 50 per cent in each sex up to 1985–89, but then ceased to rise (see Figure 17.15). At ages under 50, there was no consistent change over the study period, whereas at ages 50–64, there were increases in each sex of about a quarter until 1985–1989 and then a levelling off. At ages 70–84, the rate doubled in men and increased by two thirds in women up to 1985–89, but then levelled off or decreased slightly to 1990–91.

Incidence

Incidence rates for myeloma showed a similar pattern of slight change at young ages but large increases at the oldest ages (see Table 17.16). At ages 15–34, trends were erratic, based on small numbers; at 35–49, there were increases of around 10 per cent; at 50–69, increases of 20 per cent to 25 per cent; and at ages 70–84, there was a doubling of the rate in males and an increase of about a half in females. The increases at older ages continued until the last period of incidence data, for 1985–87, but since the incidence data did not extend beyond 1987 and survival from myeloma is poor, we were unable to determine whether the cessation of increase in mortality rates since 1985–89 had parallels in incidence rates.

The trends in myeloma in England and Wales accord with a pattern seen in whites in many Western countries, of increase in risk of myeloma at older ages, but stabilisation or even decreases at younger ages (Coleman et al., 1993; Cuzick, 1994). The increases have generally been greatest where recorded rates were initially low, and least or absent in places where diagnostic completeness is likely to have been high initially. There is no known cause of myeloma that could account for the increasing rates at older ages in England and Wales, and it is not obvious what aetiological factor might

lead to large increases in rates in each sex at older ages but not younger. Improved diagnosis, however, might plausibly affect most strongly those groups in whom underdiagnosis was initially greatest, which might well be older age-groups and populations in areas with initially low recorded rates. It is possible that the increases in rates are entirely artefactual, although the differential rate of increase for males and females argues against this (Cuzick, 1994). Alternatively, the increase (or part of it) could be a cohort effect, resulting from an increase in the prevalence of carcinogenic factors in the first half of the century, which ceased some three or four decades ago. The reason for the apparent increase is unlikely to be clear until more is known about the aetiology of this malignancy.

17.3.16 Leukaemia

Mortality

Mortality rates from leukaemia in England and Wales have decreased at younger, but not at older, ages over the period (see Figure 17.16). In males aged under 50, rates have decreased by about a quarter and, in females of this age, by about a third. At ages 50–69 in each sex, however, rates have not altered and at 70–84, rates have increased by about 15 per cent in each sex.

Incidence

Incidence data showed similar trends to those for mortality at older, but not at younger, ages (see Table 17.17). At 70–84, rates have increased by around 20 per cent and, at 50–69, they have remained little changed. At ages under 50, the changes were slight.

The rise in incidence and mortality rates from leukaemia at ages 70–84 may reflect improved diagnosis and for mortality, it partly reflects changes in ONS coding rules (see section 17.3.1). Some increase in incidence may also have

Figure 17.16

Mortality from leukaemia, by age and sex, England and Wales, 1970–91

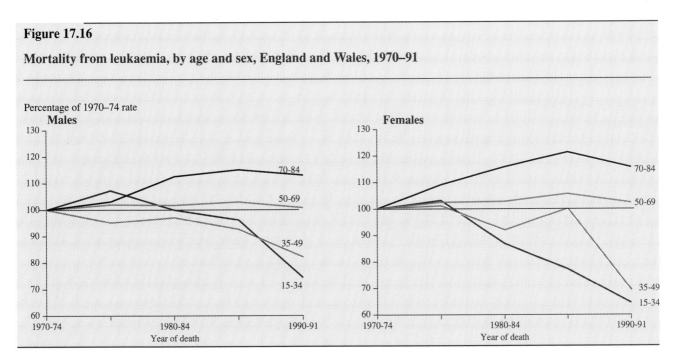

occurred, however. The substantial decreases in mortality at younger ages, without corresponding decreases in incidence, are due to improved survival from better treatment (chemotherapy and bone marrow transplantation).

17.3.17 Cancer of unspecified primary site

Mortality

Mortality certified to cancer of unspecified site has shown one of the largest increases of any 3-digit ICD cancer code over the study period, with all-age rates more than trebling in each sex (see Figure 17.17). Although an increase occurred in each age-group, its extent was greatest at older ages. In each sex and age-group, a particularly steep increase occurred from 1975–79 to 1980–84 but, except at ages 15–34 in males and 35–49 in females, the increase between these two quinquennia did not account for the full extent of the rise over the study period, and there were increases in mortality rates both before and after these dates. Examination of data by single calendar year (not presented in Figure 17.7) shows that the large increase after 1975 took place mainly over the years 1978 to 1982 and was not simply related to the change of ICD revision in 1979. Examination of data for 1978, which were double-coded to ICD8 and 9 (OPCS, 1983), also leads to the conclusion that the increase was not due primarily to the change in ICD revision.

Incidence

In incidence data too, there has been a steep increase at each age-group in cancer of unspecified site, except in women aged 35–49, for whom the increase was only 9 per cent (see Table 17.18). Unlike the mortality data, the increase between 1975–79 and 1980–84 was, in general, at no greater rate than subsequently (although it was in several instances greater than the rise up to 1975–79).

The increases in rates of cancer of unspecified primary site are large, but the reasons for them are unclear. They may reflect a diminishing tendency to investigate the site of primary cancer in patients with metastases who are terminally ill, and/or poorer specification of cancer information on death certificates and cancer registrations. It is also possible that there has been an increase in incidence of cancers that metastasise early and aggressively. The rapidity of the increase in rates over a small number of years, especially for mortality, however, argues that at the least, the majority of the apparent change must be artefactual. More information on the impact of the increase can be found in Grulich *et al.* (in press).

17.4 Conclusions

Cancer mortality has fallen over the last 20 years in men under age 70 and in women under 50, as a consequence of both improved treatment and reduced risk. Improved treatment has resulted in dramatic decreases in mortality from testicular cancer and Hodgkin's disease in a reduction in mortality from leukaemia, and has contributed to a reduction in mortality from cancers of the ovary and the large bowel. Reductions in risk have brought about large reductions in mortality from cancers of the lung and stomach. Reductions in incidence have also contributed to the reduced mortality from cancers of the ovary and large bowel. For some cancers, however, incidence rates have increased, most notably for melanoma and testicular cancer and, to a lesser extent, for non-Hodgkin's lymphoma, all of which have been increasing in incidence for several decades, and for oesophageal cancer in men and cervical cancer, which have been increasing only since 1960. All of these increases are largely real and reflect increases in risk.

Figure 17.17

Mortality from cancer of unspecified site, by age and sex, England and Wales, 1970–91

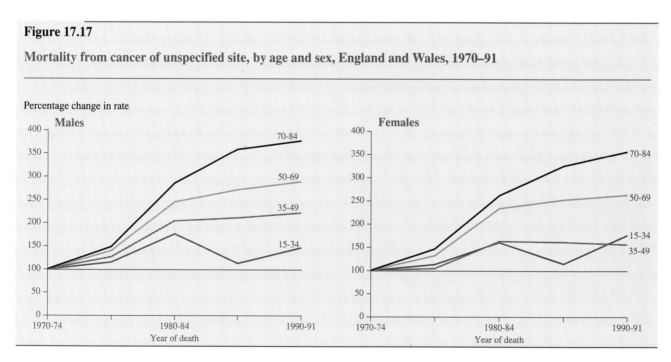

At other ages (over 70 in men and over 50 in women) mortality has risen, most markedly in women. Increases have been seen in the incidence and mortality from oesophageal cancer, lung cancer in women, melanoma, cancers of the breast, ovary, prostate, brain and nervous system, non-Hodgkin's lymphoma, myeloma and cancer of unspecified sites. With the exception of cancer of the brain and myeloma, the mortality increases must be presumed to be largely, if not wholly, real. The increases in both the incidence and mortality attributed to cancer of the brain and myeloma may, exceptionally, have been due to greatly improved methods of diagnosis. Among the types of cancer reviewed here, large downward trends in mortality have occurred only for Hodgkin's disease, as a result of improved treatment, and for stomach cancer, lung cancer in men and cervical cancer as a result of decreases in risk, reflected in decreases in incidence. Why there should have been an increase in mortality attributed to cancer of unspecified sites is unclear; it must imply that some of the decrease in the mortality of some specified cancers is artefactual and/or that the increase in some other cancers has been underestimated.

Considered by itself, the increase in mortality in the older age-groups is disturbing. It should not, however, be interpreted to mean that efforts to control the risk of cancer have failed. Cohort effects may take many years to wear off, as has been shown in the case of lung cancer and cigarette smoking, and increases in old age commonly reflect increases in the prevalence of carcinogenic hazards in the distant past.

Rates of several of the cancers that are most important in old age are decreasing at young ages and these decreases are expected to spread progressively to older ages. Although there are several types of cancer that are increasing for unknown reasons which require urgent attention, there have been major advances in both the treatment and prevention of some other cancers and the outlook for the immediate future is moderately encouraging.

Table 17.1

All cancers: mortality 1970–91 and incidence 1971–87, England and Wales
Ages 15–84

Mortality (average number of deaths per year)*

	Males					Females				
	1970–74	1975–79	1980–84	1985–89	1990–91	1970–74	1975–79	1980–84	1985–89	1990–91
All cancers	**60,381**	**63,578**	**66,115**	**68,448**	**68,198**	**49,117**	**52,143**	**55,003**	**58,190**	**57,722**
Oesophagus	1,683	1,899	2,214	2,673	2,956	1,209	1,360	1,453	1,597	1,708
Stomach	6,869	6,444	5,916	5,336	4,702	4,523	4,127	3,552	3,037	2,581
Colon and rectum	6,807	7,087	7,267	7,604	7,666	7,541	7,604	7,264	7,104	6,764
Lung	25,193	25,975	25,457	23,744	22,067	5,683	6,981	8,421	9,630	9,958
Malignant melanoma of skin	253	318	399	449	548	332	399	453	527	528
Breast (female)	-	-	-	-	-	10,390	10,963	11,454	12,089	11,761
Cervix	-	-	-	-	-	2,150	2,054	1,880	1,821	1,612
Ovary	-	-	-	-	-	3,468	3,575	3,566	3,618	3,625
Prostate	3,601	4,100	4,795	6,163	6,959	-	-	-	-	-
Testis	246	234	160	124	116	-	-	-	-	-
Nervous system	1,085	1,194	1,271	1,449	1,495	792	875	946	1,083	1,087
Hodgkin's disease	475	394	315	250	207	305	249	197	174	148
Non-Hodgkin's lymphoma	864	987	1,226	1,599	1,799	729	858	1,042	1,348	1,503
Multiple myeloma	545	682	792	986	948	574	668	757	907	907
Leukaemia	1,406	1,509	1,645	1,726	1,686	1,153	1,253	1,310	1,385	1,289
Unspecified site	1,311	1,967	3,789	4,691	5,100	1,455	2,076	3,809	4,564	4,935

Incidence (average number of cases per year)*

	Males				Females			
	1971–74	1975–79	1980–84	1985–87	1971–74	1975–79	1980–84	1985–87
All cancers	**83,812**	**90,876**	**99,509**	**101,430**	**78,284**	**84,535**	**92,444**	**95,805**
Oesophagus	1,748	1,985	2,222	2,488	1,316	1,481	1,594	1,625
Stomach	7,048	6,927	6,916	6,288	4,550	4,406	4,038	3,551
Colon and rectum	9,512	10,368	11,452	11,502	10,134	10,842	11,338	10,914
Lung	25,982	26,919	26,851	24,590	6,015	7,353	9,124	9,859
Malignant melanoma of skin	441	571	766	1,040	894	1,085	1,457	1,863
Breast (female)	-	-	-	-	19,597	20,349	21,252	22,075
Cervix	-	-	-	-	3,982	3,861	3,944	3,981
Ovary	-	-	-	-	3,985	4,163	4,477	4,508
Prostate	6,072	7,124	8,775	9,581	-	-	-	-
Testis	678	759	890	1,035	-	-	-	-
Nervous system	1,274	1,309	1,508	1,533	951	961	1,142	1,139
Hodgkin's disease	836	790	728	659	535	505	510	465
Non-Hodgkin's lymphoma	1,258	1,573	2,076	2,498	1,084	1,353	1,784	2,119
Multiple myeloma	711	890	1,044	1,165	724	850	986	1,050
Leukaemia	1,738	1,897	2,146	2,105	1,358	1,514	1,670	1,643
Unspecified site	1,353	1,538	2,132	2,559	1,356	1,681	2,277	2,591

* See Tables 17.2 to 17.18 for ICD codes of the cancer sites presented.

Table 17.2

All malignant neoplasms: mortality 1970–91 and incidence 1971–87, England and Wales

Mortality Age-group		Males					Females				
		1970–74	1975–79	1980–84	1985–89	1990–91	1970–74	1975–79	1980–84	1985–89	1990–91
15–34	n	4,139	4,281	3,906	3,651	1,381	3,465	3,793	3,994	3,702	1,389
	rate	12.24	11.86	10.45	9.61	8.81	10.91	10.96	11.08	10.28	9.20
	%	100	96.9	85.3	78.5	71.9	100	100.5	101.6	94.3	84.4
35–49	n	16,481	14,530	13,705	13,961	5,667	21,743	19,381	18,625	19,737	7,801
	rate	71.03	65.74	61.38	58.50	55.89	93.90	88.97	84.58	82.95	77.06
	%	100	92.6	86.4	82.4	78.7	100	94.8	90.1	88.3	82.1
50–69	n	159,131	155,573	147,185	142,764	55,461	114,396	117,731	117,110	116,903	44,847
	rate	606.95	593.18	573.93	554.85	534.67	389.20	405.86	418.87	427.34	414.88
	%	100	97.7	94.6	91.4	88.1	100	104.3	107.6	109.8	106.6
70–84	n	122,153	143,504	165,779	181,865	73,886	105,983	119,810	135,287	150,610	61,407
	rate	1,781.24	1,853.10	1,884.28	1,928.35	1,894.18	879.96	916.35	953.90	1,028.22	1,042.96
	%	100	104.0	105.8	108.3	106.3	100	104.1	108.4	116.9	118.5
15–84	n	301,904	317,888	330,575	342,241	136,395	245,587	260,715	275,016	290,952	115,444
	rate	350.10	351.50	347.49	345.28	335.71	255.41	264.09	272.05	284.10	281.00
	%	100	100.4	99.3	98.6	95.9	100	103.4	106.5	111.2	110.0

Incidence Age-group		Males				Females			
		1971–74	1975–79	1980–84	1985–87	1971–74	1975–79	1980–84	1985–87
15–34	n	7,073	9,693	10,177	6,609	8,412	12,123	13,537	8,823
	rate	25.94	26.73	27.21	29.04	32.78	34.82	37.53	40.9
	%	100	103.1	104.9	112.0	100	106.2	114.5	124.8
35–49	n	23,191	27,478	27,739	17,349	39,781	46,894	48,481	32,177
	rate	126.64	124.73	123.95	122.05	218.96	216.48	219.67	227.44
	%	100	98.5	97.9	96.4	100	98.9	100.3	103.9
50–69	n	180,163	229,461	229,589	132,892	149,663	195,489	201,117	118,594
	rate	855.91	875.38	895.39	874.04	634.62	673.8	719.49	728.48
	%	100	102.3	104.6	102.1	100	106.2	113.4	114.8
70–84	n	124,822	187,748	230,039	147,440	115,281	168,171	199,083	127,820
	rate	2,250.48	2,421.02	2,616.51	2,616.74	1,185.62	1,283.92	1,404.81	1,451.74
	%	100	107.6	116.3	116.3	100	108.3	118.5	122.5
15–84	n	335,249	454,380	497,544	304,290	313,137	422,677	462,218	287,414
	rate	479.51	500.27	523.6	518.06	401.48	426.33	457.59	469.53
	%	100	104.3	109.2	108.0	100	106.2	114.0	117.0

Rates: per 100,000 population, age-standardised by single year of age to the 1981 England and Wales population.
%: percentage of 1970–74 rate for mortality, 1971–74 for incidence.
All malignant neoplasms: ICD8 140.0–209, ICD9 140.0–208.9, 289.8, 298.0.

Table 17.3

Cancer of oesophagus: mortality 1970–91 and incidence 1971–87, England and Wales

Mortality

Age-group		Males					Females				
		1970–74	1975–79	1980–84	1985–89	1990–91	1970–74	1975–79	1980–84	1985–89	1990–91
15–34	n	26	35	38	50	14	14	12	10	7	8
	rate	0.08	0.10	1.10	0.14	0.09	0.05	0.03	0.03	0.02	0.06
	%	100	124.3	126.8	167.7	108.0	100	68.8	60.1	38.9	114.2
35–49	n	474	446	475	596	277	266	225	201	223	77
	rate	2.01	2.01	2.13	2.51	2.74	1.14	1.03	0.92	0.95	0.78
	%	100	99.6	105.8	124.5	135.9	100	90.2	80.6	83.7	68.5
50–69	n	4,425	4,984	5,571	6,453	2,768	2,372	2,593	2,549	2,568	1,108
	rate	16.91	19.05	21.73	25.07	26.71	8.07	8.97	9.14	9.37	10.18
	%	100	112.7	128.5	148.3	158.0	100	111.2	113.2	116.1	126.1
70–84	n	3,489	4,028	4,986	6,266	2,853	3,392	3,972	4,506	5,187	2,223
	rate	50.87	52.07	56.69	66.93	74.17	28.22	30.46	31.72	35.08	37.33
	%	100	102.4	111.5	131.6	145.8	100	108.0	112.4	124.3	132.3
15–84	n	8,414	9,493	11,070	13,365	5,912	6,044	6,802	7,266	7,985	3,416
	rate	9.77	10.47	11.66	13.61	14.75	6.44	6.98	7.17	7.71	8.22
	%	100	107.2	119.3	139.3	151.0	100	108.3	111.4	119.7	127.7

Incidence

Age-group		Males				Females			
		1971–74	1975–79	1980–84	1985–87	1971–74	1975–79	1980–84	1985–87
15–34	n	24	36	48	32	16	22	16	18
	rate	0.09	0.10	0.13	0.15	0.07	0.06	0.05	0.08
	%	100	111.0	143.9	162.3	100	91.1	64.3	118.3
35–49	n	394	486	522	355	242	252	263	147
	rate	2.11	2.18	2.35	2.53	1.30	1.14	1.20	1.05
	%	100	103.4	111.1	119.9	100	87.7	91.8	80.8
50–69	n	3,733	5,316	5,580	3,602	2,191	2,974	3,020	1,708
	rate	17.73	20.32	21.78	23.65	9.29	10.25	10.82	10.58
	%	100	114.6	122.9	133.4	100	110.4	116.4	113.9
70–84	n	2,841	4,085	4,962	3,476	2,816	4,157	4,670	3,002
	rate	51.15	52.77	56.42	61.67	29.04	31.84	32.89	33.83
	%	100	103.2	110.3	120.6	100	109.7	113.3	116.5
15–84	n	6,992	9,923	11,112	7,465	5,265	7,405	7,969	4,875
	rate	10.05	10.92	11.71	12.75	6.94	7.56	7.87	7.92
	%	100	108.7	116.5	126.9	100	109.0	113.4	114.1

Rates: per 100,000 population, age-standardised by single year of age to the 1981 England and Wales population.
%: percentage of 1970–74 rate for mortality, 1971–74 for incidence.
Cancer of oesophagus: ICD8 150; ICD9 150.

Table 17.4

Cancer of stomach: mortality 1970–91 and incidence 1971–87, England and Wales

Mortality

Age-group		Males 1970–74	1975–79	1980–84	1985–89	1990–91	Females 1970–74	1975–79	1980–84	1985–89	1990–91
15–34	n	113	100	56	84	26	98	70	74	63	27
	rate	0.35	0.29	0.15	0.23	0.17	0.31	0.20	0.21	0.17	0.17
	%	100	81.8	43.5	64.8	47.1	100	64.3	66.1	54.7	55.0
35–49	n	1,604	1,206	981	847	307	843	609	480	396	156
	rate	6.87	5.43	4.41	3.57	3.02	3.65	2.78	2.18	1.67	1.55
	%	100	79.1	64.1	52.0	43.9	100	76.2	59.6	45.6	42.5
50–69	n	18,037	15,455	12,716	10,754	3,712	7,850	6,687	5,151	4,203	1,398
	rate	68.80	58.83	49.62	41.80	35.72	26.77	23.06	18.41	15.35	12.86
	%	100	85.5	72.1	60.8	51.9	100	86.1	68.8	57.3	48.0
70–84	n	14,589	15,458	15,829	14,995	5,359	13,823	13,269	12,056	10,521	3,581
	rate	212.62	199.49	180.00	158.61	137.37	115.26	101.87	84.85	70.71	59.52
	%	100	93.8	84.7	74.6	64.6	100	88.4	73.6	61.4	51.6
15–84	n	34,343	32,219	29,582	26,680	9,404	22,614	20,635	17,761	15,183	5,162
	rate	39.97	35.68	31.09	26.84	23.08	24.41	21.28	17.48	14.54	12.26
	%	100	89.3	77.8	67.1	57.7	100	87.2	71.6	59.6	50.3

Incidence

Age-group		Males 1971–74	1975–79	1980–84	1985–87	Females 1971–74	1975–79	1980–84	1985–87
15–34	n	106	126	111	78	91	99	114	80
	rate	0.41	0.35	0.30	0.35	0.35	0.29	0.32	0.36
	%	100	85.9	73.5	85.5	100	80.9	89.9	102.3
35–49	n	1,427	1,493	1,382	697	732	716	576	362
	rate	7.72	6.75	6.21	4.95	4.00	3.28	2.62	2.58
	%	100	87.4	80.4	64.1	100	82.1	65.5	64.5
50–69	n	15,051	17,094	15,567	8,035	6,580	7,461	6,209	3,079
	rate	71.59	65.14	60.73	52.81	28.04	25.68	22.19	18.97
	%	100	91.0	84.8	73.8	100	91.6	79.2	67.7
70–84	n	11,608	15,924	17,518	10,053	10,797	13,754	13,293	7,133
	rate	209.33	205.35	199.27	177.87	111.66	105.43	93.59	79.97
	%	100	98.1	95.2	85.0	100	94.4	83.8	71.6
15–84	n	28,192	34,637	34,578	18,863	18,200	22,030	20,192	10,654
	rate	40.66	38.28	36.37	31.97	24.35	22.64	19.89	17.11
	%	100	94.2	89.5	78.6	100	93.0	81.7	70.3

Rates: per 100,000 population, age-standardised by single year of age to the 1981 England and Wales population.
%: percentage of 1970–74 for mortality, 1971–74 for incidence.
Cancer of stomach: ICD8 151; ICD9 151.

Table 17.5

Cancers of colon and rectum: mortality 1970–91 and incidence 1971–87, England and Wales

Mortality

Age-group		Males					Females				
		1970–74	1975–79	1980–84	1985–89	1990–91	1970–74	1975–79	1980–84	1985–89	1990–91
15–34	n	232	218	186	162	55	165	147	141	96	46
	rate	0.71	0.60	0.51	0.43	0.34	0.53	0.43	0.39	0.28	0.30
	%	100	85.1	72.1	60.4	48.2	100	80.4	74.3	51.8	55.6
35–49	n	1,892	1,747	1,665	1,579	576	1,776	1,487	1,313	1,364	539
	rate	8.18	7.90	7.46	6.62	5.66	7.65	6.82	5.97	5.75	5.33
	%	100	96.6	91.2	81.0	69.2	100	89.2	78.1	75.2	69.7
50–69	n	15,960	15,913	15.302	15,768	6,384	14,811	14,143	12,694	12,184	4,543
	rate	61.03	60.65	59.72	61.35	61.65	50.54	48.82	45.39	44.55	41.95
	%	100	99.4	97.8	100.5	101.0	100	96.6	89.8	88.2	83.0
70–84	n	15,952	17,556	19,182	20,513	8,316	20,954	22,245	22,174	21,874	8,399
	rate	232.23	227.29	217.67	216.06	212.71	174.51	170.84	156.08	147.81	140.68
	%	100	97.9	93.7	93.0	91.6	100	97.9	89.4	84.7	80.6
15–84	n	34,036	34,434	36,335	38,022	15,331	37,706	38,022	36,322	35,518	13,527
	rate	40.08	39.42	38.15	38.22	37.74	40.23	39.02	35.82	34.34	32.54
	%	100	98.3	95.2	95.3	94.2	100	97.0	89.0	85.4	80.9

Incidence

Age-group		Males				Females			
		1971–74	1975–79	1980–84	1985–87	1971–74	1975–79	1980–84	1985–87
15–34	n	356	452	405	217	360	435	340	248
	rate	1.36	1.26	1.10	0.98	1.42	1.26	0.95	1.16
	%	100	92.9	81.4	72.0	100	88.6	66.7	81.2
35–49	n	2,487	3,049	3,014	1,737	2,390	2,745	2,688	1,613
	rate	13.54	13.78	13.50	12.31	13.04	12.60	12.23	11.51
	%	100	101.8	99.7	90.9	100	96.6	93.7	88.3
50–69	n	19,020	24,853	25,838	15,116	17,541	22,141	21,769	12,099
	rate	90.44	94.68	100.83	99.41	74.53	76.41	77.88	74.38
	%	100	104.7	111.5	109.9	100	102.5	104.5	99.8
70–84	n	16,183	23,487	28,002	17,435	20,245	28,889	31,893	18,783
	rate	291.80	303.57	318.24	308.38	208.93	221.33	224.75	211.96
	%	100	104.0	109.1	105.7	100	105.9	107.6	101.5
15–84	n	38,046	51,841	57,259	34,505	40,536	54,210	56,690	32,743
	rate	55.08	57.33	60.22	58.60	53.22	55.31	56.00	53.17
	%	100	104.1	109.3	106.4	100	103.9	105.2	99.9

Rates: per 100,000 population, age-standardised by single year of age to the 1981 England and Wales population.
%: percentage of 1970–74 rates for mortality, 1971–74 for incidence.
Cancer of colon and rectum: ICD8 153.0–8, 154; ICD9 153, 154.

Table 17.6

Cancer of lung: mortality 1970–91 and incidence 1971–87, England and Wales

Mortality

Age-group		Males					Females				
		1970–74	1975–79	1980–84	1985–89	1990–91	1970–74	1975–79	1980–84	1985–89	1990–91
15–34	n	310	221	158	105	36	99	104	91	76	25
	rate	0.96	0.63	0.43	0.30	0.24	0.32	0.31	0.26	0.22	0.18
	%	100	65.4	45.3	30.8	24.9	100	94.9	79.7	68.1	55.2
35–49	n	5,640	4,342	3,451	3,134	1,235	2,058	1,770	1,573	1,665	701
	rate	23.89	19.43	15.54	13.26	12.24	8.73	8.01	7.18	7.07	6.92
	%	100	81.3	65.1	55.5	51.2	100	91.8	82.2	81.0	79.2
50–69	n	74,534	69,779	61,382	53,768	19,419	15,929	19,213	21,455	22,595	8,851
	rate	283.95	266.04	239.28	208.32	186.45	54.17	66.21	76.67	82.02	81.19
	%	100	93.7	84.3	73.4	65.7	100	122.2	141.5	151.4	149.9
70–84	n	45,482	55,532	62,294	61,715	23,443	10,330	13,816	18,984	23,813	10,338
	rate	665.12	715.07	709.39	662.41	610.50	85.25	105.00	134.20	165.74	180.50
	%	100	107.5	106.7	99.6	91.8	100	123.2	157.4	194.4	211.7
15–84	n	125,966	129,874	127,285	118,722	44,133	28,416	34,903	42,103	48,149	19,915
	rate	144.35	142.83	134.00	120.66	109.68	29.01	34.97	41.76	47.60	49.37
	%	100	99.0	92.8	83.6	76.0	100	120.5	143.9	164.1	170.2

Incidence

Age-group		Males				Females			
		1971–74	1975–79	1980–84	1985–87	1971–74	1975–79	1980–84	1985–87
15–34	n	303	317	223	131	130	144	152	146
	rate	1.15	0.89	0.61	0.60	0.52	0.43	0.43	0.68
	%	100	77.2	53.0	51.8	100	81.2	81.5	129.0
35–49	n	5,106	5,270	4,182	2,223	1,944	2,062	1,955	1,246
	rate	27.33	23.59	18.80	15.91	10.42	9.34	8.91	8.94
	%	100	86.3	68.8	58.2	100	89.7	85.6	85.8
50–69	n	63,171	75,225	67,445	34,779	13,944	20,900	23,899	14,322
	rate	299.87	287.07	262.95	228.51	59.11	72.06	85.43	87.57
	%	100	95.7	87.7	76.2	100	121.9	144.5	148.2
70–84	n	35,347	53,782	62,405	36,636	8,040	13,660	19,613	13,864
	rate	637.58	691.50	710.92	654.35	82.14	103.71	138.72	159.19
	%	100	108.5	111.5	102.6	100	126.3	168.9	193.8
15–84	n	103,927	134,594	134,255	73,769	24,058	36,766	45,619	29,578
	rate	147.07	147.51	141.45	126.19	30.40	36.76	45.27	48.81
	%	100	100.3	96.2	85.8	100	120.9	148.9	160.6

Rates: per 100,000 population, age-standardised by single year of age to the 1981 England and Wales population.
%: percentage of 1970–74 rates for mortality, 1971–74 for incidence.
Cancer of lung: ICD8 162; ICD9 162.

Table 17.7

Malignant melanoma of skin: mortality 1970–91 and incidence 1971–87, England and Wales

Mortality

Age-group		Males					Females				
		1970–74	1975–79	1980–84	1985–89	1990–91	1970–74	1975–79	1980–84	1985–89	1990–91
15–34	n	140	158	178	172	64	137	196	186	144	56
	rate	0.41	0.43	0.48	0.45	0.40	0.42	0.57	0.52	0.39	0.36
	%	100	104.9	117.5	110.3	96.6	100	135.9	123.8	94.5	85.4
35–49	n	284	350	447	505	242	385	364	408	488	197
	rate	1.26	1.61	1.98	2.08	2.39	1.71	1.70	1.84	2.03	1.94
	%	100	127.4	156.9	164.4	189.6	100	99.6	107.5	118.8	113.3
50–69	n	587	774	898	987	478	748	879	971	1,049	413
	rate	2.22	2.95	3.51	3.89	4.69	2.53	3.02	3.46	3.85	3.87
	%	100	133.0	158.1	175.1	211.2	100	119.3	136.7	152.3	153.0
70–84	n	253	306	473	582	312	390	555	700	954	390
	rate	3.67	3.94	5.39	6.22	7.89	3.22	4.24	4.94	6.54	6.61
	%	100	107.2	146.8	169.2	214.6	100	131.7	153.4	203.2	205.4
15–84	n	1,264	1,588	1,996	2,246	1,096	1,660	1,994	2,265	2,635	1,056
	rate	1.40	1.72	2.11	2.30	2.72	1.68	2.01	2.24	2.57	2.55
	%	100	122.4	150.4	163.8	194.0	100	119.8	133.6	153.3	152.1

Incidence

Age-group		Males				Females			
		1971–74	1975–79	1980–84	1985–87	1971–74	1975–79	1980–84	1985–87
15–34	n	251	380	475	378	492	867	1,016	754
	rate	0.91	1.04	1.28	1.67	1.83	2.45	2.80	3.43
	%	100	114.5	140.9	183.5	100	133.9	153.3	187.7
35–49	n	442	691	883	772	922	1,283	1,836	1,497
	rate	2.48	3.19	3.92	5.33	5.21	6.02	8.26	10.38
	%	100	128.6	157.6	214.5	100	115.5	158.4	199.2
50–69	n	754	1,261	1,676	1,314	1,473	2,181	2,783	2,129
	rate	3.57	4.80	6.53	8.64	6.23	7.56	9.97	13.08
	%	100	134.4	182.7	242.0	100	121.3	160.0	210.0
70–84	n	317	524	796	656	687	1,095	1,651	1,210
	rate	5.70	6.76	9.07	11.74	7.05	8.35	11.67	13.91
	%	100	118.5	159.1	206.0	100	118.4	165.6	197.2
15–84	n	1,764	2,856	3,830	3,120	3,574	5,426	7,286	5,590
	rate	2.44	3.09	4.04	5.35	4.51	5.46	7.21	9.08
	%	100	126.7	165.5	219.1	100	121.1	159.8	201.2

Rates: per 100,000 population, age-standardised by single year of age to the 1981 England and Wales population.
%: percentage of 1970–74 rates for mortality, 1971–74 for incidence
Malignant melanoma of skin: ICD8 172.0–4, 172.6–9; ICD9 172.

Table 17.8

Cancer of breast (female): mortality 1970–91 and incidence 1971–87, England and Wales

Age-group		Mortality					Incidence			
		1970–74	1975–79	1980–84	1985–89	1990–91	1971–74	1975–79	1980–84	1985–87
15–34	n	637	706	725	712	260	1,837	2,511	2,525	1,579
	rate	2.13	2.07	2.05	2.06	1.76	7.52	7.39	7.14	7.66
	%	100	97.4	96.6	97.1	83.0	100	98.3	94.9	101.9
35–49	n	7,679	7,184	7,140	7,416	2,880	17,062	20,448	20,369	13,215
	rate	33.28	33.01	32.44	31.15	28.34	94.17	94.39	92.45	93.51
	%	100	99.2	97.5	93.6	85.2	100	100.2	98.2	99.3
50–69	n	27,088	27,729	27,731	27,590	10,469	38,854	49,120	49,883	30,193
	rate	91.95	95.46	99.30	101.49	97.57	164.31	169.23	178.55	185.63
	%	100	103.8	108.0	110.4	106.1	100	103.0	108.7	113.0
70–84	n	16,546	19,195	21,675	24,728	9,913	20,636	29,665	33,481	21,238
	rate	137.09	146.54	152.93	169.22	168.10	211.61	225.97	236.48	242.53
	%	100	106.9	111.6	123.4	122.6	100	106.8	111.8	114.6
15–84	n	51,950	54,814	57,271	60,446	23,522	78,389	101,744	106,258	66,225
	rate	52.73	54.94	56.78	59.38	57.41	98.40	101.77	105.33	108.57
	%	100	104.2	107.7	112.6	108.9	100	103.4	107.1	110.3

Rates: per 100,000 population, age-standardised by single year of age to the 1981 England and Wales population.
%: percentage of 1970–74 rates for mortality, 1971–74 for incidence.
Cancer of breast (female): ICD8 174; ICD9 174.

Table 17.9

Cancer of cervix uteri: mortality 1970–91 and incidence 1971–87, England and Wales

Age-group		Mortality					Incidence			
		1970–74	1975–79	1980–84	1985–89	1990–91	1971–74	1975–79	1980–84	1985–87
15–34	n	233	402	578	600	203	1,223	2,176	3,004	1,995
	rate	0.74	1.15	1.61	1.69	1.32	4.74	6.15	8.36	9.31
	%	100	155.6	218.2	228.3	178.4	100	129.7	176.3	196.3
35–49	n	1,879	1,441	1,536	1,888	743	3,838	4,097	4,954	3,567
	rate	8.10	6.70	6.92	7.81	7.37	21.34	19.29	22.21	24.77
	%	100	82.7	85.5	96.5	91.1	100	90.4	104.1	116.1
50–69	n	5,801	5,592	4,530	3,879	1,196	8,238	9,745	8,242	4,309
	rate	19.67	19.32	16.19	14.21	11.01	34.82	33.57	29.48	26.31
	%	100	98.2	82.3	72.3	56.0	100	96.4	84.7	75.6
70–84	n	2,836	2,834	2,755	2,738	1,082	2,628	3,286	3,519	2,071
	rate	23.47	21.58	19.47	19.05	18.82	26.88	24.94	24.91	23.90
	%	100	92.0	82.9	81.2	80.2	100	92.8	92.7	88.9
15–84	n	10,749	10,269	9,399	9,105	3,224	15,927	19,304	19,719	11,942
	rate	10.78	10.27	9.32	8.92	7.76	19.81	19.26	19.55	19.42
	%	100	95.3	86.4	82.8	72.0	100	97.3	98.7	98.0

Rates: per 100,000 population, age-standardised by single year of age to the 1981 England and Wales population.
%: percentage of 1970–74 rates for mortality, 1971–74 for incidence.
Cancer of cervix uteri: ICD8 180; ICD9 180.

Table 17.10

Cancer of ovary: mortality 1970–91 and incidence 1971–87, England and Wales

Age-group		Mortality					Incidence			
		1970–74	1975–79	1980–84	1985–89	1990–91	1971–74	1975–79	1980–84	1985–87
15–34	n	254	244	207	184	73	527	673	701	426
	rate	0.81	0.70	0.58	0.5	0.49	2.04	1.92	1.93	1.96
	%	100	86.8	71.0	62.3	60.8	100	94.3	94.8	96.0
35–49	n	2,277	1,969	1,635	1,602	615	2,813	3,081	3,083	1,915
	rate	9.74	8.97	7.46	6.80	6.06	15.36	14.13	14.02	13.64
	%	100	92.1	76.6	69.8	62.2	100	92.0	91.2	88.8
50–69	n	9,669	9,777	9,473	9,224	3,610	8,582	11,256	11,655	6,761
	rate	32.86	33.72	33.88	33.81	33.70	36.35	38.71	41.68	41.63
	%	100	102.6	103.1	102.9	102.6	100	106.5	114.7	114.5
70–84	n	5,142	5,887	6,516	7,078	2,951	4,017	5,806	6,944	4,421
	rate	42.38	44.75	46.05	49.16	51.45	41.01	44.12	49.08	50.63
	%	100	105.6	108.7	116.0	121.4	100	107.6	119.7	123.5
15–84	n	17,342	17,877	17,831	18,088	7,249	15,939	20,816	22,383	13,523
	rate	17.48	17.85	17.70	17.95	18.07	19.93	20.71	22.21	22.34
	%	100	102.1	101.3	102.7	103.4	100	104.0	111.5	112.1

Rates: per 100,000 population, age-standardised by single year of age to the 1981 England and Wales population.
%: percentage of 1970–74 rates for mortality, 1971–74 for incidence.
Cancer of ovary: ICD8 183; ICD9 183.

Table 17.11

Cancer of prostate: mortality 1970–91 and incidence 1971–87, England and Wales

Age-group		Mortality					Incidence			
		1970–74	1975–79	1980–84	1985–89	1990–91	1971–74	1975–79	1980–84	1985–87
15–34	n	4	4	2	2	1	12	19	15	21
	rate	0.01	0.01	0.01	0.01	0.01	0.05	0.05	0.04	0.90
	%	100	93.1	44.6	41.1	55.4	100	116.8	87.9	198.3
35–49	n	83	56	69	79	47	135	149	180	122
	rate	0.35	0.25	0.31	0.34	0.48	0.71	0.66	0.81	0.89
	%	100	71.1	90.3	98.1	137.6	100	92.5	113.8	124.0
50–69	n	5,257	5,878	6,200	7,341	3,229	8,710	12,337	13,833	8,563
	rate	20.24	22.32	24.25	28.38	30.53	41.66	46.99	54.06	56.41
	%	100	110.3	119.8	140.3	150.9	100	112.8	129.8	135.4
70–84	n	12,662	14,561	17,702	23,395	10,640	15,429	23,114	29,847	20,036
	rate	183.87	189.49	200.26	241.65	263.97	278.48	299.88	338.44	351.02
	%	100	103.1	108.9	131.4	143.6	100	107.7	121.5	126.1
15–84	n	18,006	20,499	23,973	30,817	13,917	24,286	35,619	43,875	28,742
	rate	22.40	23.46	24.98	29.90	32.55	37.00	40.40	45.88	47.71
	%	100	104.7	111.5	133.5	145.3	100	109.2	124.0	129.0

Rates: per 100,000 population, age-standardised by single year of age to the 1981 England and Wales population.
%: percentage of 1970–74 rates for mortality, 1971–74 for incidence.
Cancer of prostate: ICD8 185; ICD9 185.

Table 17.12

Cancer of testis: mortality 1970–91 and incidence 1971–87, England and Wales

Age-group		Mortality					Incidence			
		1970–74	1975–79	1980–84	1985–89	1990–91	1971–74	1975–79	1980–84	1985–87
15–34	n	605	600	354	275	96	1,413	2,019	2,318	1,689
	rate	1.74	1.63	0.94	0.70	0.59	5.07	5.49	6.17	7.26
	%	100	93.6	53.9	40.0	33.7	100	108.4	121.7	143.2
35–49	n	314	291	214	167	63	823	1,131	1,434	1,009
	rate	1.46	1.38	0.94	0.68	0.61	4.81	5.34	6.28	6.87
	%	100	94.7	64.1	46.5	42.0	100	111.1	130.7	142.8
50–69	n	221	193	146	113	47	374	511	541	314
	rate	0.85	0.73	0.57	0.45	0.46	1.78	1.95	2.12	2.10
	%	100	85.9	67.3	53.0	54.0	100	109.7	119.3	118.4
70–84	n	91	87	86	66	25	100	134	158	92
	rate	1.31	1.11	0.98	0.98	0.60	1.80	1.72	1.80	1.64
	%	100	84.9	74.5	52.3	46.2	100	96.0	100.2	91.2
15–84	n	1,231	1,171	800	621	231	2,710	3,795	4,451	3,104
	rate	1.39	1.28	0.84	0.62	0.56	3.81	4.14	4.69	5.24
	%	100	91.8	60.4	44.8	40.2	100	108.8	123.1	137.7

Rates: per 100,000 population, age-standardised by single year of age to the 1981 England and Wales population.
%: percentage of 1970–74 rates for mortality, 1971–74 for incidence.
Cancer of testis: ICD8 186; ICD9 186.

Table 17.13

Cancer of nervous system: mortality 1970–91 and incidence 1971–87, England and Wales

Mortality

Age-group		Males 1970–74	1975–79	1980–84	1985–89	1990–91	Females 1970–74	1975–79	1980–84	1985–89	1990–91
15–34	n	500	527	508	499	215	339	387	340	363	136
	rate	1.48	1.46	1.36	1.32	1.38	1.04	1.11	0.93	0.99	0.90
	%	100	98.6	91.6	88.9	92.9	100	107.3	89.9	95.9	86.9
35–49	n	1,137	1,131	1,074	1,277	486	707	728	728	782	326
	rate	5.01	5.17	4.79	5.31	4.77	3.13	3.38	3.28	3.25	3.25
	%	100	103.2	95.6	106.1	95.2	100	108.0	105.0	104.1	104.0
50–69	n	3,329	3,611	3,702	4,053	1,588	2,452	2,583	2,652	2,922	1,085
	rate	12.58	13.80	14.44	15.87	15.65	8.34	8.92	9.48	10.72	10.19
	%	100	109.7	114.9	126.2	124.4	100	107.0	113.7	128.6	122.3
70–84	n	457	702	1,069	1,417	700	462	676	1,012	1,346	626
	rate	6.61	8.88	12.27	15.99	19.16	3.75	5.07	7.19	9.64	11.23
	%	100	134.4	185.7	242.0	289.9	100	135.4	191.8	257.3	299.7
15–84	n	5,423	5,971	6,353	7,246	2,989	3,960	4,374	4,732	5,413	2,173
	rate	5.81	6.38	6.74	7.57	7.70	3.91	4.34	4.70	5.41	5.44
	%	100	109.8	116.0	130.4	132.5	100	111.0	120.3	138.4	139.3

Incidence

Age-group		Males 1971–74	1975–79	1980–84	1985–87	Females 1971–74	1975–79	1980–84	1985–87
15–34	n	582	800	870	508	472	593	631	380
	rate	2.12	2.20	2.32	2.24	1.79	1.69	1.73	1.72
	%	100	103.9	109.8	105.8	100	94.2	96.6	95.9
35–49	n	1,053	1,331	1,378	873	707	809	926	559
	rate	5.87	6.10	6.12	6.07	3.95	3.76	4.17	3.93
	%	100	104.0	104.4	103.4	100	95.3	105.5	99.5
50–69	n	3,018	3,681	4,061	2,395	2,204	2,689	2,999	1,686
	rate	14.25	14.08	15.83	15.75	9.34	9.30	10.73	10.34
	%	100	98.8	111.1	110.5	100	99.5	114.9	110.7
70–84	n	443	733	1,229	823	421	713	1,154	793
	rate	7.86	9.27	14.09	15.12	4.24	5.36	8.19	9.21
	%	100	117.9	179.2	192.3	100	126.4	192.9	217.1
15–84	n	5,096	6,545	7,538	4,599	3,804	4,804	5,710	3,418
	rate	6.83	7.00	7.98	8.00	4.71	4.78	5.67	5.65
	%	100	102.5	116.7	117.1	100	101.4	120.4	119.9

Rates: per 100,000 population, age-standardised by single year of age to the 1981 England and Wales population.
%: percentage of 1970–74 rates for mortality, 1971–74 for incidence.
Cancer of nervous system: ICD8 191, 192.0–3, 192.9; ICD9 191, 192.

Table 17.14

Hodgkin's disease: mortality 1970–91 and incidence 1971–87, England and Wales

Mortality

Age-group		Males					Females				
		1970–74	1975–79	1980–84	1985–89	1990–91	1970–74	1975–79	1980–84	1985–89	1990–91
15–34	n	529	450	352	322	98	304	232	214	187	84
	rate	1.51	1.22	0.93	0.83	0.61	0.92	0.66	0.58	0.50	0.54
	%	100	80.6	61.9	55.2	40.5	100	71.8	63.4	54.0	58.8
35–49	n	484	402	331	290	89	248	177	136	159	36
	rate	2.18	1.87	1.47	1.19	0.90	1.13	0.84	0.61	0.66	0.37
	%	100	85.5	67.1	54.6	41.3	100	74.0	53.9	58.1	32.4
50–69	n	981	792	589	386	146	537	465	322	239	82
	rate	3.72	3.02	2.29	1.50	1.46	1.83	1.60	1.16	0.87	0.75
	%	100	81.0	61.4	40.4	39.2	100	87.7	63.2	47.4	41.2
70–84	n	379	326	304	251	81	437	371	314	286	93
	rate	5.53	4.16	3.47	2.72	2.14	3.62	2.82	2.22	1.95	1.62
	%	100	75.3	62.7	49.2	38.7	100	77.8	61.3	53.7	44.7
15–84	n	2,373	1,970	1,576	1,249	414	1,526	1,245	986	871	295
	rate	2.64	2.13	1.66	1.27	1.05	1.59	1.26	0.98	0.84	0.71
	%	100	80.7	62.9	48.2	39.8	100	79.1	61.2	52.4	44.7

Incidence

Age-group		Males				Females			
		1971–74	1975–79	1980–84	1985–87	1971–74	1975–79	1980–84	1985–87
15–34	n	1,190	1,534	1,457	851	716	958	1,087	675
	rate	4.25	4.22	3.86	3.66	2.68	2.72	2.95	2.98
	%	100	99.1	90.6	86.0	100	101.3	109.8	111.1
35–49	n	667	772	800	447	323	385	383	225
	rate	3.80	3.60	3.53	3.07	1.85	1.84	1.71	1.54
	%	100	94.6	92.9	80.8	100	99.5	92.4	83.3
50–69	n	1,144	1,210	997	479	675	724	606	285
	rate	5.40	4.61	3.89	3.16	2.85	2.52	2.15	1.77
	%	100	85.4	72.0	58.5	100	88.3	75.6	62.1
70–84	n	341	436	385	200	427	459	474	211
	rate	6.11	5.57	4.39	3.62	4.36	3.48	3.35	2.41
	%	100	91.2	71.9	59.3	100	79.8	76.8	55.2
15–84	n	3,342	3,952	3,639	1,977	2,141	2,526	2,550	1,396
	rate	4.63	4.30	3.84	3.38	2.78	2.58	2.52	2.25
	%	100	92.9	82.9	73.0	100	92.6	90.3	80.9

Rates: per 100,000 population, age-standardised by single year of age to the 1981 England and Wales population.
%: percentage of 1970–74 rates for mortality, 1971–74 for incidence.
Hodgkin's disease: ICD8 201; ICD9 201.

Table 17.15

Non-Hodgkin's lymphoma: mortality 1970–91 and incidence 1971–87, England and Wales

Mortality

Age-group		Males					Females				
		1970–74	1975–79	1980–84	1985–89	1990–91	1970–74	1975–79	1980–84	1985–89	1990–91
15–34	n	361	368	373	297	148	181	191	184	196	62
	rate	1.07	1.02	1.00	0.79	0.93	0.55	0.54	0.50	0.54	0.40
	%	100	95.2	93.1	73.4	87.2	100	97.4	91.1	97.3	72.6
35–49	n	549	531	624	793	388	345	339	388	435	218
	rate	2.43	2.44	2.79	3.30	3.80	1.52	1.57	1.76	1.82	2.14
	%	100	100.2	114.6	135.6	156.2	100	103.5	115.6	119.5	140.8
50–69	n	2,227	2,406	2,864	3,474	1,488	1,643	1,802	2,006	2,495	1,066
	rate	8.45	9.19	11.16	13.59	14.44	5.58	6.22	7.18	9.14	9.93
	%	100	108.7	132.1	160.8	170.8	100	111.5	128.7	163.9	178.2
70–84	n	1,185	1,631	2,270	3,431	1,573	1,477	1,960	2,631	3,615	1,659
	rate	17.26	21.04	25.85	36.82	40.21	12.26	14.96	18.57	24.73	28.21
	%	100	121.9	149.8	213.4	233.0	100	122.0	151.5	201.8	230.2
15–84	n	4,322	4,936	6,131	7,995	3,597	3,646	4,292	5,209	6,741	3,005
	rate	4.88	5.41	6.46	8.16	8.88	3.79	4.35	5.15	6.58	7.31
	%	100	110.8	132.3	167.1	181.8	100	114.8	135.8	173.5	192.7

Incidence

Age-group		Males				Females			
		1971–74	1975–79	1980–84	1985–87	1971–74	1975–79	1980–84	1985–87
15–34	n	475	700	760	456	299	366	450	303
	rate	1.77	1.92	2.03	2.01	1.13	1.04	1.24	1.36
	%	100	108.8	114.7	113.6	100	91.9	109.4	119.9
35–49	n	793	1,075	1,471	1,057	496	763	967	707
	rate	4.43	4.94	6.56	7.37	2.76	3.56	4.37	4.99
	%	100	111.6	148.1	166.4	100	129.1	158.5	180.8
50–69	n	2,535	3,916	4,844	3,358	2,030	3,099	3,759	2,586
	rate	12.01	14.98	18.86	22.10	8.64	10.67	13.43	15.88
	%	100	124.8	157.1	184.0	100	123.4	155.4	183.7
70–84	n	1,229	2,175	3,304	2,622	1,510	2,539	3,746	2,762
	rate	22.15	27.97	37.65	46.91	15.49	19.36	26.46	31.50
	%	100	126.3	170.0	211.8	100	125.0	170.8	203.4
15–84	n	5,032	7,866	10,379	7,493	4,335	6,767	8,922	6,358
	rate	7.05	8.58	10.94	12.85	5.58	6.82	8.83	10.39
	%	100	121.7	155.2	182.3	100	122.3	158.3	186.3

Rates: per 100,000 population, age-standardised by single year of age to the 1981 England and Wales population.
%: percentage of 1970–74 rates for mortality, 1971–74 for incidence.
Non-Hodgkin's lymphoma: ICD8 200, 202; ICD9 200, 202.

Table 17.16

Multiple myeloma: mortality 1970–91 and incidence 1971–87, England and Wales

Mortality

Age-group		Males					Females				
		1970–74	1975–79	1980–84	1985–89	1990–91	1970–74	1975–79	1980–84	1985–89	1990–91
15–34	n	13	12	11	16	5	7	6	5	2	3
	rate	0.04	0.03	0.03	0.04	0.04	0.02	0.02	0.01	0.01	0.02
	%	100	87.4	76.9	115.5	96.5	100	74.2	62.2	26.1	76.7
35–49	n	159	184	163	182	63	104	121	123	112	44
	rate	0.68	0.83	0.73	0.77	0.62	0.45	0.55	0.56	0.48	0.43
	%	100	120.8	107.3	113.4	90.1	100	122.5	126.0	107.5	97.1
50–69	n	1,588	1,848	1,852	2,082	802	1,343	1,448	1,435	1,570	617
	rate	6.06	7.02	7.19	8.09	7.82	4.60	4.99	5.12	5.73	5.71
	%	100	115.9	118.7	133.5	129.0	100	108.5	111.3	124.6	124.2
70–84	n	966	1,365	1,933	2,648	1,025	1,416	1,764	2,220	2,851	1,149
	rate	14.06	17.62	21.98	28.10	25.97	11.73	13.46	15.65	19.43	19.59
	%	100	125.3	156.3	199.8	184.7	100	114.7	133.4	165.6	167.0
15–84	n	2,726	3,409	3,959	4,928	1,895	2,870	3,339	3,783	4,535	1,813
	rate	3.12	3.74	4.16	4.98	4.67	3.02	3.39	3.73	4.41	4.42
	%	100	119.9	133.4	159.7	149.8	100	112.2	123.5	145.9	146.3

Incidence

Age-group		Males				Females			
		1971–74	1975–79	1980–84	1985–87	1971–74	1975–79	1980–84	1985–87
15–34	n	18	31	20	12	13	16	11	23
	rate	0.06	0.09	0.06	0.05	0.05	0.05	0.03	0.11
	%	100	140.8	86.5	86.2	100	95.1	60.0	220.4
35–49	n	212	300	278	174	144	205	179	124
	rate	1.15	1.35	1.25	1.25	0.78	0.93	0.82	0.89
	%	100	117.1	108.2	108.0	100	119.2	104.7	113.6
50–69	n	1,726	2,392	2,481	1,519	1,416	1,896	1,935	1,218
	rate	8.18	9.10	9.69	9.95	6.03	6.56	6.95	7.51
	%	100	111.3	118.5	121.6	100	108.8	115.3	124.6
70–84	n	889	1,725	2,441	1,789	1,321	2,131	2,807	1,784
	rate	15.99	22.23	27.76	31.84	13.52	16.26	19.81	20.20
	%	100	139.0	173.6	199.1	100	120.2	146.5	149.3
15–84	n	2,845	4,448	5,220	3,494	2,894	4,248	4,932	3,149
	rate	3.99	4.87	5.50	5.94	3.75	4.31	4.88	5.14
	%	100	122.0	137.8	148.8	100	114.9	130.1	137.0

Rates: per 100,000 population, age-standardised by single year of age to the 1981 England and Wales population.
%: percentage of 1970–74 rates for mortality, 1971–74 for incidence.
Multiple myeloma: ICD8 203; ICD9 203.

Table 17.17

Leukaemia: mortality 1970–91 and incidence 1971–87, England and Wales

Mortality

Age-group		Males					Females				
		1970–74	1975–79	1980–84	1985–89	1990–91	1970–74	1975–79	1980–84	1985–89	1990–91
15–34	n	717	815	800	778	243	506	548	489	443	152
	rate	2.12	2.28	2.12	2.04	1.58	1.54	1.59	1.34	1.19	0.99
	%	100	107.3	100.0	96.2	74.4	100	103.2	86.9	77.3	64.5
35–49	n	747	687	727	741	276	596	569	538	631	186
	rate	3.33	3.16	3.23	3.08	2.73	2.64	2.66	2.42	2.64	1.82
	%	100	95.1	97.0	92.5	82.0	100	101.0	91.8	100.0	69.1
50–69	n	3,004	3,065	2,998	3,029	1,193	2,174	2,207	2,122	2,132	816
	rate	11.47	11.70	11.68	11.82	11.56	7.39	7.58	7.60	7.81	7.57
	%	100	102.0	101.8	103.0	100.8	100	102.5	102.8	105.7	102.4
70–84	n	2,560	2,977	3,700	4,081	1,660	2,488	2,942	3,400	3,717	1,423
	rate	37.31	38.48	41.98	42.92	42.12	20.69	22.54	23.94	25.08	23.89
	%	100	103.1	112.5	115.0	112.9	100	109.0	115.7	121.2	115.5
15–84	n	7,028	7,544	8,225	8,629	3,372	5,764	6,266	6,549	6,923	2,577
	rate	8.17	8.37	8.63	8.69	8.28	6.08	6.41	6.47	6.68	6.20
	%	100	102.4	105.6	106.3	101.3	100	105.5	106.4	109.9	102.0

Incidence

Age-group		Males				Females			
		1971–74	1975–79	1980–84	1985–87	1971–74	1975–79	1980–84	1985–87
15–34	n	611	859	873	516	462	626	599	350
	rate	2.26	2.39	2.32	2.29	1.77	1.80	1.64	1.59
	%	100	105.7	102.5	101.1	100	101.9	92.7	89.8
35–49	n	699	837	851	506	515	639	633	459
	rate	3.91	3.84	3.78	3.54	2.88	2.98	2.86	3.24
	%	100	98.3	96.7	90.4	100	103.6	99.5	112.9
50–69	n	3,205	3,997	4,217	2,286	2,151	2,779	2,810	1,545
	rate	15.25	15.29	16.46	14.96	9.13	9.56	10.07	9.51
	%	100	100.3	107.9	98.1	100	104.7	110.2	104.1
70–84	n	2,435	3,790	4,788	3,006	2,304	3,527	4,307	2,574
	rate	43.87	48.96	54.36	53.08	23.74	27.00	30.35	28.89
	%	100	111.6	123.9	121.0	100	113.7	127.8	121.7
15–84	n	6,950	9,483	10,729	6,314	5,432	7,571	8,349	4,928
	rate	10.00	10.51	11.28	10.68	7.12	7.73	8.25	7.96
	%	100	105.1	112.8	106.9	100	108.5	115.9	111.7

Rates: per 100,000 population, age-standardised by single year of age to the 1981 England and Wales population.
%: percentage of 1970–74 rates for mortality, 1971–74 for incidence.
Leukaemia: ICD8 204–207; ICD9 204–208.

Table 17.18

Cancer of unspecified site: mortality 1970–91 and incidence 1971–87, England and Wales

Mortality

Age-group		Males 1970–74	1975–79	1980–84	1985–89	1990–91	Females 1970–74	1975–79	1980–84	1985–89	1990–91
15–34	n	103	124	194	130	70	62	80	117	84	53
	rate	0.30	0.34	0.52	0.34	0.44	0.20	0.23	0.32	0.23	0.36
	%	100	115.4	176.2	113.0	146.8	100	113.3	160.6	114.7	176.3
35–49	n	376	451	739	820	364	439	434	680	726	302
	rate	1.62	2.05	3.31	3.43	3.60	1.90	1.98	3.09	3.06	2.96
	%	100	126.3	203.9	210.9	221.7	100	104.2	162.8	161.1	156.0
50–69	n	3,363	4,722	8,079	8,964	3,858	3,131	4,086	6,994	7,395	3,050
	rate	12.83	18.02	31.51	34.88	37.13	10.67	14.11	24.99	26.98	28.10
	%	100	140.4	245.5	271.7	289.3	100	132.3	234.3	252.9	263.4
70–84	n	2,713	4,537	9,934	13,539	5,908	3,642	5,782	11,252	14,613	6,465
	rate	39.51	58.58	112.81	141.73	149.03	30.30	44.34	79.25	98.58	107.98
	%	100	148.2	285.5	358.7	377.2	100	146.3	261.6	325.4	356.4
15–84	n	6,555	9,834	18,946	23,453	10,200	7,274	10,382	19,043	22,818	9,870
	rate	7.62	10.89	19.90	23.41	24.77	7.68	10.62	18.79	21.99	23.63
	%	100	143.0	261.3	307.4	325.3	100	138.3	244.7	286.4	307.8

Incidence

Age-group		Males 1971–74	1975–79	1980–84	1985–87	Females 1971–74	1975–79	1980–84	1985–87
15–34	n	75	73	113	93	57	71	104	60
	rate	0.28	0.20	0.30	0.42	0.22	0.21	0.29	0.28
	%	100	72.3	108.0	147.7	100	94.2	130.3	127.7
35–49	n	297	373	417	314	333	363	406	274
	rate	1.62	1.69	1.87	2.19	1.80	1.65	1.85	1.95
	%	100	104.2	115.1	135.2	100	92.1	102.8	108.8
50–69	n	2,730	3,620	4,532	2,988	2,282	3,272	4,015	2,446
	rate	12.95	13.80	17.64	19.69	9.71	11.27	14.34	14.98
	%	100	106.6	136.2	152.1	100	116.1	147.7	154.2
70–84	n	2,310	3,622	5,597	4,282	2,750	4,701	6,861	4,994
	rate	41.63	46.81	63.56	75.19	28.41	36.05	48.31	56.12
	%	100	112.4	152.7	180.6	100	126.9	170.1	197.6
15–84	n	5,412	7,688	10,659	7,677	5,422	8,407	11,386	7,774
	rate	7.83	8.52	11.18	12.93	7.13	8.60	11.23	12.51
	%	100	108.8	142.8	165.0	100	120.5	157.4	175.4

Rates: per 100,000 population, age-standardised by single year of age to the 1981 England and Wales population.
%: percentage of 1970–74 rates for mortality, 1971–74 for incidence.
Cancer of unspecified site: ICD8 195, 199; ICD9 195, 199.

Chapter 18

Cardiovascular diseases

By
John Charlton, Mike Murphy, Kay-tee Khaw,
Shah Ebrahim and George Davey Smith

Summary

- In the nineteenth century infectious diseases were the major cause of death. Circulatory diseases are now the most important. They accounted for 45 per cent of all deaths in Britain in 1994.

- There has been a marked rise in ischaemic heart disease in Britain since the 1920s, which peaked in the 1970s, and fell subsequently.

- The trend in ischaemic heart disease mortality this century is similar for men and women, although female mortality has always been lower than male, particularly at younger ages, and the rise and fall was less marked.

- There have been substantial changes in diagnostic coding practices affecting ischaemic heart disease this century, but it is unlikely that observed changes in mortality can be attributed to such artefacts alone.

- Social environment and lifestyle have been the main driving forces behind trends in ischaemic heart disease. The best researched candidates are diet (especially saturated fat) and cigarette smoking.

- There has been a steady decline in stroke mortality this century, with similar rates of decline in all ages under 75. Although changes in diagnostic coding practices have also affected levels of stroke mortality, the downward trend is likely to be real.

- The decline in stroke mortality is associated with declines in case fatality and incidence.

- The fall in stroke mortality during this century is probably explained by reductions in exposure to risk factors, improvements in nutrition and non-specific effects of socio-economic development.

- There are both period and cohort effects in the stroke mortality trends, but the period effect is far stronger. There is growing evidence that the decline in mortality at younger ages is now over.

18.1 Background

While in the nineteenth century infectious diseases were the major cause of death in Britain, circulatory diseases are now the most important, accounting for 45 per cent of all deaths in 1993 (OPCS, 1995a). Of these diseases ischaemic heart disease (IHD, also termed coronary heart disease) and stroke (or cerebrovascular disease) account for 25 and 11 per cent of all deaths respectively. Although strokes account for fewer deaths, they have a major impact on sufferers through chronic and distressing disability – they are the single most important cause of hospital admission after mental disorders, and place a heavy burden on patients' relatives and friends (Anderson, 1992). The incidence of stroke is strongly related to blood pressure, where each 10 mm Hg increase in diastolic blood pressure multiplies the stroke risk by 1.84 (95 per cent CI 1.80–1.90) (Prospective Studies Collaboration, 1995). IHD is caused by the obstruction of coronary artery blood flow by atherosclerosis and its complications, including thrombotic events. The process begins progressively from early adult life with the formation of cholesterol-rich fibro-fatty deposits under the intima of the larger arteries. Thrombosis complicating atherosclerosis may produce a myocardial infarction, half the cases of which are so mild that the heart attack is not recognised (Rose, 1991). In 20 per cent of heart attacks the first manifestation of disease is sudden death. About a quarter of all attacks are fatal before the arrival of a doctor, and these constitute 60 per cent of all IHD deaths. Only a quarter of deaths occur in hospital (Rose, 1991). The commonest chronic effect of myocardial ischaemia is angina – chest pain brought about by increased cardiac work. Thrombolytic treatment immediately after a heart attack can reduce the mortality risk by some 25 per cent (Rose, 1991; Rawles, 1996).

The relationship between IHD and blood cholesterol is strong: based on cohort studies it has been estimated that a difference in plasma cholesterol of 0.6 mmol/l (10 per cent) lowers the risk of IHD by 50 per cent at age 40, falling to 20 per cent at age 70 (Law et al., 1994a). Such a reduction could be difficult to achieve through clinical dietary intervention (Hunninghake et al., 1993; Neil et al., 1995), although trends from the USA suggest that changes in social attitudes towards diet can lead to changes of this magnitude. Randomised controlled trial evidence shows that the effects of lowering cholesterol can be seen within 2 years (Law et al., 1994b). There is no evidence that low serum cholesterol increases mortality from any cause other than haemorrhagic stroke, and even the risk association with haemorrhagic stroke is at best suggestive (Davey Smith et al., 1992). The benefits from low risk of IHD outweigh any possible detrimental effects on haemorrhagic stroke among people with low cholesterol levels, even if the association between haemorrhagic stroke and cholesterol were causal (Law et al., 1994c). Overall stroke incidence is unrelated to blood cholesterol, except possibly among those aged under 45 (Prospective Studies Collaboration, 1995), but there may be different associations for different stroke types, namely thromboembolitic and haemorraghic strokes that cancel out in the overall figures. Only 1 per cent of stroke deaths occurred in those aged less than 45 in England and Wales in 1993, and 51 per cent of these were coded as subarachnoid haemorrhage, compared with only 4 per cent of all strokes (OPCS, 1995a).

IHD and stroke share many risk factors: cigarette smoking (Kuller et al., 1991); obesity (Gronbaek et al., 1994); high blood pressure (Martin et al., 1986); diabetes; and family history of the disease. Fibrinogen, a circulating blood protein involved in the formation of blood clots, is also a major risk factor for IHD and stroke (Ernst and Res, 1993). Fibrinogen levels are increased by smoking (De Bouver et al., 1995), and may also be determined by factors operating throughout life – adverse childhood environment and lower socio-economic status as measured by employment grade are associated with higher fibrinogen concentrations (Brunner et al., 1996), which may partly explain why individuals with lower socio-economic status are at greater risk of IHD (Kaplan and Keil, 1993). For IHD, moderate alcohol consumption, which may lower fibrinogen levels (Brunner et al., 1996), appears to confer some protection (Jackson and Beaglehole, 1991).

In spite of sharing a number of risk factors, stroke and IHD are two distinct disorders. The first part of the chapter mainly considers IHD, with some reference to stroke, and the second part concentrates on stroke. IHD and stroke are relatively uncommon below the ages of 35 years; over 75 years of age there may be more of a problem in diagnostic accuracy since there are likely to be multiple contributors to death. Thus most of our analysis is concentrated on ages 35–74, over the full period for which comparable data are available. Trends from 1911–1994 for circulatory diseases as a whole are described in Chapter 4. The emphasis is on mortality data for England and Wales – hospitalisation and other health service utilisation data for circulatory diseases are more difficult to interpret (see Chapter 5).

There are notable differences between IHD and stroke: firstly, time trends in mortality rates differ; secondly, men have similar rates to women for stroke but a three to sixfold excess for IHD; and thirdly, the rankings of different countries on IHD and stroke mortality, although weakly correlated, can vary considerably as Figure 18.1 (all ages) shows (Zarate, 1994). Among the 36 countries described here the United Kingdom has the seventh highest IHD mortality and tenth highest stroke mortality, but France is the 34th highest on IHD and 5th on stroke. The most striking features in this century in Britain have been the rise and decline in IHD mortality especially at younger ages, and the marked sex differences in patterns of mortality. Stroke has declined since the early part of the century for both sexes.

PART 1 – IHD

18.2 Introduction and definitions

ONS data for the group of diseases affecting the cardiovascular system as a whole have been greatly affected by changes in nomenclature, methods of diagnosis, classification and coding instructions. Table 18.1 shows the classifications

Figure 18.1

Comparison of age adjusted mortality rates for IHD and stroke for 36 countries
Stroke mortality rate per 100,000

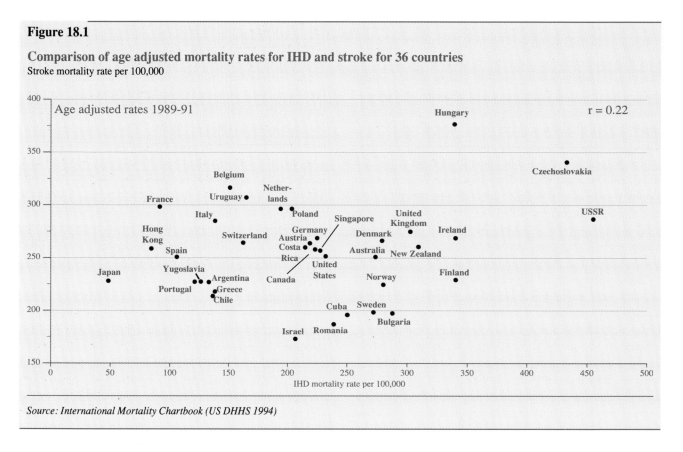

Source: *International Mortality Chartbook (US DHHS 1994)*

Table 18.1

ICD codes used to describe trends in ischaemic heart disease (coronary heart disease) between 1901 and 1992

	ICD 1&2 1901–20	ICD 3 1921–30	ICD 4 1931–39	ICD 5 1940–49	ICD 6 1950–57	ICD 7 1958–67	ICD 8 1968–78	ICD 9 1979 current
Darby and Doll (Chapter 9)	N/A				420, 422.1 (+422.0, 422.2, 450)	420, 422.1 (+422.0, 422.2, 450)	410-414 (+428, 440)	410-414 (+429, 440)
Alderson and Ashwood (1986)	N/A				420-422	420-422	395.9 410-414 410-414	424, 429.0 424, 428 429.1
Campbell (1965)	N/A		94	94	420	420		
Halliday and Anderson (1979)	N/A		93, 94	93, 94	420, 422	420, 422	410, 413	
Ryle and Russell (1949)	N/A	90 (5) 90 (7) 91(b) (2) 89	93b 93c 97 (3)	93c 93d				
Taylor and Dauncey (1955)	N/A		93, 94	93, 94				
Clayton (1977) et al.					420, 422	420, 422	410-414 (+428)	
This chapter; (see Appendix A for descriptions)	N/A	90 (5) 90 (7) 91(b) (2) 89	93, 94	93, 94	420, 422	420, 422	410-414	410-414

* Clayton et al. quote various options for IHD but do not finally believe it best defined alone.

others have used and those we have chosen to use in the comparisons of various revisions of the International Classification of Diseases (ICD) in England and Wales. Appendix 21.1 gives the descriptions of the codes that we have used. Bridge coding across the different revisions is thought to be least successful in the older age-groups. There have also been shifts, particularly for the older age-groups, from poorly specified causes of deaths (including symptoms and signs) to more precisely specified ones, including heart disease (see Chapter 4). We thus focus on trends in those aged under 75 years. Coding artefacts between 1921 and 1961 have been discussed in detail by Ryle and Russell (1949) and Campbell (1963a, 1965). For example, between the 4th and 5th revisions Campbell (1965) reported that, for all ages combined, largely because of assignment for stroke, there was an 8 per cent (–16,000) reduction in deaths attributed to diseases of the coronary arteries, and a 61 per cent (–17,000) reduction in deaths attributed to arteriosclerosis. Between the 5th and 6th revisions, there was a 10 per cent increase (+4,000) in deaths assigned to diseases of the coronary arteries and an increase (+815) in deaths attributed to the verticular lesions affecting the CNS. Between the 4th and 5th revisions (in 1939–40) there was a large shift in coding from arteriosclerosis to cerebrovascular disease and from myocardial disease and endocarditis to bronchitis. Alterations from the 5th revision to the 6th (1949–50) resulted in a small shift from respiratory diseases back to heart diseases, and a large increase in hypertension at the expense of arteriosclerosis and nephritis.

These problems of classification may be overcome by broadening the group of codes used. Figures 18.2 and 18.3 show trends for ages 35–74 for IHD (our definition), stroke and other circulatory diseases, as well as respiratory diseases, ill defined and all other diseases. Also shown in Figure 18.3 are

the first year of each coding revision, including the adoption of automatic cause coding by ONS in 1993. It can be seen that, for example, there were major increases in respiratory and stroke mortality with the adoption of the 5th revision of the ICD in 1940, and a corresponding reduction in 'other circulatory diseases' at the same time. Ill defined causes declined to negligible levels by the 1950s; such deaths would have been transferred to other categories, including circulatory diseases. The introduction of automatic cause coding in 1993 resulted in increases in mortality classified as 'other circulatory diseases' and respiratory diseases, but had little effect on the trends for other causes. It is thus unlikely that the trends in IHD as defined in this chapter could be accounted for in the main by changes in coding or diagnosis, and there are no sharp discontinuities for IHD with different coding revisions.

As indicated above, a major problem in reconstructing trends in coronary heart disease mortality is the change in diagnostic ability and death certification practice that has occurred over the course of the century. IHD mortality could not have been recorded in 1900, as it was not included in the disease classification. There was a category 'angina pectoris', but its use was uncommon, with only 1.5 per cent of all deaths attributed to heart disease falling into this category (Campbell, 1963a). In retrospect it seems clear that IHD deaths occurred before the term was introduced (Fye, 1985; Lawrence, 1992). The initial description of angina pectoris is generally attributed to William Heberden in 1768, who detailed the pattern of symptoms and the fact that sudden death occurred as a complication. The concept was further developed by others, including Allan Burns in 1809 (Proudfit, 1983), and in the middle of the nineteenth century Richard Quain described 'fatty disease of the heart' (Fye, 1985). A retrospective re-

Figure 18.2

Mortality from IHD and other causes, 1921–94, ages 35–74

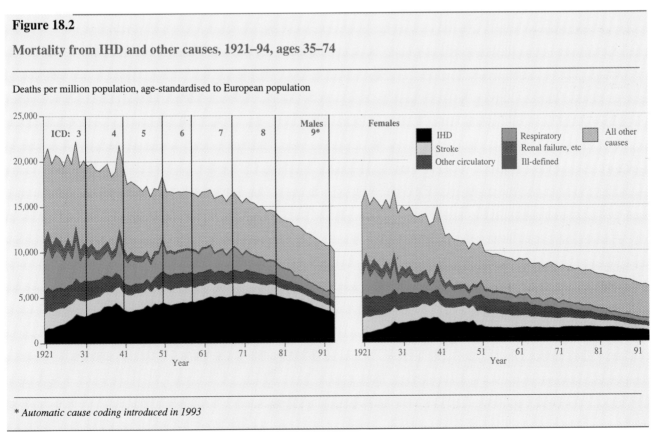

Deaths per million population, age-standardised to European population

* Automatic cause coding introduced in 1993

Figure 18.3

Mortality from IHD and other causes, 1921–94, ages 35–74

Deaths per million population, age standardised to European population

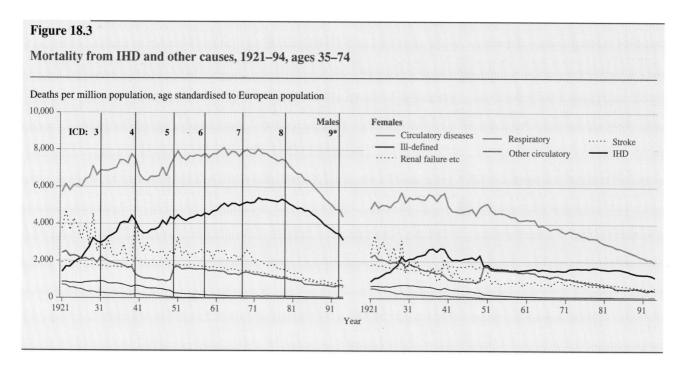

view of his case reports suggests that 52 out of 83 cases represented IHD (Morgan, 1968). The pathologist Carl Weigert and clinician Carl Huber in Leipzig described the myocardial lesions induced by acute ischaemia and developed the notion that myocardial infarction and angina both reflected underlying coronary artery disease (Fye, 1985). Before the turn of the century myocardial infarction and coronary thrombosis were described as terminal events (Acierno, 1994), with the diagnosis of acute coronary thrombosis in the living patient being generally first attributed to two Russian doctors, Obrastzow and Straschesko in 1910 (Krikler, 1987). By 1918 Herrick was able to link clinical information with electrocardiogram evidence from experimental canine and human subjects, since when the occurrence of coronary thrombosis was increasingly recognised (Lawrence, 1992).

Atherosclerosis has retrospectively been demonstrated in Egyptian mummies, but the first contemporary descriptions occurred in the sixteenth century (Acierno, 1994). The main theories relating to its origins date from the mid-nineteenth century. Its thrombogenic basis was proposed by Karl Freiherr von Rokitansky of Vienna but disputed by Rudolph Virchow who considered it to be an inflammatory lesion (Acierno, 1994). The notion that lipid infiltration was the key character of atherosclerosis dates back to Vogel, who identified cholesterol as the major component of atherosclerotic lesions in 1847 (Acierno, 1994). However, the major developments of interest in the lipid accumulation theory resulted from animal feeding experiments around the turn of the century.

As coronary heart disease is generally associated with advanced coronary atherosclerosis it would be expected that the dramatic increase in coronary heart disease mortality in the first half of this century would be accompanied by increasing evidence of severe coronary atheroma. However, studies of post-mortem records of the London Hospital (Morris, 1951) suggest that there was no such increase between 1908 and 1949; in fact the degree of coronary atheroma declined. In a review of post-mortem records from St

Bartholomew's Hospital there was no major change in the degree of atheroma of the abdominal aorta over the same period (Finlayson, 1985). Morris interpreted his data as indicating that an increase in the tendency to thrombose was responsible for the increase in coronary heart disease incidence and mortality. It had, however, earlier been suggested that not all myocardial infarctions were due to coronary thrombosis (Friedberg and Horn, 1939), although the fundamental role of thrombosis has been re-established more recently (DeWood et al., 1980). A recent study in the United States covering the period 1980–89, when ischaemic heart disease was declining rapidly, found no reduction in the prevalence of atherosclerosis (Enriquez-Sarano et al., 1996). The relative contribution of atherosclerosis and thrombotic tendency to trends in IHD mortality remain difficult to elucidate, but the studies by Enriquez-Sarano and Morris suggest that the trends were not due to changes in atherosclerosis alone.

18.3 IHD mortality trends

18.3.1 IHD and other cardiovascular disease mortality

Table 18.2 shows annual death rates for selected causes of death in men and women between 1921 and 1994 in four age-standardised age-groups: 35–44, 45–54 and 55–64 and 65–74. Figure 18.3 shows the trends in IHD, stroke, and all circulatory diseases mortality rates that have been age standardised to the European population (Waterhouse et al., 1976) for ages 35–74 years over 1921–94. This is the age-group where diagnoses are most likely to be accurate over the period. Changes in ICD revision are indicated on the graph. For men and women there was a marked rise in IHD mortality until 1939, and then a decline, which lasted for only a few years for men, but continued longer for women. The validity of the decline in IHD mortality during the war in men has been challenged by Barker and Osmond (1986). This possible decline was followed by a sustained rise for both sexes, with mortality peaking in the mid-1970s for women and the late 1970s for men. Since then mortality has been declining sharply. While some of the rise in IHD could be attributed to coding transfer from other heart diseases categories, which have shown a dramatic drop between 1939 and 1951, coding changes are unlikely to account for all the rise in IHD mortality as total circulatory mortality has increased overall (see also Chapter 4). Transfers from respiratory and poorly specified causes of death could also have increased the numbers of deaths attributed to more specific causes such as heart disease, but trends for respiratory diseases, (see Figure 4.13) and symptoms, signs and ill-defined causes (see Figure 4.17), are not consistent with this explanation for all age-groups. For women, total circulatory disease has, in contrast, shown an overall downward trend this century, and the trend in stroke mortality has been similar to men's, with a steady decline over this century, apart from the 1940s when the decline appeared to stagnate. The change from ICD4 to ICD5 raised the apparent level of stroke mortality considerably in 1941.

The contrast in patterns for total circulatory disease mortality between men and women over this century can thus largely

Table 18.2

Ischaemic heart diseases trends, 1921–1994
Age-standardised rates per million

Year	Males Definition x				Males Definition y Defn a codes			
	35–44	45–54	55–64	65–74	35–44	45–54	55–64	65–74
1921	77	397	1,569	5,601	77	397	1,569	5,601
1931	241	1,012	3,342	11,625	241	1,012	3,342	11,625
1941	263	1,267	4,457	13,901	263	1,267	4,457	13,901
1951	282	1,490	4,397	9,752	314	1,675	5,576	16,472
1961	482	2,063	6,072	13,350	493	2,103	6,370	15,725
1971	–	–	–	–	664	2,733	6,927	16,064
1981	–	–	–	–	526	2,509	6,882	15,563
1991	–	–	–	–	326	1,508	4,873	12,796
1994	–	–	–	–	268	1,182	4,061	11,200

Year	Females Definition x				Females Definition y Defn a codes			
	35–44	45–54	55–64	65–74	35–44	45–54	55–64	65–74
1921	50	277	929	3,571	50	277	929	3,571
1931	164	573	2,314	8,676	164	573	2,314	8,676
1941	144	583	2,304	9,705	144	583	2,304	9,705
1951	45	265	1,225	4,389	80	382	1,846	7,893
1961	66	328	1,626	5,879	76	368	1,647	6,391
1971	–	–	–	–	96	455	1,819	5,604
1981	–	–	–	–	77	472	1,860	6,083
1991	–	–	–	–	56	244	1,516	5,228
1994	–	–	–	–	53	236	1,198	4,794

Year	Sex ratio M:F death rates Definition x				Definition y			
	35–44	45–54	55–64	65–74	35–44	45–54	55–64	65–74
1921	1.5	1.4	1.7	1.6	1.5	1.4	1.7	1.6
1931	1.5	1.8	1.4	1.3	1.5	1.8	1.4	1.3
1941	1.8	2.2	1.9	1.4	1.8	2.2	1.9	1.4
1951	6.3	5.6	3.6	2.2	3.9	4.4	3.0	2.1
1961	7.3	6.3	3.7	2.3	6.5	5.7	3.9	2.5
1971	–	–	–	–	6.9	6.0	3.8	2.9
1981	–	–	–	–	6.8	5.3	3.7	2.6
1991	–	–	–	–	5.8	6.2	3.2	2.4
1994	–	–	–	–	5.1	5.0	3.4	2.3

Definition x: ICD4 94; ICD5 94a,b; ICD6 420; ICD7 420
Definition y: ICD4 94; ICD5 94a,b; ICD6 420,422; ICD7 420,422; ICD6 420, 422; ICD7 420,422; ICD8 410-414; ICD9 410-414

Figure 18.4

Ratio of male to female mortality, 1921–94, ages 35–74 (based on rates age-standardised to European population)

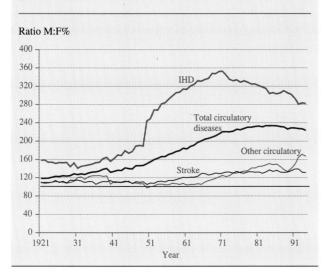

be attributed to the differing absolute contributions of stroke and IHD mortality in men and women. For both sexes at the turn of the century stroke mortality predominated and IHD was uncommon. However, the rise in IHD has been much greater, in absolute terms, in men compared to women. The most recent crossover between IHD predominating over stroke as cause of death occurred in the 1920s in men and in the 1960s in women. Thus, total circulatory disease mortality trends this century have been dominated more by trends in IHD in men and more evenly balanced between stroke and coronary heart disease in women. This is summarised in the mortality sex ratio (see Figure 18.4), and considered further in the next section.

18.3.2 Age- and sex-specific trends 1921–92 for IHD

To examine trends in more detail, we used sex- and age-specific rates for the age-groups 35–44, 45–54, 55–64 and 65–74 years to look at changing patterns and sex ratios. Within these groups the data have been age standardised to the European population, based on 5-year age-groups. Data for IHD mortality were available from 1921 to 1994. Table 18.2 shows IHD mortality trends for sex-specific age-groups, and the sex ratios. Two coding schedules were used so that the differences between using Campbell's definition (which left out myocardial degeneration, code 422) and ours could be examined. The trends for 1921–94 are shown in Figure 18.5, which also shows the substantial effect of missing out myocardial degeneration. The difference is greatest for men above age 55, and for women. All other alternative coding choices described inTable 18.1 have small effects, greatest at older ages.

For men in all age-groups IHD rates increased steadily from 1921 apart from an apparent temporary fall during the Second World War, reaching a peak in the late 1970s, and thereafter declining. There is a strong period-of-death effect, since the rises and falls occurred more or less at the same time at all ages. However, the falls in the 1970s began some years

earlier in the youngest age-groups. The rise was greatest during the years 1921–39, and the fall was steepest between 1981 and 1994. For women, IHD rates followed a similar pattern to males but with a longer and more pronounced fall from 1940, and a more gradual rise until the 1970s. Thereafter, rates began to decline, in the 1970s for ages 35–44 but only in the 1980s for ages 65–74. It is of interest that the pattern of changes in IHD mortality resemble those of men in that the relative rises occurred at about the same time in all age-groups, although female mortality has always been lower than male. Table 18.2 shows that this sex differential is greatest at younger ages. Between the 1920s and 1960s the ratio of male to female mortality rates has risen considerably, from around 1.5 to around 6 for those under the age of 54, 3 for ages 55–64 and 2.5 for ages 65–74. The sex ratios have remained relatively constant since the 1960s.

It is difficult to identify whether trends are best described in terms of influences around the time of death (period effects) or those accumulated over a life time (generation or cohort effects – see Chapter 2). Period of death and period of birth are related, since given the age and date at death it is possible to derive the date of birth arithmetically. If mortality rates followed a linear trend then it would be impossible to distinguish whether this was due to cohort of period influences. Variations associated with coding changes are more likely to appear as period effects, as are changes in incidence and efficacy of treatment. Methods have been developed to identify whether period or cohort effect are more important, but all these methods are fallible (see Chapter 2). In order to test rigorously whether there could be a cohort effect we modelled death rates for each sex, age (5-year grouping), period of death (5-year grouping) and period of birth (5-year grouping) using the GLIM4 package (Francis et al., 1993), and data for 1921–92 (see Figure 18.5, our definition). We adopted the usual approach of a log-linear model with Poisson error structure, with age, period and cohort as factored explanatory variables (Clayton and Schifflers, 1987). When period terms are constrained to be linear the resulting explanatory variable is called 'drift'. Comparisons between the comparative explanatory power of cohort and period effects are made relative to the variation explained by 'drift', which could be due to cohort effects, period effects, or both. A summary of the results of these analyses is given in Table 18.3.

The analyses show that a model based on age and period of death is substantially better at explaining variance (deviance) than one based on age and cohort (even though the latter has more parameters). However, there is statistically significant evidence for a smaller 'cohort effect' as well. A further analysis was undertaken by Osmond (1996, personal communication) using the same data but a different model. For males the log-linear model shown in Table 18.3 was a better fit to the data (the reverse was true for females), but the overall conclusion remained the same. Figure 18.6 shows the data plotted by generation (year of birth). Death rates in each successive generation born during or after the Second World War have been lower. The major part of this reduction will be due to period effects, but part will be due to factors operating from around

Figure 18.5

Trends in ischaemic heart disease deaths, England and Wales, 1921–94

Death rates per million population (log scale)

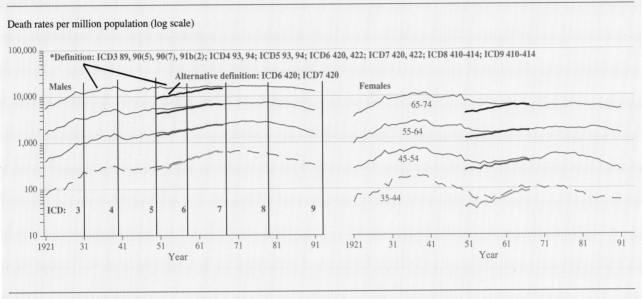

Source: ONS historic deaths file

Standardised to European* population

Table 18.3

Deviances and degrees of freedom of statistical models applied to the coronary heart disease rates

Model	Deviance		Degrees of freedom
	Men	Women	
Age+drift	112,076	42,333	125
Age+cohort	100,299	22,134	104
Age+period	31,202	7,613	112
Age+period+cohort	2,801	4,205	91

the time of birth (in-utero and/or in childhood) over the lifetime of each cohort. Osmond (1995) examined heart disease for 1952–91 but using a much broader grouping that included IHD, hypertensive disease and 'other forms of heart disease'. He also found evidence for both period and cohort effects, with the period effects explaining the greater part of the variance.

18.3.3 Socio-economic and geographical differences

The Registrar General's occupational supplements showed a marked social class differential in IHD mortality in 1931 and 1951 with highest rates in the professional classes. In 1931

Figure 18.6

Trends in ischaemic heart disease deaths, England and Wales, 1921–94, by central year of birth, 1846–1961

Death rates per million population (log scale)

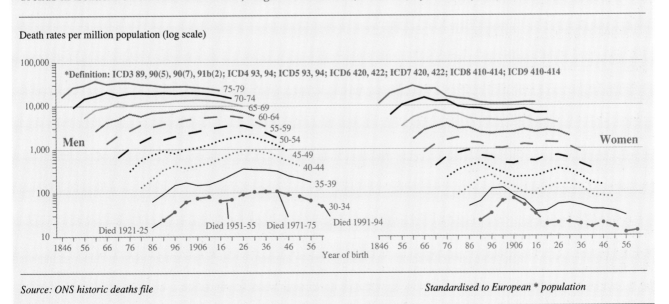

Source: ONS historic deaths file

Standardised to European * population

Table 18.4

IHD and stroke, by county district: 1985–94, county districts ranked by male IHD rate
Rates per 100,000 population, age standardised to European population

	IHD, males 35–74			IHD, females 35–74			Stroke, males 35–74			Stroke, females 35–74		
	Deaths	Rate	95% CI	Deaths	Rate	95% CI	Deaths	Rate	95% CI	Deaths	Rate	95% CI
20 lowest IHD rates												
Elmbridge CD	702	245	(227 264)	264	74	(65 83)	139	47	(39 55)	143	41	(34 48)
Chichester CD	740	246	(228 264)	329	81	(72 90)	180	57	(48 65)	167	42	(35 49)
East Dorset CD	638	253	(232 273)	234	73	(63 83)	129	49	(40 58)	106	33	(26 39)
Vale of White Horse CD	634	256	(236 276)	279	98	(86 110)	132	52	(43 61)	86	30	(24 37)
Runnymede CD	483	264	(240 287)	193	90	(77 103)	101	54	(43 64)	76	36	(27 44)
West Oxfordshire CD	532	265	(242 287)	218	90	(78 102)	107	52	(42 62)	103	42	(34 50)
South Cambridgeshire CD	706	266	(246 285)	297	97	(85 108)	123	45	(37 53)	108	36	(29 42)
Cotswold CD	535	266	(243 289)	204	78	(67 90)	137	64	(53 75)	124	46	(37 54)
Woking CD	503	268	(244 291)	217	95	(82 108)	88	45	(36 55)	110	49	(40 58)
Waverley CD	743	271	(252 291)	339	95	(84 105)	130	45	(37 53)	163	47	(40 55)
Wealden CD	967	272	(254 289)	362	75	(67 84)	202	54	(46 62)	179	39	(33 45)
Horsham CD	707	272	(252 292)	259	80	(70 90)	142	53	(44 62)	148	45	(37 52)
South Oxfordshire CD	824	274	(255 293)	328	94	(84 104)	188	62	(53 71)	130	37	(30 43)
Wokingham CD	693	274	(254 295)	211	76	(66 87)	140	57	(47 66)	118	42	(35 50)
South Bucks CD	447	275	(249 300)	183	98	(84 112)	93	57	(45 69)	106	57	(46 69)
South Norfolk CD	785	278	(258 298)	304	91	(81 102)	171	57	(48 66)	153	46	(39 54)
Christchurch CD	417	279	(250 308)	182	83	(70 96)	91	60	(46 73)	84	45	(34 56)
North Norfolk CD	829	279	(259 299)	297	81	(71 91)	189	61	(52 70)	167	45	(38 52)
Kensington and Chelsea LB	762	280	(260 300)	287	85	(75 95)	194	71	(61 81)	155	46	(39 53)
Lewes CD	713	280	(259 301)	271	80	(70 90)	149	58	(48 67)	150	44	(36 52)
20 highest IHD rates												
Middlesbrough CD	1,620	509	(484 534)	798	205	(190 219)	336	105	(93 116)	279	75	(66 84)
Merthyr Tydfil CD	752	509	(473 546)	373	204	(182 225)	157	105	(88 122)	122	67	(55 80)
Oldham MCD	2,485	510	(490 530)	1,216	200	(188 211)	528	105	(96 114)	471	75	(68 82)
Liverpool MCD	5,541	511	(497 524)	2,859	201	(194 209)	1,089	98	(92 104)	1063	74	(69 79)
Rochdale MCD	2,278	511	(490 532)	1,157	211	(198 223)	427	94	(85 103)	376	68	(61 75)
Blackburn CD	1,514	512	(486 538)	713	191	(177 206)	296	97	(86 109)	250	67	(59 76)
Sedgefield CD	1,127	513	(482 543)	575	217	(199 235)	227	101	(88 115)	169	63	(53 73)
Knowsley MCD	1,698	515	(490 539)	850	209	(195 223)	327	98	(88 109)	284	70	(61 78)
Gateshead MCD	2,645	515	(495 535)	1,446	222	(210 234)	499	94	(86 103)	448	70	(63 77)
Rossendale CD	742	517	(480 555)	377	214	(191 236)	123	83	(68 98)	136	73	(61 86)
Rhondda CD	1,044	517	(486 549)	559	208	(190 226)	197	92	(79 105)	206	76	(65 87)
Sunderland MCD	3,486	518	(501 536)	1,811	219	(209 229)	749	109	(101 117)	572	68	(63 74)
Manchester MCD	4,892	522	(507 537)	2,332	195	(187 204)	993	102	(95 108)	837	71	(66 76)
Salford MCD	2,898	523	(504 542)	1,410	196	(185 207)	587	102	(94 110)	551	77	(71 84)
Stoke-on-Trent CD	3,262	530	(511 548)	1,479	195	(185 206)	549	85	(78 93)	563	74	(67 80)
Easington CD	1,298	531	(502 560)	689	239	(221 257)	282	113	(100 126)	267	95	(84 107)
Burnley CD	1,102	536	(504 568)	525	197	(180 215)	220	104	(90 118)	199	77	(66 88)
Blaenau Gwent CD	1,067	538	(505 571)	520	217	(198 236)	189	93	(80 107)	164	65	(54 75)
Wear Valley CD	895	540	(504 576)	431	216	(194 237)	160	94	(79 108)	163	79	(67 92)
Scunthorpe CD	823	542	(505 580)	319	179	(159 199)	169	108	(91 124)	133	72	(60 85)

Social Class I had an approximately fourfold greater standardised mortality ratio than Social Classes IV and V. This gap had narrowed to a less than twofold difference in 1951 (Martin, 1956). The large gradient for coronary heart disease around the 1931 Census was likely to be over-estimated by differential misclassification with myocardial degeneration, which was more common than coronary heart disease at the time, and has consistently shown a strong inverse gradient. Analysis in England and Wales using area-based measures of socio-economic status have not shown inverse gradients (Martin, 1956), and data from the US found much less consistent evidence (Guralnick, 1963; Lilienfeld, 1956; Antonovsky, 1968). Whether there were ever substantially greater IHD rates among higher socio-economic groups in the USA and United Kingdom remains unresolved. Studies with objective measures of disease, or in which classificatory methods were standardised across classes, show much less evidence than those where data sources are more liable to differential categorisation according to socio-economic position (Antonovsky, 1968; Davey Smith, 1997). Men in physically active occupations do tend, other things being equal, to have a lower incidence of disease and a lower case fatality (Fox and Naughton, 1972), and a large necroscopy study suggested that differences in physical activity accounted for any tendency for higher disease rates among the non-manual classes earlier this century (Morris and Crawford, 1958). Since about 1960 IHD mortality in Social Classes I and II was static, whereas for semi-skilled and unskilled men it continued to rise (Rose and Marmot, 1981). By 1971 non-manual groups tended to have higher IHD mortality rates, and widening socio-economic differentials have been seen since, (Devis, 1993; Davey Smith and Marmot, 1991), with data from the ONS Longitudinal Study showing increasing gradients in ischaemic heart disease up till 1989 (Harding, 1995).

The wide geographical disparities in IHD mortality in England and Wales have remained relatively constant over time (Ryle and Russell, 1949; Martin, 1956; Britton, 1990). Figure 18.7 shows how IHD and stroke mortality for 1985–94 varied for males by local authority. Although stroke and IHD are highly correlated geographically, even in areas with similar stroke mortality (around 70 per 100,000) there are almost twofold variations in IHD mortality. The correlation between male and female IHD mortality is much greater (see Figure 18.8). This suggests that the environmental and lifestyle factors that influence IHD mortality operate on men and women alike. Some of the highest mortality areas are geographically close together, e.g. Manchester and Salford. Table 18.4 shows the 20 highest and lowest mortality areas. Further analysis of small area mortality data was undertaken to establish what types of area have highest IHD mortality rates. Table 18.5 shows that in 1990–92, among those aged 0–74, based on the ONS classification of 1991 census wards (Charlton, 1996), IHD mortality was up to 40 per cent above

Table 18.5

Hypertension and stroke SMRs, 1990–92, ages 0–74, by ward classification
England and Wales = 100

ONS ward classification	IHD*, Males 0–74			IHD*, Females 0–74			Stroke**, Males 0–74			Stroke**, Females 0–74		
	Obs	Expected	SMR	Obs	Expected	SMR	Obs	Expected	SMR	Obs	Expected	SMR
A Prosperous areas	5,929	8,473	70	2,112	3,394	62	1,274	1,691	75	1,107	1,394	79
B Rural areas	4,166	5,096	82	1,522	2,004	76	839	1,034	81	664	816	81
C Established Owner-occupiers	13,067	16,659	78	4,896	6,968	70	2,572	3,338	77	2,266	2,869	79
D Armed forces bases	543	636	85	212	252	84	95	130	73	103	106	97
E Mature populations	11,132	12,359	90	4,889	6,058	81	2,420	2,582	94	2,270	2,452	93
F Rural areas with mixed economies	10,662	11,485	93	4,363	4,835	90	2,024	2,325	87	1,886	1,980	95
G Suburbia	14,694	15,686	94	6,072	6,754	90	2,851	3,166	90	2,515	2,791	90
H Metropolitan professionals	3,836	4,265	90	1,567	2,010	78	930	875	106	812	832	98
I Middling England	19,666	18,429	107	9,133	8,084	113	3,817	3,750	102	3,510	3,308	106
J Deprived city areas	4,745	4,413	108	2,032	1,890	108	1,058	896	118	838	785	107
K Industrial & manufacturing towns	17,312	13,946	124	8,339	6,252	133	3,360	2,851	118	2,999	2,546	118
L Lower status owner occupiers	12,307	10,071	122	5,816	4,561	128	2,623	2,064	127	2,254	1,870	121
M Purpose-built, inner city estates	3,186	2,540	125	1,421	1,066	133	772	517	149	530	437	121
N Deprived industrial wards	9,825	7,011	140	4,815	3,061	157	2,012	1,426	141	1,680	1,248	135

*   *ICD 410-414*
** *ICD 430-438*

the national average level in 'deprived industrial areas', 'inner city estates', 'low status areas' and 'industrial and manufacturing towns', and around 70 per cent of the national average in 'prosperous' and 'rural' areas. In Scotland between 1981 and 1991 there have been increasing relative and absolute differences in IHD mortality between deprived and non-deprived areas (McLoone and Boddy, 1994).

18.4 Possible explanations for the trends in IHD mortality

IHD is pathologically the interaction between two processes, atheroma of the vessels and the thrombotic event. The present public health approach in the United Kingdom and the USA is based on the hypothesis that a diet high in saturated fatty acids leads to raised levels of blood cholesterol in individuals and populations. This is responsible in the main for the increased susceptibility to atherosclerosis and IHD observed in such populations. Raised blood pressure, cigarette smoking, physical inactivity and diabetes mellitus are major aggravating factors. Raised cholesterol levels are not an essential factor, however – South Asians have relatively low cholesterol levels, but high prevalence of insulin resistance, and high myocardial infarction mortality (McKeigue et al., 1989), demonstrating that raised cholesterol levels in a population are not an essential prerequisite for high IHD rates. Satisfactory explanations have to account for both the rise in coronary heart disease observed since the 1920s and the subsequent decline in the 1970s.

The trends in IHD mortality will reflect changes in incidence and case fatality. Incidence was likely to have been increasing over the period when mortality was increasing. The question must be asked: what factors can cause changes in incidence? Diet, raised blood pressure, cigarette smoking, and lack of exercise are recognised risk factors. Exercise and diet may act through altering cholesterol levels and other physiological factors. Other documented risk factors include haemostatic (blood clotting) factors, diabetes, respiratory function, white cell count, infection and homocysteine levels. While genes predisposing to atherosclerotic disease have been identified, genetic differences may explain some individual susceptibility but are unlikely to explain the time trends observed. Among the many factors influencing the risk of IHD, a central issue is which of them best account for the population mortality trends. Any explanation would have to account for both the rise and fall in mortality in all age-groups and men and women. It should also explain differing time trends observed in different countries – for example in the US the decline in IHD mortality began a decade before that observed in Britain, whereas several Eastern European countries such as Poland and Romania are still experiencing increases (Zarate, 1994).

Of related interest is the disjunction between time trends for stroke and IHD. While IHD and stroke share many of the same risk factors, raised low density and decreased high density lipoprotein cholesterol levels are strong risk factors for IHD mortality (Law et al., 1994a), but not for stroke where raised blood pressure is the most important related risk factor (Prospective Studies Collaboration, 1995). Blood cholesterol is strongly related to dietary saturated fatty acids and can be altered by changing diet (Cox et al., 1995). Blood pressure is related to body weight, alcohol consumption, and dietary sodium and potassium, among other factors. Thus, differences in trends between these two conditions could be explained by divergent trends for lipids and blood pressure, and the lifestyle factors most strongly related to these two risk factors.

Table 18.6

Mean intake of total fat as a percentage of energy for all studies divided into 10-year periods from 1900 to 1985

Time period	UK data			US data		
	No. of studies	No. of subjects	Fat (% energy)	No of studies	No of subjects	Fat (% energy)
1900–09	1	57	24.6	-	-	-
1910–19	3	348	24.1	-	-	-
1920–29	13	5,220	25.9	2	148	35.5
1930–39	8	916	33.1	2	37	41.2
1940–49	15	2,385	33.2	20	4,178	37.6
1950–59	13	1,568	38.4	46	20,993	40.5
1960–69	10	3,873	40.1	28	11,239	39.9
1970–79	4	2,294	40.3	53	73,499	37.8
1980–85	20	7,384	38.2	20	1,492	37.5

Source: Stephen and Seber (1994)
Note: Means are weighted according to the number of subjects in each study.

18.4.1 Changes in diagnostic fashion or changes in classification

Burnand and Feinstein (1992) have shown that changes in diagnostic practices have accelerated the apparent decline in IHD mortality rates in the US. It is unlikely, however, that changes in investigations, diagnostic fashion or classification can completely explain either the rise or the decline in IHD in England and Wales. Several investigators have examined the rise in IHD mortality in the 1920s and found that this cannot be explained by changing diagnostic practices or coding (Campbell, 1963a,b, 1965; Anderson and Le Riche, 1970). This exercise was repeated with respect to the continued increase among men from 1950 to 1962 (Record and Whitfield, 1964). The increase in coronary heart disease mortality was greater than the decrease in other heart disease categories in every age-group from 30 to 64. Additionally, the decline in all cause mortality rates levelled off between 1920 and 1940, despite a continuing decline in causes of death other than IHD (Morris, 1960; Davey Smith and Marmot, 1991). The rise in IHD mortality was also seen in all age-groups (Ryle and Russell, 1949). Though it is likely there was some transfer between categories, the rise in IHD mortality far outstripped the decline in mortality from valvular and other heart diseases (Ryle and Russell, 1949). Similarly, it is also unlikely that the decline in mortality seen from the 1970s was due to changing diagnostic fashion or coding practice as all cause and total circulatory mortality also declined (see Figures 18.2 and 18.3). Autopsy rates for deaths finally certified as IHD may influence the figures (Stehbens, 1987a, b), and have changed considerably, rising steadily from around 22 per cent of deaths in 1959 to around 43 per cent in 1979, but since then have remained relatively constant (see Chapter 2, Figure 2.2), so this cannot explain any changes since the late 1970s.

Thus the changes in mortality appear to be real, but are these due to changing incidence of IHD or changing case fatality? The increase in mortality in the 1920s is likely to be explained by increasing incidence, if only because clinical literature indicates that the classical clinical presentations of IHD were uncommon at the beginning of the twentieth century (Fye, 1985; Acierno, 1994). There is more debate over the decline in IHD mortality occurring in the late 1970s, which has been attributed to both declining incidence and to declining case fatality (possibly due to less severe disease or better treatment of IHD). Inadequate data exist from the United Kingdom to distinguish between trends in incidence and mortality. However, detailed studies from the US suggest that declines in IHD mortality have been much greater than declines in incidence (Sytkowski et al., 1996; McGovern et al., 1996). In the Framingham Study, incidence and mortality were compared for cohorts aged 50–59 in 1950, 1960 and 1970. For women, IHD mortality declined by 51 per cent while incidence declined by only 20 per cent. For men the contrast was even more stark: a 44 per cent decline in mortality compared with a 2 per cent decline in incidence (Sytkowski et al., 1996). Among women stroke incidence declined more than stroke mortality, but for men the reverse was true. On the basis of their analyses the authors could not determine whether the 20-year decline in cardiovascular disease incidence among men was so small because of increased detection, a delay and compression of morbidity, or a real small reduction in disease, but the analyses did indicate that among men and women mortality was not delayed or shifted to other causes. Recent trends from 1985 to 1990 in the Minneapolis-St Paul metropolitan area reveal similarly greater declines in mortality than incidence rates for IHD (McGovern et al., 1996).

18.4.2 Improvements in treatment

Reduced incidence may be the result of reductions in risk factors, in which primary prevention has a part to play. Medical interventions can influence incidence, presentation and case fatality rates (Kaplan et al., 1988). Improvements in treatment, management and care of IHD may decrease case fatality and increase survival, leading to a decline in mortality even without a real change in incidence. However, it is unlikely that a large proportion of the observed decline in mortality from the late 1970s can be attributed to improvements in treatment. Some 25 per cent of attacks lead to death before the arrival of a doctor, accounting for 60 per cent of all deaths. Comparisons of mortality and incidence in different communities and over time have shown that case fatality overall has changed little in males aged 35–44 (Traven et al., 1995). Beaglehole (1986) concluded that the majority of the IHD decline in Auckland up to the early 1980s was attributable to factors other than medical intervention. However, the recent introduction of thrombolysis and aspirin post-myocardial infarction would be expected to lead to decreases in case fatality. Their usage is now widespread enough to influence overall population mortality rates – in 1993–94 some 49 per cent of hospital patients in the United Kingdom received thrombolytic drugs (European Secondary Prevention Study Group, 1996). The effect of treatment is demonstrated in recent data from the Minneapolis Heart Survey of 25–74-year-olds covering the period 1985–92 (McGovern et al., 1996). This showed that hospital mortality declined by 41 per cent between 1985 and 1990, while out-of-hospital mortality declined by 17 per cent. Survival of hospitalised patients increased substantially. After adjustment for age and previous myocardial infarction the relative risk of dying within 3 years of hospitalisation (for the 1990 cohort as compared with the 1985 cohort) was 0.76 for men and 0.84 for women.

18.4.3 Lifestyle

There is little argument that modifiable lifestyle factors, such as diet, cigarette smoking and physical activity have considerable influences on IHD in individuals and populations. These conclusions are based on data from laboratory and prospective population studies and clinical trials. The question is how far these can satisfactorily explain the mortality trends observed.

Diet
Morris (1951) suggested that the rise in IHD up to 1950 was unlikely to be explained by increasing atheroma, as necropsy

studies indicated that the prevalence of atheroma did not change substantially between 1908–13 and 1944–49. He postulated that additional factors were required to precipitate the acute event, possibly through increasing the tendency towards thrombosis. Meta-analyses of recent cohort and clinical trial data have shown that there is a strong relationship between serum cholesterol and IHD – a difference in plasma cholesterol of 0.6 mmol/l (10 per cent) lowers the risk of IHD by 50 per cent at age 40, falling to 20 per cent at age 70 (Law *et al.*, 1994a). Randomised controlled trial evidence shows that the effects of lowering cholesterol can be seen well within 5 years (Law *et al.*, 1994b). Indeed angiographic regression trials have shown a very rapid reduction in event rates following cholesterol lowering (Brown *et al.*, 1993), suggesting that cholesterol lowering also affects processes related to acute events other than atheroma.

The dietary factor most strongly implicated in IHD from laboratory and epidemiological studies has been high saturated fat intake. Low intake of nutrients found most commonly in plant foods, such as vitamin E, vitamin C, carotenoids and flavonoids, or low intake of nutrients affecting haemostasis (clotting), such as alpha-linolenic acid and omega-3 fatty acids, may also be important. Intervention studies indicate that dietary factors may influence both atherogenesis and thrombosis. Most studies would suggest that dietary changes tend to have more or less concurrent effects on several IHD risk factors.

Though few data are available on dietary intake early this century there is evidence that fat intake has increased since the nineteenth century (see Table 7.5 and Figures 7.7 and 7.13 of Chapter 7) up to the 1970s, and that the ratio of polyunsaturated to saturated fats (P/S ratio) has increased since the 1970s. Total fat intake as a proportion of total energy intake has altered little since the 1970s, but energy intake has declined (MAFF, 1993). A recent meta-analysis of data from all published surveys undertaken in the United Kingdom and US between 1900 and 1985 (97 UK surveys) showed that fat represented 30 per cent or less of dietary energy until the 1930s, when it began to rise – see Table 18.6 (Stephen and Sieber, 1994). National per capita consumption of saturated fats, particularly of butter and lard, declined after 1970 (see Figure 7.7).

The ratio of polyunsaturated fats to saturated fats has increased considerably since the 1970s. In the USA consumption of saturated fats and eggs fell about a decade before the fall in Britain, as did their fall in IHD (Friend *et al.*, 1979). These trends seem to mirror the trends in IHD in both countries. The rise in saturated fats was curtailed by rationing during and after the Second World War, after which the rise continued. It reached a plateau of about 40 per cent in the late 1950s, and has since declined, most sharply since the 1970s (see Figure 7.13). This may have contributed towards the observed rise in IHD mortality and its subsequent decline from the late 1970s. Heller *et al.* (1983) observed that the decline in IHD in the late1970s in the United Kingdom was preceded 5 years earlier by a decline in saturated fat intake and suggested this could be the explanation.

As most dietary influences tend to affect the whole of a community this theory would be consistent with the patterns observed, where overall changes are seen in all age-groups and in men and women. Heller *et al.* also examined regional variations and suggested these were compatible with differential changes in fat intake. Table 18.7 shows regional variations in diet for 1970–93, and also some national trends, all taken from the National Food Survey (MAFF, 1990, 1993). While all regions have reduced egg consumption and increased fruit consumption there remain variations, with the highest fruit consumption in the South East and East Anglia and the lowest in the North, Scotland and North West. The differences between regions are not substantial, and unlikely to explain fully the geographic variations. The ONS survey of adult diets (Gregory *et al.*, 1990) similarly found only small differences between regions. There are also three to fourfold variations in IHD and stroke mortality in 1990–94 among men and women aged 35–74, when analysed by county district of England and Wales. Figures 18.7 and 18.8 show the variation for 1990–94. An analysis of fat intake using the National Food Survey and data for the two years 1974 and 1981 did not find significant differences in trends by social class (Morgan *et al.*, 1989). This contrasts with survey data from 1902 which showed marked contrasts between social classes, with almost threefold differences between upper and working class consumption of butter and meat (see Table 7.10 of Chapter 7). Data in Chapter 7 shows that in the 1950s the higher income group had the highest fat and egg consumption, but by 1993 it had the lowest (see Figures 7.3 and 7.4). This reversal of eating habits, although by income group and not social class, is consistent with the possible reversal of social class differences for IHD mortality and the more recent widening mortality gap found by Harding (1995).

Numerous other investigators have examined trends in IHD internationally. Epstein (1989), in an extensive review of the relationship of lifestyle to international trends in IHD, concluded that marked declines or increases in mortality were correlated respectively with reductions or increases in the intake of animal fats. Saturated fat intake is believed to have an effect largely through blood lipids. British data are limited, but national surveys have been conducted in 1986/7 and 1991–93 (OPCS, 1990, 1995b). Over this limited period there has been little evidence of change in average lipid levels in the English population. In the USA data from the National Health and Nutrition Examination Surveys showed that between 1960 and 1980 age-adjusted mean serum cholesterol levels decreased by 3 to 4 per cent (NCHS, 1987). The secular trend continued between 1980 and 1987, which was attributed to changes in lifestyle, such as diet and exercise, and to a lesser extent to more aggressive intervention with lipid lowering drugs by clinicians (Burke *et al.*, 1991). Cox *et al.* (1995) have shown in a double crossover trial that alterations in diet can alter blood cholesterol consistently in about two thirds of people. Thus dietary interventions aimed at susceptible individuals as well as populations have the potential to reduce IHD mortality.

It has been suggested that high intake of dietary antioxidant nutrients, such as carotenoids, flavonoids and vitamin C,

Table 18.7

Food consumption per person per week – regional comparison

	Eggs (no. per week)			Fruit (oz per week)			Vitamin C (mg)	Potassium (g)	Saturated fatty acids (g)	% Energy from fat (%)
	1970	1990	1993	1970	1990	1993	1993	1993	1993	1993
England	4.7	2.2	1.9	24.8	32.2	33.9	53	2.55	32.9	41.2
Scotland	4.8	2.6	2.0	21.8	29.0	28.2	44	2.31	32.1	42.3
Wales	4.6	2.1	1.9	26.8	26.8	29.0	47	2.43	31.5	40.5
North	5.5	2.9	2.0	21.4	29.3	25.4	46	2.48	32.6	41.3
Yorkshire/Humberside	4.6	2.4	2.1	22.7	30.3	30.4	49	2.5	33.7	41.3
North West	4.2	2.3	1.9	21.8	25.6	28.8	49	2.54	32.4	40.3
West Midlands	4.3	1.9	2.0	25.6	24.2	32.7	50	2.52	33.5	41.7
East Midlands	4.9	2.2	1.8	26.2	31.0	29.4	49	2.55	32.5	40.9
SouthEast&East Anglia	4.5	2.0	1.8	30.0	37.7	39.1	58	2.58	32.7	41.2
South West	5.0	2.3	1.9	26.2	33.6	33.6	53	2.61	33.4	41.9

Nutritional value of household foods, national (GB) averages 1959-1993

	Energy (Kcal)	Fatty acids			% Energy from fat (%)
		Saturated (g)	Mono-unsaturated (g)	Poly-unsaturated (g)	
1959	2,620	53.0	43.0	9.2	38.8
1969	2,570	56.7	46.5	11.0	42.0
1972	2,430	52.0	42.9	11.5	41.5
1975	2,290	51.7	39.8	10.1	42.2
1980	2,230	46.8	39.6	11.3	42.6
1985	2,020	40.6	34.7	13.1	42.6
1990	1,872	34.6	31.8	13.9	41.6
1991	1,840	33.7	31.5	13.8	41.4
1992	1,860	33.6	31.8	14.4	41.7
1993	1,830	32.7	31.0	14.1	41.3

Source: National Food Survey Committee (1990); Household Food Consumption and Expenditure 1990; National Food Survey 1993

found mainly in fresh fruit and vegetables, is protective for cardiovascular disease. Trials of carotene have, however, shown very inauspicious results (Rapola *et al.*, 1996; Greenberg *et al.*, 1996). There was no reduction in total mortality in a trial of vitamin E and carotene in male smokers (Alpha-Tocopherol Beta Carotene Cancer Prevention Study Group, 1994). The CHAOS study found that vitamin E reduced non-fatal MIs but, if anything, increased fatal MIs (Stephens *et al.*, 1996). The epidemiological associations that have been observed in prospective studies (Meydani, 1995) may be confounded by other 'lifestyle' and environmental factors (Davey Smith and Ben Shlomo, 1996). Cohort studies of elderly people have suggested that in people aged 65–74 vitamin C is protective against stroke (Gale *et al.*, 1995) and lowers fibrinogen levels, possibly partly through the response to infection (Khaw and Woodhouse, 1995). There is experimental evidence that a large dose of vitamin C increases

fibrinolytic activity (Bordia, 1980). However, until controlled trials have been conducted the results need to be treated with caution. Estimates of population intakes of dietary antioxidants over this century are only available from 1955 onwards, since when fruit intake, especially fruit juice, has increased (see nutrition, Chapter 7). There has been a rise in intake of canned, refrigerated and frozen food, and improved distribution, which may have resulted in an increased intake of these nutrients, which are now also more evenly distributed throughout the year. Many forms of processed foods are currently fortified with vitamins.

Cigarette smoking

The rise in IHD coincided with the increase in cigarette smoking habit, where tar-weighted per capita cigarette consumption among men grew from negligible levels around 1900 to a peak of around 11 kg per person per year during the Second

Figure 18.7

IHD and stroke mortality rate, local authority districts of England and Wales, 1990–94, males aged 35–74

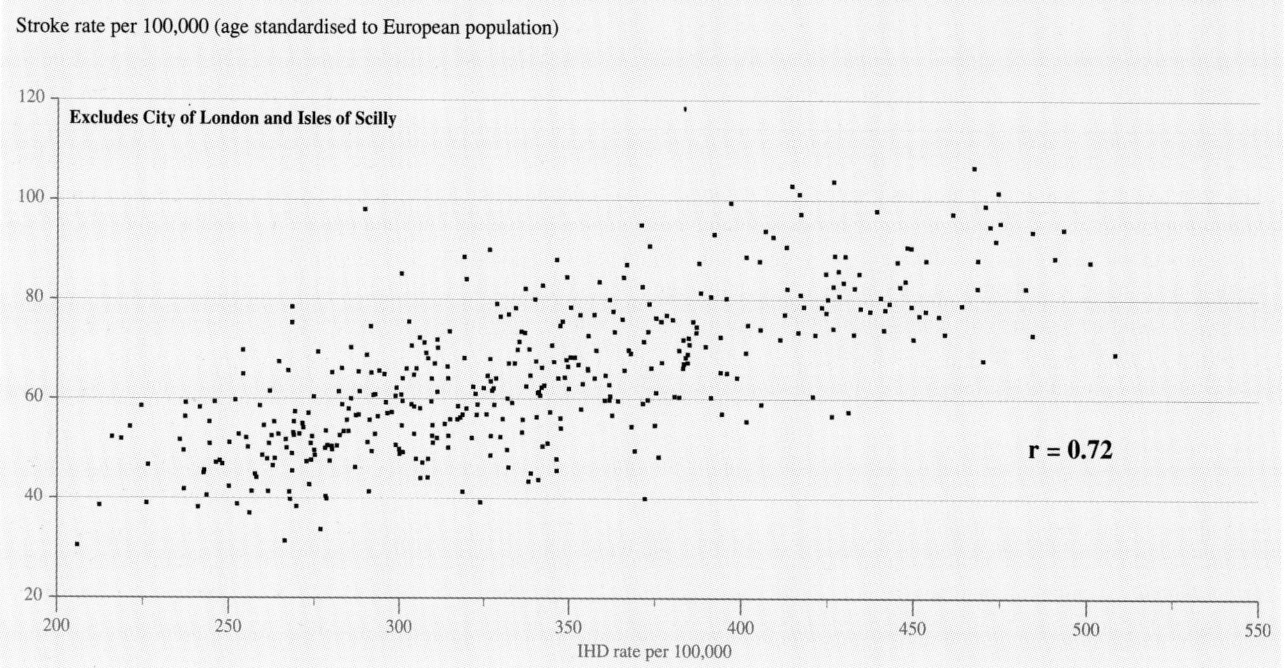

Stroke rate per 100,000 (age standardised to European population)

Figure 18.8

IHD and stoke mortality rate, local authority districts of England and Wales, 1990–94, males and females aged 35–74

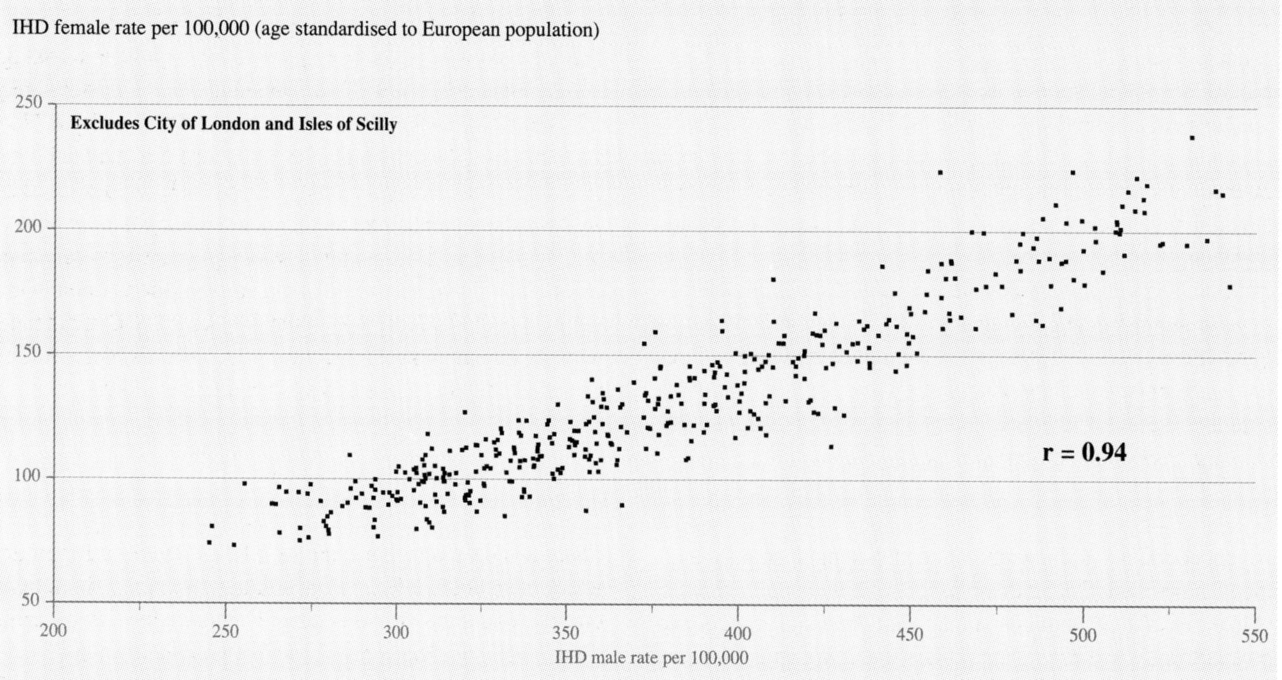

IHD female rate per 100,000 (age standardised to European population)

World War, stabilised until the early 1960s and then declined (see Chapter 9). The decline in consumption was some 10 years later in women, who began smoking some 20 years after men. The number of cigarette smokers has also been falling since the 1970s, when the General Household Survey began collecting such information, from 52 per cent of men in 1972 to 29 per cent in 1992 (41 and 28 per cent for women) (OPCS, 1994). Cigarette smoking is a well demonstrated risk factor for IHD in the presence of other risk factors such as atheroma, and has acute and chronic effects on thrombosis. A lagged effect might be expected between cigarette smoking and the risk of IHD, both in the process of initiating atherosclerosis and thrombosis, and in the process involved in giving up smoking and the slow decline in risk thereafter (Ben-Shlomo *et al.*, 1994). The continuing increase in mortality after 1960 while cigarette consumption was declining could not have been due to cigarette consumption alone, because consumption was declining. The Health Education Authority estimates that currently 24 per cent of deaths from IHD in men and 11 per cent of the deaths in women are due to smoking (HEA, 1991). At least some of the sex differential in coronary heart disease may be explained by the differing prevalence of cigarette smoking in men and women. However, women did not take up smoking until the 1920s, 20 years after men, and it would be hard to explain why IHD rates rose in women at the same time as men, albeit to a smaller extent. The decline in cigarette consumption may have contributed to the decline in IHD, but cannot be the sole explanation (see also Chapter 9). Despite high prevalence of smoking, Japanese men have low IHD mortality rates (see Figure 18.1). It is likely that these results are due to an interaction between cigarette smoking and other factors such as diet.

Early life influences

'The Barker hypothesis' postulates that intrauterine nutrition and growth profoundly affects IHD risk in later life through early life 'programming' of metabolism. Barker and colleagues related birth weights, placental weight and weight at one year in individuals to subsequent mortality rates from IHD (Barker, 1992). According to this hypothesis the decline in IHD risk might be explained by improved intrauterine nutrition occurring decades earlier. This model would predict strong birth cohort effects related to year of birth. However, the data on mortality trends indicate concurrent changes in rates in all age-groups, which is more easily understandable as a period affect, although there is weaker evidence of a cohort effect, particularly at younger ages (see section 18.3.2). Other influences in early life, such as nutrition in childhood, could have influences on later IHD risk.

Interactions between early life and later life may occur (Leon et al., 1996) and these would lead to no clear predictions regarding the importance of period and cohort effects. For example, if poor nutrition in-utero or in early childhood leads to increased risk of IHD when associated with obesity in adulthood (Frankel et al. 1996), then contradictory trends of decreasing prevalence of poor early-life environments in successive cohorts but increasing levels of obesity could occur, masking associations with the risk factors.

Other factors

Psychosocial stress, for example unemployment and bereavement, have been found to be associated with heart disease (Moser et al., 1986; Jones, 1987), but these are unlikely to provide a satisfactory explanation for the time trends observed for IHD. There is evidence that emotional stress may precipitate cardiac events in people who are predisposed to such events through underlying IHD (Leor et al., 1996; Muller and Verrier, 1996). Socio-economic factors appear to increase risk of cardiovascular disease independently of conventional risk factors, suggesting additional environmental influences on disease risk (Davey Smith et al., 1990). Obesity is another postulated risk factor for IHD, associated with raised blood pressure, raised blood cholesterol and low levels of physical activity. About 44 per cent of men and 32 per cent of women are overweight, and the proportion obese or overweight has been increasing since 1980 (see Chapter 7). A DH report suggests that if half those people taking some moderate activity increased it to moderate activity at least five times a week there would be a 7 per cent reduction in deaths from IHD (DH, 1995). The Health Survey for England did not detect any change in the level of physical activity between 1991 and 1993, with 18 per cent of men and 20 per cent of women not taking part in any activity of a moderate level or above (OPCS, 1995b). There has also been a decrease in work activity, partly as a result of raised unemployment levels in the 1980s and 1990s (see Chapter 6).

There is evidence that for every 5 mm Hg reduction in diastolic blood pressure the risk of IHD is reduced by about 16 per cent (MacMahon et al., 1990; Colins et al., 1990). This could be achieved by drug treatment, weight loss, an increase in physical activity, and a reduction in salt and alcohol intake. Blood pressure levels in the United Kingdom are high, and a Health of the Nation target is to reduce mean systolic blood pressure by at least 5 mm Hg by 2005 from the 1991/92 baseline of 138 mm Hg (DH, 1992). While the mean systolic blood pressure of all adults was lower in 1993 than in 1991/92, the difference was not statistically significant (OPCS, 1995b), but the time period during which nationally representative measurements have been available is short.

It is likely that a number of factors may well interact, rather than the trends being due to single factors. For example, high saturated fat intake and concomitant high prevalent levels of blood lipids may be a pre-condition for IHD, but the effect may be potentiated or precipitated by cigarette smoking. Jackson and Beaglehole (1987) estimated that approximately 30–50 per cent of the overall decline in IHD mortality in New Zealand could be accounted for by changes in serum cholesterol and tobacco consumption. Many risk factors for IHD act over the entire life course. Low birthweight, for example, only leads to high blood pressure and poor insulin resistance among people who become obese in adulthood (Leon et al., 1996). Similar effects may exist for actual IHD incidence, with factors at two different times, at birth and determining the risk of IHD at middle age (Frankel et al., 1996).

18.5 Conclusions

There has been a rise and fall of IHD in Britain this century which resembles a long-term epidemic curve. It is notable that the rise and decline occurred more or less at the same time in all age-groups and in both men and women and the evidence for period effects is much stronger than that for birth cohort effects. There is a striking male excess which diminishes with age. However, the male-female ratio for IHD mortality has remained relatively constant since the 1960s. Though the relative increases and declines were similar in men and women, the magnitude of the changes was substantially greater in men compared to women because of different absolute rates. The relative changes were also similar in all age-groups but the absolute magnitude of changes was greatest in older ages where rates were highest.

While there have been substantial changes in diagnostic and coding practices, it is unlikely that the observed changes can be attributed to such artefacts. The disjunction in time trends between stroke and IHD rates is explained by changing diagnostic or coding practices. Together with the lack of sex differential trends observed for stroke, they suggest differing contributions of the etiologic factors which are responsible for these two conditions, possibly including different dietary factors more related to blood pressure and blood cholesterol. This is considered further in the next section.

The increase in social class differences (Harding, 1995) and the different trends in different countries are broadly compatible with the central model that social environment and lifestyle have been the main driving forces behind the IHD trends. The pattern suggests some environmental factor or factors that had an impact on the whole population, though clearly men appear more susceptible than women as far as IHD is concerned. The best researched candidates are diet (especially saturated fat) and cigarette smoking or an interaction of these.

Determining the reasons for the IHD epidemic in Britain this century may help ensure that present favourable trends continue or are accelerated, and that appropriate intervention strategies may be defined and implemented for those population groups not experiencing a decline or experiencing increasing rates of IHD. An understanding of the factors underlying the trends in IHD in Britain over this century is particularly important in relation to the advice that can be given to newlyindustrialising countries where IHD rates are currently increasing.

PART 2 – Stroke

18.6 Overview

Stroke mortality rates have shown a steady decline in many countries, although in Eastern Europe rates have increased (Zarate, 1994). In the USA, the rate of decline has accelerated during the last century from 0.5 per cent per year in 1900–20 to 4–5 per cent per year since the 1970s (Ostfeld, 1980). In England and Wales mortality rates have been declining throughout the twentieth century (see Figure 18.9).

Data from the ONS historical mortality file from 1901–94 were used for the relevant International Classification of Diseases (ICD) codes for the 1st to the 9th revisions. Trends were examined for all causes of stroke and no attempt was made to distinguish between diagnostic categories. ICD manuals were reviewed for each of the revisions to examine differences in coding rules for stroke. We have chosen to represent cerebrovascular deaths in a way that is broader than the usual definition, including codes that might encompass multi-infarct dementia as well as codes for conditions such as hemiplegia that are largely, but not exclusively, due to stroke. This was to approximate closely the less specific terms coded for in the earlier part of the century. Some of these codes should not have been used for primary death certification, but we have included them if they were. The codes used are shown in Table 18.8. Figure 18.9 shows trends in stroke mortality in 4 age-standardised 10-year-age bands between 35 and 75 years of age, where certification is most accurate. Death rates were

---

Table 18.8

ICD codes used to describe trends in cerebrovascular disease between 1901 and 1992

	ICD 1&2 1901–20	ICD 3 1921–30	ICD 4 1931–39	ICD 5 1940–49	ICD 6 1950–57	ICD 7 1958–67	ICD 8 1968–78	ICD 9 1979– current
Wolfe and Burney (1992)	N/A		82	83	330-334	330-334	430-438	430-438
Campbell (1965)	N/A		82, 97.1	83	330-334	330-334		
Halliday and Anderson (1979)	N/A		82 97.1 97.2		330-334	330-334	430-438	
This chapter (see Appendix A for descriptions)	ICD1: 840, 1060-1070 ICD2: 64a-64e, 65, 66A	74, 83 75a 91b (j)	82 97.1 97.2	83 97	330-334 352	330-334 352	430-438 293.0-293.1 344	430-438 290.4 342 344

Figure 18.9

Trends in cerebrovascular disease* deaths, England and Wales, 1901–94

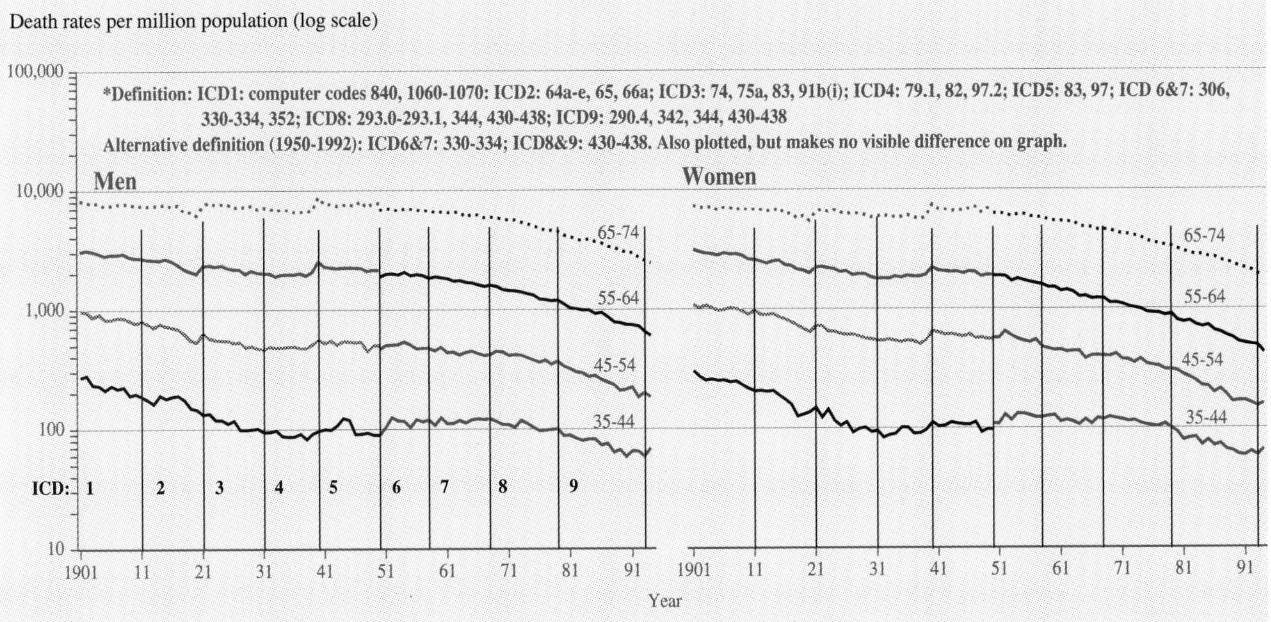
Death rates per million population (log scale)
100,000
10,000
1,000
100
10
*Definition: ICD1: computer codes 840, 1060-1070: ICD2: 64a-e, 65, 66a; ICD3: 74, 75a, 83, 91b(i); ICD4: 79.1, 82, 97.2; ICD5: 83, 97; ICD 6&7: 306, 330-334, 352; ICD8: 293.0-293.1, 344, 430-438; ICD9: 290.4, 342, 344, 430-438
Alternative definition (1950-1992): ICD6&7: 330-334; ICD8&9: 430-438. Also plotted, but makes no visible difference on graph.
Men
Women
65-74
55-64
45-54
35-44
ICD: 1 2 3 4 5 6 7 8 9
1901 11 21 31 41 51 61 71 81 91
Year

Source: OPCS

*Standardised to European population***

also summarised as annual percentage change figures, using regression analysis, for age-groups 15–44, 45–54, 55–64, 65–74 and three time periods, corresponding to the early fall (1901–39), plateau phase (1940–67) and the later fall (1968–91) observed in Figure 18.9 (see Table 18.10). Two alternative definitions of stroke were used from 1950 onwards, but the additional codes have almost no impact on the trends compared with the more usual definition (430-438 for ICD8 and 9) – the number of additional deaths introduced by the wider definition is negligible .

18.7 Age-and sex-specific trends for stroke

Table 18.9 shows the figures at 10-year intervals. A steady decline occurred at all ages and for both men and women from 1901 to 1936–39 (see Figure 18.9). The Second World War and the introduction of the 5th ICD revision in 1940 were associated with an increase in death rates, especially in ages 35–44. Rates continued to decline at a slower rate at younger ages compared with before the introduction of the 5th revision, although from a higher base line. This decline continued at a faster rate at all ages and both sexes, from the 1970s through to 1994, apart from age-group 35–44, where the decline may have ceased.

Table 18.10 shows percentage changes obtained from linear regressions on age and sex for three time periods consistent with ICD revisions and determined by observing changes in the trends: 1901–39, 1940–67 and 1968–91. During the first time period, the rates of decline were greatest at younger ages for both men and women. In the middle time period, the rates of decline are smaller in middle-age and show increases at younger ages. During the most recent period, the rates of decline are similar to 1901–39 for ages 15–44, but greater for ages 45–74 and for women.

18.8 Artefact or real effect?

Stroke mortality has declined throughout the twentieth century. Previous reports of the secular changes in cerebrovascular diseases have focused on changes over much more recent and shorter time periods (Bonita *et al.*, 1990), which has resulted in only a partial view, and a focus on the declining trend since the 1960s to 1970s. The decline in stroke mortality slowed just after the second world war and accelerated again after 1978. In interpreting these trends it is important to ask whether they could be due to:

a) changes in coding practices associated with ICD revisions
b) changes in diagnostic fashion
c) changes in diagnostic technology leading to greater accuracy
d) real effects of reductions in risk of death due to lower case-fatality or falling incidence

18.8.1 Coding changes

The pattern of decline in stroke in both men and women suggest that changes in ONS coding with the introduction of the

Table 18.9

Stroke mortality rates 1901–94, England and Wales
Age-standardised rates per million

ICD1: computer codes 840, 1060-1070; ICD2 64a-64e, 65, 66A; ICD3: 74, 75a, 83, 91b(i); ICD4: 79.1, 82,97.2; ICD5: 83,97; ICD6&7: 330-334; ICD8&9: 430-438

Year	Males 35–44	45–54	55–64	65–74	Females 35–44	45–54	55–64	65–74	Ratio M:F death rates 35–44	45–54	55–64	65–74
1901	275	991	3,061	8,215	307	1,094	3,136	7,360	0.9	0.9	1.0	1.1
1911	191	815	2,696	7,468	207	982	2,584	6,800	0.9	0.8	1.0	1.1
1921	134	646	2,324	7,427	151	728	2,202	6,419	0.9	0.9	1.1	1.2
1931	96	473	2,014	7,152	96	550	1,778	5,888	1.0	0.9	1.1	1.2
1941	101	534	2,292	7,743	104	641	2,076	6,762	1.0	0.8	1.1	1.1
1951	105	511	2,038	7,249	110	577	1,922	6,386	1.0	0.9	1.1	1.1
1961	113	442	1,866	6,638	114	455	1,437	5,512	1.0	1.0	1.3	1.2
1971	111	418	1,482	5,732	119	380	1,117	4,294	0.9	1.1	1.3	1.3
1981	90	323	1,054	4,163	80	282	789	3,077	1.1	1.1	1.3	1.4
1991	66	226	762	3,056	60	170	522	2,220	1.1	1.3	1.5	1.4
1994	70	188	620	2498	67	162	435	1,903	1.0	1.2	1.4	1.3

Alternative definition:
ICD6&7: 306, 330-334, 352; ICD8: 293.0-293.1, 344, 430-438; ICD9: 290.4, 342, 344, 430-438

Year	Males 35–44	45–54	55–64	65–74	Females 35–44	45–54	55–64	65–74
1951	105	513	2,054	7,304	110	581	1,935	6,441
1961	113	443	1,882	6,694	114	456	1,446	5,559
1971	111	419	1,500	5,820	119	382	1,127	4,347
1981	90	326	1,069	4,263	80	284	797	3,148
1991	67	229	764	3,192	60	173	525	2,303
1994	70	188	620	2,498	67	162	435	1,903

Table 18.10

Annual percentage changes in stroke mortality, 1901–91 England and Wales

Age-group	Males 1901–39 (%)	1940–67 (%)	1968–91 (%)	Females 1901–39 (%)	1940–67 (%)	1968–91 (%)
15–44	-2.2	0.6	-2.0	-2.2	1.0	-2.1
45–54	-2.0	-0.5	-2.4	-1.9	-1.3	-2.8
55–64	-1.8	-0.7	-2.4	-1.8	-1.4	-2.5
65–74	-1.5	-0.1	-2.2	-1.4	-0.7	-2.4

5th revision of the ICD (see Chapter 2) had considerable impact, raising the apparent mortality level. In the USA, recoding of deaths to a single revision shows a consistent decline from the turn of the century (Ostfeld, 1980). It is clear from Figure 18.9 that the broader definition makes a negligible difference to the figures compared with the conventional definition. With the introduction of the 8th revision of the ICD in 1967 it was estimated that deaths were 0.4 per cent more likely to be attributed to stroke than in the 7th revision (Haberman *et al.*, 1978). The duplicate coding exercise undertaken when the 9th revision was introduced was associated with a 0.7 per cent reduction in attribution of deaths to stroke and a 1.9 per cent reduction in deaths attributed to myocardial infarction (OPCS, 1983). Thus coding changes, especially the introduction of ICD5, had an impact on stroke mortality levels, but the overall trend was nevertheless downward.

18.8.2 Diagnostic fashion

Changes in diagnostic fashion in stroke have largely affected the use of diagnostic terms within the broad category of cerebrovascular diseases. There was a marked increase in the use of 'acute, ill-defined and unspecified' (ICD 436, 437) following the introduction of the 8th ICD revision and a commensurate reduction in the rates for cerebral haemorrhage (Acheson and Sanderson, 1978; Baum and Goldstein, 1982). Clinico-pathological correlation studies were published in the mid-1960s and demonstrated how poor clinical diagnosis was, which may have moved diagnostic fashion further towards simply recording stroke (or cerebrovascular accident) as the underlying cause of death rather than a more specific diagnosis (Heasman and Lipworth, 1966). However, post-mortem evidence from Manchester hospitals does suggest that the ratio of cerebral haemorrhage to cerebral thrombosis declined over the period 1877–1961 (Yates, 1964). With the advent of modern geriatric medicine and increased investigation of older people, it is likely that more rather than fewer diagnoses of stroke would occur and that deaths in older age-groups would be ascribed to more specific diagnoses. It is, therefore, unlikely that diagnostic fashion has had a major effect on the trends observed.

18.8.3 Diagnostic technology

A major innovation of the twentieth century was the widespread use of the sphygmomanometer, which enabled blood pressure to be recorded, and consequently the importance of hypertension as an underlying cause of brain, heart and kidney damage was realised. Early revisions of the ICD placed great emphasis on coding to the underlying cause, and it is possible that application of this general rule during the century was responsible for the decline in deaths attributed to stroke, because of a tendency to classify deaths of this type to hypertension and heart disease. However, mortality rates from hypertensive disease have also declined during the century making this explanation for the observed trend untenable.

The other major advance in stroke diagnosis was the relatively recent introduction of computerised tomographic (CT) scanning. However, even today, the proportion of stroke patients who are scanned is small in England and Wales, and it is unlikely that the increased diagnostic accuracy associated with scanning will have had even a minor impact on recent trends.

18.8.4 The effect of the Second World War

The introduction of the 5th revision in 1940 increased recorded mortality rates for stroke at all ages for both men and women. The change in coding practice by ONS was to use the underlying cause of death as described by the attendant doctor rather than an arbitrary set of precedence rules. During the Second World War stroke mortality rates increased for men (but not women) aged under age 45, and although these fell imediately after the war, rates for men and women under 45 did not decline subsequently until the 1970s (see Table 18.9, Figure 18.9). The data for the war years relate to the civilian population, and substantial reductions in the healthy population at risk (particularly for men) occurred as a result of conscription. The civilian population would have thus been less healthy on the whole than the total population, and thus may account to some extent for the observed raised mortality levels during the war. Selection effects might be expected to have a stronger impact on men than women and this is supported by the gender differences in younger people. However, health selection due to conscription cannot explain the increased rates among older men and women.

18.8.5 Real effects

Reviewing the overall trend this century it appears that a steady reduction in stroke mortality has occurred but that coding changes have been responsible for major shifts in the baseline in 1940 and in 1979. The greatest declines occurred among ages 45–64, but the trends appear to have affected people of every age-group at the same time, suggesting that cohort effects are likely to be less important, and pointing towards environmental aetiological factors affecting the whole population. It is unlikely that this steady downward trend is an artefact because of its consistency, and because it follows the downward trend in all-cause mortality this century. It is in accord with the pattern described in the USA, although the United Kingdom did not enjoy the same steady decline during the 1940s and 1950s observed in the USA (Ostfeld, 1980).

There is evidence that case-fatality improved over the century making it much less likely that people suffering from a stroke would die from it (Garraway *et al.*, 1983; Tanaka *et al.*, 1981). The reduction in incidence reported by several investigators (Baum and Goldstein, 1982; OPCS, 1983; Tanaka *et al.*, 1981; Ueda *et al.*, 1981) together with reductions in case fatality almost certainly explain the overall downward trend this century. Data from the Royal College of General Practitioners Weekly Returns Service, available from 1976 onwards, shows that stroke incidence has continued to decline (RCGP, 1993). Since the 1970s the decline in stroke mortality has been more rapid, and explanations have been sought in the use of antihypertensive treatment which became available from the 1950s (Klag *et al.*, 1989; Nicholls and

Johansen, 1983; Tuomilehto *et al.*, 1985; Whisnant, 1984), changes in smoking rates (see also Chapter 9) (Bonita *et al.*, 1986), secular changes in blood pressure distributions (Joosens *et al.*, 1979), changes in atmospheric pollution (Knox, 1981) and increases in the amount of anti-oxidant-containing foods eaten (Acheson and Williams, 1983; Khaw and Barrett-Connor, 1987). Reduction in salt intake could also reduce the risk of stroke (Intersalt Research Group, 1988). Average sodium intake in Britain has fallen slightly since it was first measured in 1985 (MAFF, 1993) but is still high. The COMA Report on Nutritional Aspects of Cardiovascular Disease recommended that average population intake of salt should be reduced to 6 g/day (a one third reduction). Average potassium intake is currently some 20 per cent below recommended nutrient intake (RNI), but national trend data are not available.

It has been suggested that maternal and infant health is of major importance in determining risk of cardiovascular disease in later life (Barker, 1992) and that this may explain the declining trend in stroke mortality (Editorial, 1988). If this were an important factor, cohort effects should be prominent, with progressively greater rates of decline in consecutive birth cohorts, but the changes occurred at the same time in all age-groups, suggesting that period effects dominate. Wolfe and Burney (1992) showed that there are both significant period and cohort effects in the trends for stroke mortality, with the period effects being greater. The accelerated decline in mortality since the 1970s may be related to the introduction of treatment for hypertension, and the deceleration in risk for cohorts born between 1870 and 1910 may be due to a reduction in various risk factors for stroke. Wolfe and Burney found evidence that recent younger (45–64) cohorts are showing increased risk of stroke mortality, once period declines are taken into account, which may eventually slow down the long-term decline in mortality (Wolfe and Burney, 1992). They suggested that this could be associated with increased survival of those with IHD or diabetes, increases in heavy use of alcohol, and immigration from the West Indies, where the risk of stroke is high (Balarajan, 1991). These cohort trends are not readily explained by early life influences or 'programming' hypotheses. Figure 18.9 suggests that the downward tend in stroke mortality may now have ceased for ages 35–44.

18.9 Conclusions

Although coding changes have affected the levels of stroke mortality, the downward trend is likely to be real. There is now good evidence that interventions in the form of antihypertensive therapy can reduce the risk of stroke (MacMahon *et al.*, 1990; Collins *et al.*, 1990; Mulrow *et al.*, 1995). A reduction in salt consumption may also reduce population blood pressure (Intersalt Co-operative Research Group, 1988), although evidence from randomised trials suggests only a small effect should be expected (Midgley *et al.,* 1996). Reduction in cigarette smoking and an increase in physical activity, reduction of overweight and obesity, and keeping alcohol consumption below sensible limits would benefit the population (Wannamethee *et al.*, 1995; Wannamethee and Shaper, 1992). If these could be achieved then further declines should be possible. It is most likely that much of the observed decline in stroke since the beginning of this century, as for mortality generally, has been due to a range of improvements including nutrition and non-specific effects of socio-economic development (McKeown *et al.*, 1975). Thus the need to maintain socio-economic development and reduce inequality in the population also deserves attention.

Acknowledgements

The authors are grateful to Gerry Shaper for his helpful comments and suggestions on a previous draft.
The Stroke Association provided funds to support Olia Papacosta who carried out regression analysis of the stroke data provided by ONS.

Appendix 18.1: Descriptions of codes used for cardiovascular diseases 1901–92

Ischaemic heart disease

1921-30: ICD3
90(5)	Fatty heart
90(7)	Other unspecified myocardial disease
91(b)(2)	Arteriosclerosis without record of cardiovascular lesion
89	Angina pectoris

1931-39: ICD4
93a	Acute myocarditis
93b(1)	Fatty heart
93b(2)	Cardio-vascular degeneration
93b(3)	Other myocardial degeneration
93c	Myocarditis, not returned as acute or chronic
94	Diseases of the coronary arteries, Angina pectoris
97(3)	Arterio-sclerosis without record of cerebral lesion

1940-49: ICD5
93a	Acute myocarditis
93b	Chronic myocarditis specified as rheumatic
93c(1)	Cardio-vascular degeneration
93c(2)	Myocardial degeneration described as fatty
93c(3)	Other myocardial degeneration
93d	Myocarditis not distinguished as acute or chronic
94a	Diseases of the coronary arteries
94b	Angina pectoris without mention of coronary disease

1950-57: ICD6
420.0	Arteriosclerotic heart disease, including coronary disease
420.1	Heart disease specified as involving coronary arteries
420.2	Angina pectoris without mention of coronary disease
422.0	Other myocardial degeneration
422.1	With arteriocslerosis
422.2	Other
450	Arterio-sclerosis

1958-67: ICD7
420.0	Arteriosclerotic heart disease, including coronary disease (as stated)
420.1	- specified as involving coronary arteries
420.2	- Angina pectoris withoput mention of sclerosis or cerebral haemorrhage)
422.0	Other myocardial degeneration - Fatty degeneration
422.1	- With arteriosclerosis
422.2	- Other
450	Arterio-sclerosis

1968-78: ICD8
410	Acute myocardial infarction
411	Other acute and subacute forms of ischaemic heart disease
412	Chronic myocardial infarction
413	Angina pectoris
414	Asymptomatic ischaemic heart disease

1979-92: ICD9
410	Acute myocardial infarction
411	Other acute and subacute forms of ischaemic heart disease
412	Chronic Old myocardial infarction
413	Angina pectoris
414	Other forms of chronic ischaemic heart disease

Cerebrovascular disease

1901-10: ICD1
1070*	Apoplexy, hemiplegia
1060*	Cerebral haemorrhage, cerebral embolism
840*	Softening of brain

1911-20: ICD2
64A	Apoplexy
64B	Serous apoplexy & oedema of brain
64C	Cerebral congestion
64D	Cerebral atheroma
64E	Cerebral haemorrhage
65	Softening of brain
66A	Hemiplegia

1921-30: ICD3
74a(1)	Cerebral haemorrhage so returned
74a(2)	Apoplexy (lesion unstated)
74b(1)	Cerebral embolism
74b(2)	Cerebral thrombosis
75a	Hemiplegia
83	Cerebral softening
91b(1)	Arterio-sclerosis with cerebral vascular lesion

1931-39: ICD4
82a(1)	Cerebral haemorrhage so returned
82a(2)	Apoplexy (lesion unstated)
82b(1)	Cerebral embolism
82b(2)	Cerebral thrombosis
82b(3)	Cerebral softening
82c(1)	Hemiplegia
82c(2)	Other paralysis of unstated origin
97(1)	Arterio-sclerosis, with cerebral haemorrhage
97(2)	Arterio-sclerosis with record of other cerebral vascular lesion

1940-49: ICD5
83a	Cerebral haemorrhage
83bc	Cerebral embolism, thrombosis and softening
97	Arteriosclerosis (ex. coronary or renal disease)

1950-57: ICD6 and 1958-67: ICD7
330	Subarachnoid haemorrhage
331	Cerebral haemorrhage
332	Cerebral embolism and thrombosis
333	Spasm of cerebral arteries
334	Other and ill-defined vascular lesions affecting central nervous system
352	Other cerebral paralysis

1968-78: ICD8
293.0	
293.1	
430-438	Cerebrovascular disease
344	Other cerebral paralysis

1979-92: ICD9
430-438	Cerebrovascular disease
290.4	Arteriosclerotic dementia
342	Hemiplegia
344	Other paralytic syndromes

* No numbering was used for ICD1. The codes given are the computer codes used in the ONS historic deaths database.

Chapter 19

Neurological diseases

By
Robert Swingler and Christopher Martyn

Summary

- Demographic changes in the past 150 years have led to an increase in the numbers of people suffering from chronic neurological disease. Recent estimates suggest that 2 per cent of the population has some persistent neurological disability.

- Since 1920 it has been possible to collect routine mortality data for Parkinson's disease. These data provided an opportunity to re-evaluate previous epidemiological studies.

- Evidence from age-period cohort analysis shows that since 1920 Parkinson's disease has declined by about two thirds in the younger age-groups while increasing fivefold in those over 80.

- L-dopa became available for the treatment of the symptoms of Parkinson's disease in the late 1960s. Although the drug has improved the quality of life for sufferers there is little evidence that it has had any effect on mortality.

- Surveys of incidence show that rates of motor neurone disease are increasing. Mortality rates from motor neurone disease in England and Wales have doubled over the past 30 years.

- Only limited inferences can be made about trends in mortality rates from dementia over time. This is due to variations in diagnostic terminology and recording issues. The results of longitudinal studies of ageing and cognitive impairment are awaited.

- The incidence of epilepsy is falling in Britain today. The decrease is greatest in younger age-groups. Rising life expectancy has been associated with an increase in new cases among elderly people.

- Evidence for the genetic aetiology of multiple sclerosis is presented in ecological studies, case-control studies and linkage studies. Epidemiological studies provide evidence that environmental factors are also important in determining the prevalence of the disease.

19.1 Introduction

One of the consequences of the demographic changes of the last 150 years is an increase in the numbers of people suffering from chronic neurological illnesses. The continuing improvement in life expectancy has meant that a greater proportion of the population survive to an age when the risk of neurodegenerative conditions is high. It is now estimated that 2 per cent of the general population have some persistent neurological disability (Wade and Langton-Hewer, 1987). Each year 9.5 per cent of the United Kingdom population consult a general practitioner about neurological symptoms (Hopkins, 1989). Many neurological conditions require inpatient care and, even when psychiatric disorders are excluded, diseases of the nervous system account for 1 in 5 admissions to hospital (Morrow and Patterson, 1987).

Whether changes in the incidence of diseases of the nervous system have also contributed to the increase in numbers of patients is less clear. The incidence of even the most prevalent chronic neurological illnesses is low and to derive an estimate that is precise enough to be worthwhile, large populations must be studied over a considerable period. Very few such studies have been carried out.

In this chapter, we have attempted to describe the current state of five neurological conditions that cause high levels of disability and place great demands on health service resources. Mortality data for England and Wales supplied by ONS have been used to explore how the frequency of occurrence of some of these diseases has changed over time. Three of these diseases, Parkinson's disease, Alzheimer's disease and motor neurone disease, affect older people and are becoming increasingly important. The other two, multiple sclerosis and epilepsy, are responsible for a considerable amount of morbidity in young people. Stroke, cerebral neoplasms and infections of the nervous system are covered in other chapters.

19.2 Parkinson's disease

The first comprehensive description of Parkinson's disease in western medical literature appeared in 1817 with the publication of James Parkinson's celebrated *Essay on the shaking palsy*. We do not know whether the disease was a recent occurrence at the beginning of the nineteenth century or whether Parkinson was simply the first person to have realised that its signs and symptoms represented a distinct neurological condition. The nineteenth century was a period of rapid progress in physiology and neurology and many diseases of the nervous system were being delineated for the first time in a way that a modern physician can recognise. Descriptions of patients with a syndrome similar to that of Parkinson's disease are said to exist in ancient Chinese medical writings, although no English translation of these documents has been published, and it may be that Parkinson described a disease that had been in existence for many hundreds of years. On the other hand, except in the earliest stages of the disease, the features of Parkinson's disease are usually so striking that the only problem in diagnosis is distinguishing idiopathic Parkinson's disease from rarer causes of a parkinsonian syndrome. It cannot be ruled out that the disease that now bears Parkinson's name arose for the first time in Europe around the beginning of the nineteenth century.

19.2.1 Aetiology

The causes of Parkinson's disease are poorly understood. Carbon monoxide intoxication, chronic manganese poisoning and exposure to phenothiazine drugs are known to produce symptoms and signs that resemble those of idiopathic Parkinson's disease and a parkinsonian syndrome may also occur following an encephalitic illness. A large number of people developed such a syndrome in the years following the epidemics of von Economo's disease (encephalitis lethargica) which swept the world between 1918 and 1926. More recently, a clinical syndrome indistinguishable from Parkinson's disease has been described in a small number of people who injected themselves parenterally with a synthetic opiate that had been inadvertently contaminated with 1-methyl-4-phenyl-1,2,3,6-tetrahydropyridine (MPTP). This observation led to the development of an animal model of Parkinson's disease and stimulated a search for chemical analogues of MPTP that might be present in the environment.

Despite several large case-control studies, no strong environmental risk factors for Parkinson's disease have been identified. Positive associations of the disease with rural residence, drinking water from wells, and exposure to herbicides and pesticides have been reported, but the associated relative risks were small and the findings of different studies have not always been consistent (Tanner, 1992). Nor has the search for powerful genetic determinants of the disease yet been successful. The prevalence of the condition in first-degree relatives of cases is not significantly different from controls (Duvoisin *et al.*, 1969) and concordance rates in mono- and dizygotic twins are similar (Ward *et al.*, 1983). Although the CYP2D6 allele associated with slow metabolism of desbrisoquine is over-represented in patients with Parkinson's disease, its prevalence is low and the proportion of cases that can be attributed to this polymorphism is small (Armstrong *et al.*, 1992).

There is a long-running and still unresolved argument about whether the differences between idiopathic Parkinson's disease and other parkinsonian syndromes are qualitative or quantitative. Poskanzer and Schwab (1963) reported the results of an analysis of cases of a parkinsonian syndrome seen at the Massachusetts General Hospital between 1875 and 1961. All but 24 cases had been seen after 1918. Between the group of cases with onset of disease in the period 1920–24 and the group with onset in the period 1955–59, a gap of 35 years, the mean age of cases had risen by 27 years. To explain this increase in the age of patients at the time of the onset of symptoms, they suggested that parkinsonism was a disease largely restricted to the cohort of people aged between 5 and 59 years in 1920 and postulated that both idiopathic Parkinson's disease and post-encephalitic parkinsonism were the result of a single aetiology related to an event that occurred about that time. They thought that the most likely candidate for this event was the pandemic of encephalitis lethargica. Because only 11 per cent of their cases gave a history of encephalitis, Poskanzer and Schwab conjectured that, while a severe, clinically apparent episode of encephalitis would be followed by a rapidly developing parkinsonian syndrome, milder, subclinical and undiagnosed attacks of the same infection might lead to parkinsonian symptoms only after an interval of many years. In their paper they pointed out that this hypothesis had been constructed to fit their data and emphasised the need for it to be tested in studies of other populations. Some support came from a later study in England (Brown and Knox, 1972) that investigated 76 cases of parkinsonism seen at neurological out-patient departments in Birmingham between 1953 and 1963. Once again, the age at onset of symptoms in these cases increased over time. This result reproduced Poskanzer and Schwab's data from Massachusetts in a strikingly close way (see Table 19.1).

The cohort hypothesis of the aetiology of idiopathic Parkinson's disease has never been widely accepted among clinical neurologists. One reason is that the hypothesis does not adequately explain the existence of Parkinson's disease before 1918 or cases of the disease in people born after the epidemic of encephalitis lethargica subsided in 1926. Another objection is derived from the view that post-encephalitic parkinsonism and idiopathic Parkinson's disease are different entities and can be distinguished clinically by their different signs and symptoms and histologically by their different pathological features. It has been pointed out that the rise in the mean age of cases observed in Massachusetts and Birmingham can be explained if post-encephalitic parkinsonism is associated with a younger age at onset than idiopathic Parkinson's disease and if the relative frequencies of the two diseases has changed with time. Another possibility is that improvement in access to medical care has led to more complete ascertainment of elderly cases and that this has tended to increase the mean age of cases.

The time trends of Parkinson's disease are therefore potentially extremely interesting. No new information is available that casts any light on the matter of whether the disease occurred for the first time in the nineteenth century but, since the 3rd revision of the International Classification of Diseases (ICD), mortality data for Parkinson's disease (paralysis agitans) as a separate entity have been collected routinely. These data provide an opportunity to re-evaluate the cohort hypothesis.

19.2.2 Time trends in mortality from Parkinson's disease

The results described here are all derived from analysis of mortality data on Parkinson's disease for England and Wales made available by ONS. Using data from the beginning of the 3rd revision of the International Classification of Diseases (ICD3 code 84.4, 4th and ICD5 code 87c, ICD6, ICD7 code 350, ICD8 code 342, and ICD9 code 332.0), we calculated age- and sex-specific mortality rates by 5-year age-groups for each year from 1921 to 1992 using the corresponding mid-year population estimates. We then used an age-period-cohort analytical approach to examine the trends in mortality over time.

Age-period-cohort analysis, which is described in the chapter on methods at the beginning of this book, and in detail elsewhere (Osmond and Gardner, 1982), is a statistical technique that attempts to dissect the trends in mortality data into the three components described in the previous paragraph — the separate effects of age at death, period of death and cohort of birth. Its purpose is to provide a more profound insight into the influences that determine changes over time than could be gained by a simple inspection of age-specific death rates. Diseases in which long intervals elapse between exposure to the cause of the disease and death from that disease tend to show changes between successive generations. Such changes are known as birth cohort effects. Diseases whose causes operate with a shorter latency are likely to affect all age-groups more synchronously, even if different age-groups are affected to a different extent, and reveal themselves as period of death effects. Table 19.2 is a summary of mortality from Parkinson's disease in England and Wales for the period 1959–92. Each descending diagonal in the table running from left to right, therefore, refers to the deaths of people born in the same 10-year-period, and describes the experience of mortality from Parkinson's disease of a particular birth cohort.

In the age-period-cohort analyses, we have used mortality data from 1959 onwards only because, before then, data for people older than 80 years were aggregated. Fewer than 1 per cent of deaths from Parkinson's disease occurred in people under the age of 55 years and they have been excluded from the analysis. One limitation of these data is that numbers of deaths were only available after grouping into 5-year age categories. A corollary is that the age-specific death rates in the individual cells in Table 19.2 are derived from deaths that occurred in people whose year of birth is distributed over a

---

Table 19.1

Mean age of cases of parkinsonism in 1920 according to date of onset of symptoms

Date of onset of parkinsonism symptoms	England		Massachusetts,USA	
	No. of cases	Mean age in 1920	No. of cases	Mean age in 1920
1940–44	1	23.5	149	26.5
1945–49	3	28.5	278	24.5
1950–54	28	22.2	331	24.8
1955–59	38	22.2	226	21.9
1960–64	6	21.7	13	14.8
Total	79	22.4	997	24.2

Table 19.2

Mortality (per million person-years) from Parkinson's disease by age according to quinquennuim of death for men and women combined in England and Wales

Period of death	Age of death						
	55–59	60–64	65–69	70–74	75–79	80–84	85+
1959–63	21.6	50.5	129.2	241.0	378.1	441.9	394.1
1964–68	16.8	39.5	108.0	215.5	356.1	427.8	419.3
1969–73	13.1	35.2	96.1	194.9	359.6	453.9	473.9
1974–78	10.5	27.8	72.8	165.8	290.8	416.0	464.1
1979–83	7.9	23.6	61.1	170.0	326.5	481.0	574.4
1984–88	6.8	27.5	91.3	264.7	590.4	1,047.4	1,470.1
1989–92	7.0	21.5	82.4	229.5	557.1	1,030.6	1,510.2

10-year period. This lack of precision might blur or obscure any birth cohort effect. To overcome this potential difficulty, we obtained data that classified deaths occurring during the period 1959–92 by individual year of birth rather than by 5-year age-group at death. Unfortunately, age-specific death rates cannot readily be calculated from these data. We, therefore, adopted a proportional mortality approach in this analysis, calculating not a mortality rate but the proportion of all deaths that were due to Parkinson's disease. Information on year of birth was missing for a small number of people who died in the first quarter of 1969 and they were omitted from the analysis. As in the previous age-period-cohort model, we excluded deaths from Parkinson's disease in people under the age of 55 years (0.8 per cent). We also excluded deaths in people over the age of 95 years (0.6 percent). The analysis was based on 76,976 deaths from Parkinson's disease in people whose year of birth was known.

19.2.3 Age-specific mortality

Age-specific death rates, plotted on a logarithmic scale, for Parkinson's disease for men and women over the period 1921–92 are shown in Figure 19.1. The trends are different at different ages. In all age-groups under 75 years, there has been a steady decline in mortality in recent decades. The point at which the decline starts is not sharply defined but, from around 1930, there has been a consistently falling rate. In the age groups 75–79 years and 80 years and older, mortality has tended to increase. Rates are slightly lower in women than in men, but the changes over time are similar in both sexes. The diverging trends in mortality from Parkinson's disease at different ages are worth emphasizing. In 1929, rates of death from this disease in people aged 80 years and over were 11 times higher than in people aged 55–59 years. By 1992 this differential had increased to 175-fold.

Two inflexions can be seen in all the curves. The first is the sudden decrease in mortality that occurred in 1940, which can be attributed to the adoption of ICD9 and the abandoning of the convention under which chronic conditions, such as Parkinson's disease, were selected as the cause of death when more than one cause was recorded by the doctor certifying death. The second is the abrupt rise in mortality in 1984 that coincided with a policy change in the application of WHO rule 3. This rule concerns the selection of the underlying cause of death from the conditions listed in parts 1 and 2 of the death certificate. The change affected how the underlying

Figure 19.1

Parkinson's disease in England and Wales, 1921–92

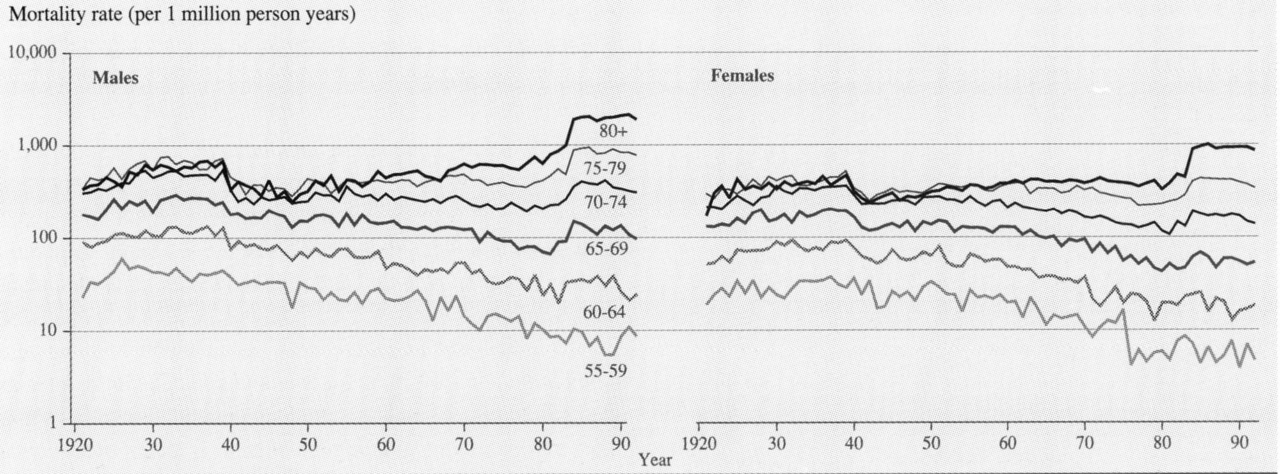

cause of death was determined from death certificates where the proximate cause of death had been recorded as broncho-pneumonia, pulmonary embolism, cardiac arrest or a number of other events that might have been no more than incidental to the primary pathology. Before 1984, the underlying cause of death in a patient with Parkinson's disease whose terminal event was bronchopneumonia was likely to be coded as bron-chopneumonia even if Parkinson's disease was mentioned under part 2. From 1984 onwards, in such circumstances, the disease mentioned in part 2 was taken as the underlying cause of death.

19.2.4 Age-period-cohort analyses

The results of the age-period-cohort analysis based on death rates are summarised in Figure 19.2. The age effect is shown on the left of the figure. It may be thought of as the equiva-lent of an age-specific death rate that has been adjusted for birth cohort and period-of-death effects. There is a nearly exponential rise in mortality from Parkinson's disease with increasing age in both men and women. Only in the very eld-erly is the rise less than exponential. At all ages mortality for women is slightly less than mortality for men.

Cohort and period effects, plotted on a logarithmic scale, were standardised to have a mean value of one for the data as a whole. Strong trends over time are apparent for both effects. Risk of death from Parkinson's disease increases steeply in successive birth cohorts from 1869–78 to a peak in the co-horts born 1899–1908 and then falls equally sharply. People born in the first decade of the twentieth century are more than twice as likely to die from Parkinson's disease as people born before 1888 or after 1924.

There is also a pronounced period-of-death effect. Independ-ently of the effects of age and birth cohort, likelihood of death from Parkinson's disease fell from 1959 to around 1979. An abrupt increase occurred in 1984 that coincided with the change in the way WHO rule 3 was applied.

The second age-period-cohort analysis was carried out using the data in which deaths from Parkinson's disease were clas-sified by year of birth. These data, as we noted previously, cannot be used to calculate age-specific mortality rates and the results shown in Figure 19.3 refer to proportional mortal-ity. Because of the rising numbers of deaths from competing causes of mortality as age increases, the age effect in this proportional mortality model is not exponential. The birth cohort and period of death effects are estimated for each year separately and the trends are less smooth than in the analysis based on age-specific rates in which the data were aggre-gated over 5-year periods. The estimates at the beginning and end of the curves that describe the cohort effect are derived from small numbers of deaths and are unstable. Overall, how-ever, the trends for both birth cohort, and period-of-death effects are very similar to those obtained in the previous analy-sis and confirm that a cohort of people born around 1905 experienced the greatest risk of death from Parkinson's dis-ease.

Figure 19.2a

Parkinson's disease in England and Wales: age effect

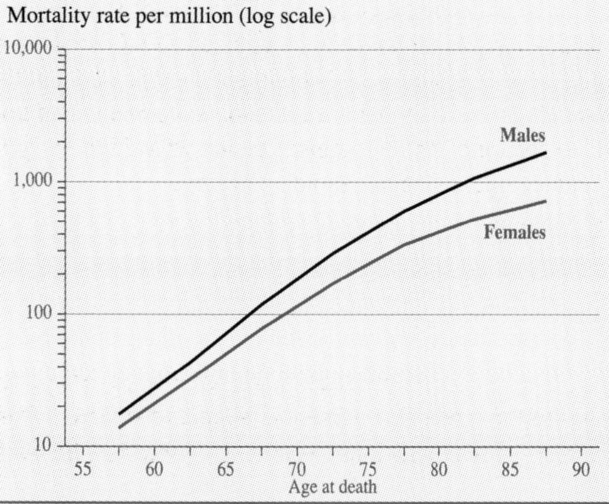

Mortality rate per million (log scale)

Figure 19.2b

Parkinson's disease in England and Wales: cohort and period effects

Mortality rate per million

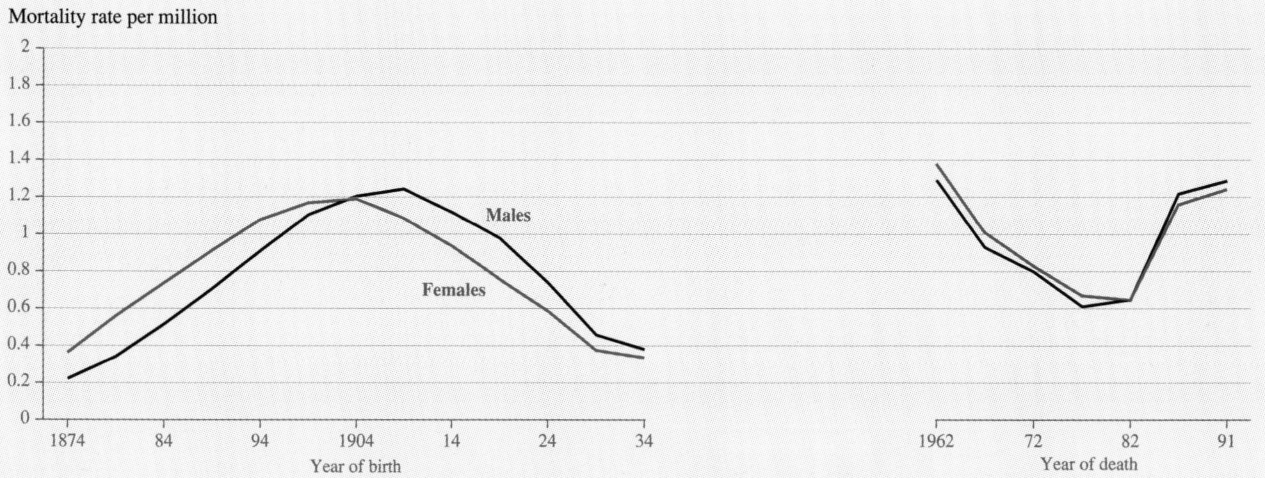

To summarise, since 1920, mortality from Parkinson's disease has declined by about two thirds in the younger age-groups while increasing fivefold in those 80 years and older. The cohort of people born around the turn of the century experienced a risk of death from Parkinson's disease two or three times greater that of cohorts born a decade earlier or later. From 1959 to 1983, there was a decline in the period of death effect. This indicates a reduction in risk of death in all age- groups, after adjusting for the effects of age and birth cohort. Trends in the period of death effect after 1983 are difficult to interpret because of the influence of the change in application of WHO rule 3.

One problem that must be addressed in attempting to interpret these findings concerns the validity of mortality data. There is little doubt that Parkinson's disease is under-reported on death certificates at present and the degree of under-reporting may have been more severe in the past (Kessler, (1972a, b) Williams, 1966). This misclassification may affect different age-groups to different extents. Artefactual changes in mortality certainly occurred with the change in implementation of WHO rule 3 and with the introduction of the 5th revision of the International Classification of Diseases. However, the consistency of the trends in mortality from Parkinson's disease within and between all revisions of the International Classification of Diseases, except the 4th and 5th, makes it hard to believe that the trends we have demonstrated can be accounted for by artefacts and inadequacies in death certification. It seems particularly unlikely, as Marmot (1980) has pointed out, that cohort effects can be explained in this way. To produce the cohort effect that we have described, doctors certifying deaths in 1960 would need to have been biased towards a diagnosis of Parkinson's disease in a 60-year-old person but against this diagnosis in an 80-year-old. In 1980, they would need to have been biased towards the diagnosis in an 80-year-old but against it in a 60-year-old.

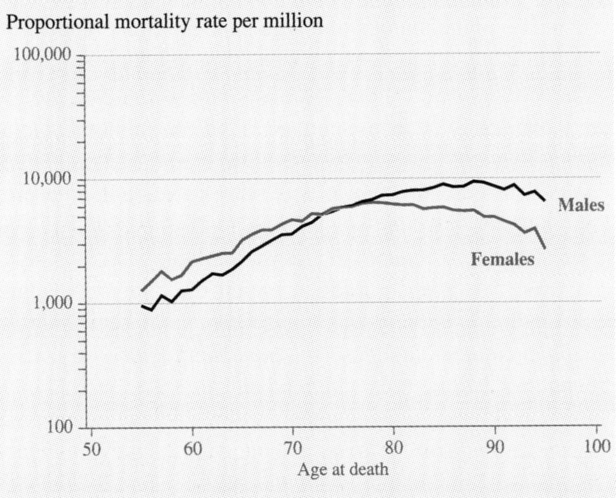

Previous analyses of mortality data for England and Wales, carried out over a decade ago, produced evidence of a birth cohort effect in Parkinson's disease (Li *et al.,* 1985; Marmot, 1980). With an additional 10 years of data we have been able to confirm the strength of the effect and identify the cohort at greatest risk more precisely. The findings fit the hypothesis first formulated by Poskanzer and Schwab over 30 years ago. One simple and economical explanation of the time trends of mortality from Parkinson's disease is that levels of exposure to an aetiological factor were high early in this century but have since rapidly declined.

19.2.6 The impact of treatment with L-dopa on mortality

Within the last three decades there have been important changes in the medical treatment available to sufferers from Parkinson's disease. L-dopa became available for the treat-

Figure 19.3a

Parkinson's disease in England and Wales: age effect

Proportional mortality rate per million

Figure 19.3b

Parkinson's disease in England and Wales: cohort and period effects

Proportional mortality rate per million

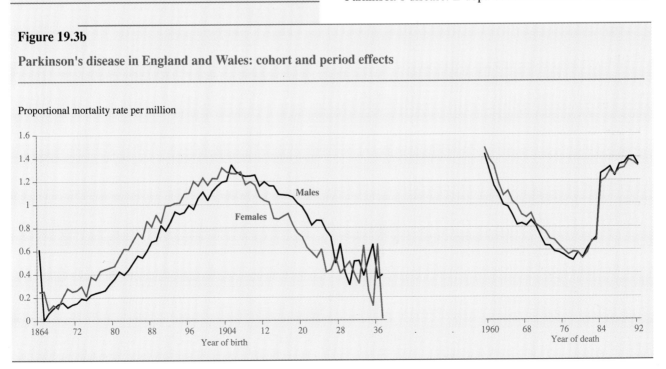

ment of the symptoms of Parkinson's disease in the late 1960s. It provided one of those few examples where the benefit to the patient, in the short term at least, was so remarkable that no randomised controlled trial was necessary to demonstrate the drug's efficacy. Since then, other drugs have been developed but L-dopa remains the mainstay of drug treatment of the disease. Nonetheless, while there can be no doubt that the drug has improved the quality of life of people with Parkinson's disease, there is less certainty about the effect that the drug has had on longevity.

Figure 19.2 shows that the period of death effect for Parkinson's disease declined from 1959–83. Although the data are not shown, the beginning of this decline actually occurred around 1940. The fact that the downward trend in the period of death effect antedated the introduction of L-dopa by 20 years and remained stable during the following decade suggests that it has had little effect on mortality.

19.3 Motor neurone disease

In the United Kingdom, the term motor neurone disease is used to refer to a syndrome of progressive muscular wasting and weakness that results from degeneration of upper and lower motor neurones in the brain and spinal cord (Leigh and Ray-Chaudhuri, 1994). The worldwide distribution of the disease has recently been the subject of a systematic review (Chancellor and Warlow, 1992). In the nine surveys of incidence judged to have achieved complete or nearly complete ascertainment of cases, crude rates ranged from 0.6 per 100,000 population per year in Sardinia to 2.6 per 100,000 population per year in Sweden. Statistically significant differences in incidence rates between these surveys remained after direct age-standardisation to a single population. Exceptionally high levels of a degenerative neurological syndrome that resembles motor neurone disease have been recorded in the Western Pacific on the island of Guam, in the Kii peninsula in Japan and in parts of New Guinea. In contrast to almost all other countries, where rates of motor neurone disease seem to be increasing, the incidence of the Guamanian form of the disease has declined from 87 per 100,000 population per year in 1962 to 5 per 100,000 population per year in 1985 (Rodgers-Johnson et al., 1986).

Since 1989, the Scottish Motor Neurone Disease Research Group has tried to identify all incident cases in Scotland using multiple sources of case ascertainment. 535 patients were registered between 1989 and 1993 giving an crude incidence of 2.1 per 100,000 population per year. 298 (56 per cent) were men (incidence 2.42 per 100,000 population per year) and 237 (44 per cent) were women (incidence 1.8 per 100,000 population per year). The mean age at registration was 64.8 years. 367 (69 per cent) patients have died; mean survival was 24 months from onset of symptoms and 12 months from diagnosis. The prognosis was worse in older people and in those with symptoms affecting the bulbar musculature at the onset of the disease (Chancellor et al., 1993).

19.3.1 Aetiology

Motor neurone disease is familial in 5–10 per cent of cases, usually with a dominant pattern of transmission. Further evidence that genetic factors may contribute is provided by the recent discovery of mutations in the Cu-Zn superoxide dismutase (SOD1) gene in some pedigrees (Rosen et al., 1993). Cu-Zn superoxide dismutase is a cytoplasmic enzyme which binds and eliminates superoxide free radicals and this discovery has lent support to the hypothesis that these reactive oxygen species may be crucial to pathogenesis. However, the precise mechanisms remain unclear for, while there is some evidence of reduced superoxide dismutase activity in patients who carry these mutations, studies of transgenic mice with overexpression of the superoxide dismutase gene indicate that motor neurones are selectively affected (Brown, 1995).

Motor neurone disease is sporadic in 90–95 per cent of cases. A study of a cohort of patients from the Scottish motor neurone disease register has demonstrated one particular mutation in the superoxide dismutase gene in 3 out of 56 unrelated patients without a family history of the disease (Jones et al., 1995). But in the majority of patients, there is no identifiable genetic defect and superoxide dismutase function is normal. Other studies indicate that toxic levels of glutamate, the primary excitatory neurotransmitter in the central nervous system, can lead to increased levels of intracellular calcium and free radical-mediated neuronal death (Rothstein et al.,1994). This raises the possibility that exogenous agents may cause motor neurone disease by stimulating glutaminergic receptors.

It is hard to explain the rapidly declining incidence of motor neurone disease on Guam except in terms of diminishing exposure to a causal environmental factor. Suspicion fell on a dietary excitotoxin, beta-N-methylamino-L-alanine (L-BMAA), present in cycad flour obtained from false sago palm (*Cycas circinalis*), but it now seems likely that levels in the diet are too low to be toxic.

Clusters of sporadic motor neurone disease have occasionally been reported in developed countries but their significance is unclear. None of these clusters has generated hypotheses about aetiology. Motor neurone disease was associated with affluence in a study in Scotland (Chancellor et al., 1992) but this may be due to under-ascertainment of older patients in less affluent areas. Although numerous case reports link the onset of symptoms of motor neurone disease to physical trauma, the results of case-control studies are inconsistent. Kurland et al., (1992) concluded, after a comprehensive review of published studies, that there was no association of the disease with antecedent trauma.

19.3.2 Time trends in motor neurone disease

Mortality from motor neurone disease is increasing rapidly in most industrialised countries. In England and Wales, rates have doubled over the past 30 years. It was previously thought that mortality from motor neurone disease declined in the very elderly but recent studies from the USA, Sweden, and England and Wales have shown that this is no longer true (Yoshida *et al.*, 1986; Gunnarsson *et al.*, 1990; Martyn, 1994). For people born after 1900, mortality rates increase with age continuously.

It has been suggested that the rising motor neurone disease mortality rates may be a delayed consequence of increased rates of asymptomatic poliovirus infection during the epidemics that occurred before immunisation (Martyns *et al.*, 1988). A prediction from this hypothesis is that rates of motor neurone disease will begin to decline from about the year 2010, when the first cohort of people to have been immunised against poliovirus in childhood will reach the age at which the disease usually presents. A study in Scotland provided no evidence that mortality is yet declining in immunised populations (Swinglers *et al.*, 1992) but, as this cohort is still too young to be at high risk of motor neurone disease, it will be some time before the hypothesis can be tested conclusively.

Neilson *et al.*, (1992), have offered a different interpretation. They found that age- and sex-specific mortality rates from motor neurone disease fitted a Gompertzian model for deaths occurring below the age of 64 years. After this age, observed mortality rates were much lower than predicted by the model. They interpreted this deviation as indicating the presence of a subgroup of people susceptible to motor neurone disease within the population, some of whom have died from other causes before they could develop the disease. They suggest that the increasing mortality from motor neurone disease over time can simply be explained by the decreasing mortality from competing causes.

19.4 Dementia

The ageing populations of almost all countries in the developed world, the rapidly increasing prevalence of dementia with age and the demands that people suffering from the condition make on health care resources combine to make dementia a public health issue of global importance. Alzheimer's disease has recently been redefined. Until a few years ago it was a diagnostic label for a rare form of pre-senile dementia affecting young and middle-aged people. With the recognition that the underlying pathology was similar in many elderly demented people, Alzheimer's disease has become the commonest cause of dementia accounting for more than half of all cases of deterioration in cognitive function of late onset. The other major cause of dementia in the elderly is cerebrovascular disease. A clinical syndrome of intellectual decline is a frequent accompaniment of ischaemic, hypoxic or haemorrhagic brain lesions resulting from disease of cerebral blood vessels.

Studies that presented age-specific prevalence rates for Alzheimer's disease have been conducted in Europe, the USA and Japan; the geographical differences in rates are not strik-
ing. Although prevalence was lowest in Japan, where vascular dementia predominated, differences in the application of diagnostic criteria may be at least part of the explanation (Breteler *et al.*, 1992). The results of a survey of an elderly population in Nigeria (Osuntokun *et al.*, 1990) in which no demented individuals were found are intriguing and suggest that, if standardised diagnostic criteria can be applied, cross-cultural studies may be of great importance in the search for aetiology.

A combined analysis of 12 European studies of the prevalence of dementia shows that rates increase exponentially with age (Hofman *et al.*, 1991), although it is possible that very elderly survivors may be at diminishing risk (Ritchie and Kildea, 1995).

Important progress has been made in understanding the genetic determinants of familial Alzheimer's disease, which accounts for 5–10 per cent of all cases. But the vast majority of late onset cases are sporadic. The inheritance of the E4 allele of the gene encoding apolipoprotein E is a strong risk factor, but the results of epidemiological investigations of environmental determinants of the disease have so far been disappointing. Attention has fallen on increasing parental age, head trauma, exposure to aluminium and educational level, but no consistently strong associations have emerged.

One crucial question yet to be answered is whether the risk of dementia or of particular forms of dementia has changed over time. It is certain that the numbers of people suffering from dementia are increasing, but it may be that this increase can be accounted for demographically by the increasing numbers of elderly people.

19.4.1 Time trends in dementia

Unfortunately, routinely collected mortality data for dementia are unable to provide much useful information about time trends. Part of the difficulty arises from the fact that a diagnosis of dementia may be recorded in a number of ways. Even in the 9th revision of the International Classification of Diseases, the rubrics 290, 298.9, 331 and 797 may all be used to code dementia. The potential problems that this may cause in interpreting time trends are exemplified in Figure 19.4. While deaths from dementia (ICD 290) have been gradually increasing over recent decades, deaths from senility (ICD8 794; ICD9 797) have been slowly falling. It is probable that these divergent trends reflect a changing preference in diagnostic labels. A further problem in interpretation of mortality data arises because only a small proportion of people diagnosed in life as having dementia eventually receive this diagnosis as the underlying cause of death. A study of patients diagnosed as having dementia at a psychogeriatric clinic in Newcastle upon Tyne revealed that less than 25 per cent of those who had died had this diagnosis coded as the underlying cause of death (Martyn and Pippard, 1988). Cases who had died in a psychiatric hospital were more likely to have dementia recorded than those dying in general hospitals or at home.

Figure 19.4

Deaths from dementia

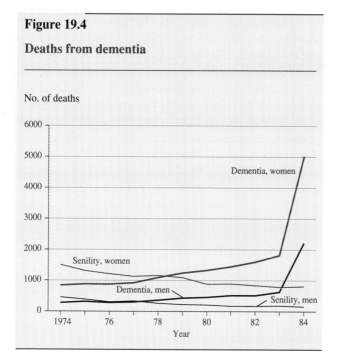

The policy change in the application of WHO rule 3, discussed above in the section on Parkinson's disease, led to a sudden increase in numbers of deaths from dementia. The effects can be seen in Figure 19.4. Mortality from dementia apparently doubled as a result of the more stringent application of this rule.

The geographical distribution of mortality from dementia is seriously distorted by patterns of long-term care. Mortality from dementia in England and Wales tended to be highest in areas where large psychiatric hospitals were located. Hospitals with long-stay beds are considered to be the patient's usual address by ONS if the patient has been living there for more than 6 months before the date of death. Local authority areas which contain a hospital with a large number of long-stay beds are likely to show elevated mortality for chronic neuropsychiatric disorders.

The variations in diagnostic terminology, the influence of WHO rule 3 and the low rate of recording of dementia as a cause of death limit any inferences that can be drawn from changes in mortality rates from dementia over time. We must await the results of the longitudinal studies of ageing and cognitive impairment that are now in progress.

19.5 Epilepsy

Epilepsy, a tendency to recurrent seizures, is a common condition, with an incidence of 70 per 100,000 population per year and a prevalence of 500–1000 per 100,000 per year, after the exclusion of patients with febrile convulsions, single seizures and people in remission. The cumulative lifetime prevalence of non-febrile epileptic seizures is between 2 and 5 per cent (Goodridge and Shorvon, 1983). Epilepsy occurs worldwide, but geographical variation is hard to assess because of the lack of agreed diagnostic criteria and differences in methods of case ascertainment. Some studies suggest that

the incidence is higher in developing countries and in the non-white and less affluent populations of developed countries (Haerer et al.,1986; Gomez et al.,1978).

A US Government-sponsored commission assessed the services of patients with epilepsy assuming a 1 per cent prevalence. Applying these figure to the United Kingdom gives estimates of 22,400 people (0.04 per cent of the population) institutionalised because of epilepsy and a similar number living in residential care in the community. Active epilepsy is likely to be present in about 185,000 people (0.33 per cent of the population) who probably require continual medical treatment, usually in hospital clinics. Occasional medical treatment will be required by a further 145,600 people and there are probably a further 160,000 people who are in remission or undiagnosed and are not receiving medical attention.

The cost of epilepsy is difficult to estimate because of the wide spectrum of disease and changes in expenditure at different times in the course of the condition. However, recent studies from Dundee indicate an average annual cost of over £2,000 for each patient attending a specialist clinic. More than 40 per cent of these patients were unemployed (Swingler et al., 1994). Using a more comprehensive population-based approach, Cockerell et al., (1994b) able to confirm the high indirect costs of epilepsy and suggested that total annual expenditure on this condition might be as much as £1,930 million in the United Kingdom.

19.5.1 Aetiology

Community-based studies in the United Kingdom indicate the following aetiologies: cerebrovascular disease in 15 per cent, cerebral tumours in 6 per cent, alcohol related in 6 per cent and post-traumatic causes for a further 2 per cent. Primary generalised epilepsy syndromes, genetic and rare congenital conditions account for some of the remainder but no clear cause is found in 60–70 per cent of cases, which are labelled cryptogenic (Sander et al., 1990). Death rates in patients with newly diagnosed epilepsy are high, mainly due to the underlying cause (Cockerell et al., 1994a).

19.5.2 Time trends

While the prevalence of epilepsy does not seem to be changing, there is evidence that the incidence of epilepsy is falling in the United Kingdom and USA (Sander et al., 1993). The change is greatest in younger age-groups. Rising life expectancy has been associated with an increase in new cases among the elderly and some 25 per cent of new cases are now over the age of 65 years (Sander et al., 1990). In the elderly, epilepsy is more likely to be symptomatic of underlying neurological disease and the prognosis for remission is poorer.

19.6 Multiple sclerosis

Multiple sclerosis is an inflammatory disease affecting the myelin sheaths of neurones in the central nervous system.

The disease usually starts with a phase of relapses and remissions but the long-term outcome is very variable. Occasionally, evidence of the disease is found unexpectedly at autopsy in a person who had no symptoms of multiple sclerosis during life. In others the condition remains latent after the initial attack. For many, there is a pattern of progressive disability (Matthews, 1991).

Multiple sclerosis is common among Caucasian populations in Europe and their descendants in America and Australasia, but within each region there are latitudinal gradients of increasing disease frequency with distance from the equator. In Europe the prevalence is approximately 60 per 100,000 population per year in the south, rising to 100 per 100,000 population per year in the north. The distribution of multiple sclerosis in the United Kingdom has been the subject of intense scrutiny because, although rates in England and Wales seem comparable to those observed elsewhere in Northern Europe, the disease seems to be more common in the northeast Scottish mainland, Orkney and Shetland (prevalence 150–200 per 100,000 population per year) (Compston, 1990; Martyn, 1991) than anywhere else in the world. Williams and McKeran (1986) have argued that the difference might be artefactual because the Scottish prevalence estimates are based on serial studies using the diagnostic criteria of Allison and Millar rather than single surveys that have used the more specific criteria proposed by Poser. Nevertheless, recent surveys of south east Scotland have confirmed the high prevalence using the Poser criteria (Rothwell P, personal communication). Independent sources of morbidity data also provide evidence of a north-south difference within Britain. A case-finding study using the GPASS database of 527,736 patients registered in 80 practices in Scotland yielded a standardised prevalence ratio which was 37 per cent (95 per cent C.I. 26–48 per cent) higher than a similar study of the VAMP database of 3,617,890 patients registered with 524 practices in England and Wales (SMRs 158 vs 116; Swingler RJ, Rothwell P, unpublished observations).

19.6.1 Aetiology

It has been suggested that multiple sclerosis might be more prevalent in Scotland because of genetic factors (Sutherland, 1956; Swingler and Compston, 1986; Robertson and Compston, 1995). And it is possible that genetic variations may also explain the differences in the frequency of the disease seen in neighbouring regions such as Sicily and Malta, Sardinia and mainland Italy, and the Magyar and Gypsy peoples of Hungary (Compston et al., 1994). In North America, rates are higher in the north-west USA and southern Canada, which are heavily populated by migrants from north Germany and Scandinavia, than in the south, where more people originate from Africa and the Caribbean. Multiple sclerosis is more prevalent in white South Africans than in orientals, Asiatics and African blacks and the disease is also commoner in whites in Australia and New Zealand than in Aborigines or Maoris.

The nature of the putative susceptibility genes remains obscure but the clearest associations are with polymorphisms of human leucocyte antigens (HLA). These proteins are known to stimulate immune responses by presenting foreign antigen to T lymphocytes and they are encoded by genes in the major histocompatibility complex on chromosome 6q21.1-21.3. There is an allelic association with the DR15 and DQ6 subtypes of HLA-DR2 and DQW6, respectively. But, there are difficulties in reconciling ecological studies of genetic gradients, case-control studies of allelic association and linkage studies in families. For example, while the distribution of multiple sclerosis in the United Kingdom has been related to the frequency of HLA-DR2 in the population, a case-control study in north-east Scotland (Francis et al., 1987), where the disease is particularly prevalent, showed no increased risk associated with this allele. Nor, in studies of affected sibling pairs, is there any evidence of increased sharing of HLA haplotypes. Twin studies have shown that the majority of monozygotic twins are discordant for the disease, which unambiguously demonstrates the powerful effect of non-heritable factors (Sadovnick et al., 1993).

Epidemiological studies also provide evidence that environmental factors are important. Studies of US veterans show a north-south gradient in risk of multiple sclerosis in both white and black Americans and there is evidence that people born in the north have a lower risk if they move south during the first two decades of life (Kurtzke et al., 1979). Within Australia and New Zealand there are also gradients of declining prevalence of disease with decreasing latitude but the cause of the variation is unclear (Hammond et al., 1988; Miller et al., 1990).

Further evidence for an environmental aetiology comes from the study of multiple sclerosis in migrant populations. The disease is virtually unknown in the black populations of Africa, but is found in African-Americans. In second generation descendants of immigrants to the United Kingdom from the West Indies, Africa and the Indian subcontinent rates are the same as in the white population of Britain (Elian et al., 1990). Migrants from northern Europe who have moved to South Africa or Australasia experience lower rates of multiple sclerosis than occur in their countries of origin. Although interpretation of migrant studies may be difficult, the findings are remarkably consistent. They suggest either that exogenous aetiological factors are operating in the developed temperate regions of both hemispheres or that there are protective factors in countries nearer the equator.

Within the United Kingdom there are variations in distribution which point to environmental influences on the risk of disease. In a recent study of the place of residence of 8,066 multiple sclerosis patients discharged from Scottish hospitals there was evidence of higher ages and sex-standardized discharge ratios in the most affluent areas (SDR =1.17, 95 per cent C.I. 1.13–1.21), falling to 0.84 (95 per cent C.I. 0.81–0.88) in the most deprived areas (Chi-squared test P<0.001). (Swingler RJ, unpublished observations). It is unusual for chronic disabling diseases to be more prevalent among affluent populations and comparisons have been made between multiple sclerosis and poliomyelitis, which is more common in affluent communities with better sanitation who tend to be infected at a later age, when neurological sequelae are more common (Poskanzer *et al.*, 1963). Alter *et al.* (1986) have pointed out that the world distribution of multiple sclerosis can be correlated with late childhood infection. A similar mechanism might explain the apparent outbreaks of multiple sclerosis in isolated island populations where childhood infections typically occur later. There is evidence that infection with measles, mumps, rubella and Epstein-Barr virus tend to occur later in multiple sclerosis than in genetically matched controls (Compston *et al.*, 1986; Martyn *et al.*, 1993). However, it has proved remarkable difficult to incriminate any particular agent. It seems likely that the world distribution of multiple sclerosis reflects an interaction between genetic and exogenous factors.

Chapter 20

Diseases of the respiratory system

By
Guy Marks and Peter Burney

Summary

- Mortality due to chronic obstructive pulmonary disease (COPD) in under-55-year-olds has declined since 1921. In 55–74-year-old men it reached a peak in those born around 1900 and has declined in successive cohorts born since then.

- Separate epidemics of smoking in men and women have had important effects on COPD mortality during this century.

- Changes attributable to smoking are superimposed on a declining trend since the middle of the nineteenth century in lifetime risk of death due to COPD.

- There has been no overall trend in asthma mortality rates in 5–35-year-olds during this century.

- A major epidemic of asthma mortality in the period 1960–70 can probably be attributed to an adverse effect of treatment that was in use at that time.

- In children and young adults the frequency of severe exacerbations of asthma is highest in late summer and early autumn.

- The declining trend in mortality due to pneumonia in the early part of this century accelerated in the late 1930s with the introduction of antimicrobial chemotherapy.

- The current age differential in mortality due to pneumonia may, in part, be a cohort effect, with those born in the early part of this century being at greatest risk.

20.1 Introduction

Three diseases form the focus of this chapter: chronic obstructive pulmonary disease (COPD), asthma and pneumonia. Pulmonary tuberculosis, influenza and lung cancer are covered in Chapters 14, 15 and 17. COPD is also referred to as 'chronic obstructive lung disease' (COLD). The chapter starts with an overview of changes in the burden of illness attributable to respiratory diseases during this century. This is followed by a discussion of the framework for interpreting changes in observed mortality and morbidity, and an outline of the methods used to construct the plots and analyse the data. In sections dealing separately with the three principal diseases, a description of the details of the relevant ICD codes and the impact of changes in these codes is outlined, followed by a description of the temporal pattern of mortality and morbidity. Finally, changes in morbidity and mortality are discussed in the context of changes in risk factors, diagnosis and treatment.

20.1.1 Changes in the burden of illness

The change in the pattern of premature adult mortality (ages 15–74) attributed to respiratory causes is shown in Figure 20.1.

In 1901, pulmonary tuberculosis was a major contributor to adult mortality, and other infectious respiratory diseases, particularly pneumonia, were also important. Asthma and lung cancer were not coded as separate entities at this time. By 1951, the proportion of all deaths caused by respiratory disease had decreased, largely as a result of substantial reductions in death resulting from infectious causes. Two forms of respiratory disease which are related to smoking, lung cancer and COPD, were the major causes of respiratory mortality at this time, although pulmonary tuberculosis was still important. In 1991, respiratory diseases were an even smaller proportion of total deaths. Lung cancer is now the most im-

portant respiratory cause of death whereas pulmonary tuberculosis is a very rare cause of death.

Premature mortality attributable to infectious respiratory diseases, has declined throughout the century (see Figure 20.2). This decline was apparent before the introduction of effective chemotherapy, and is steeper for influenza, (for which no specific therapy is available) than for non-tuberculous pneumonia. Only for tuberculosis is the sudden impact of an effective treatment obvious from the change in trend. There has been a small decline in mortality attributable to obstructive airway diseases since the beginning of the century. The trend is disturbed by a major change in coding practice in 1940 (see Chapter 2). The trend for death resulting from asthma is not uniform over the century, with short-term increases in the mid-1910s and mid-1960s and a short-term decrease before 1960.

Mortality from lung cancer rose steeply between 1931 (when a separate code was first introduced routinely) and 1960. Since 1952 it has been a greater cause of premature adult mortality than COPD. Since 1960 mortality from both these causes has levelled off, then declined, although the decline in deaths resulting from lung cancer occurred later than for COPD.

20.1.2 Interpreting changes in mortality and morbidity

In explaining trends in mortality over a span of 90 years, those changes that are more apparent than real must first be identified, as indicated in Chapter 2. Where changes in the International Classification of Diseases (ICD) or the coders' instructions are important, they usually result in sudden changes in reported mortality, around the years of introduction, of the new revisions.

Fluctuations attributable to changes in diagnostic trends are more gradual and hence more difficult to identify. They may result in reciprocal changes with an alternative diagnosis but

Figure 20.1

The burden of respiratory diseases in the 20th century: ages 15–74, proportion of all deaths due to respiratory diseases

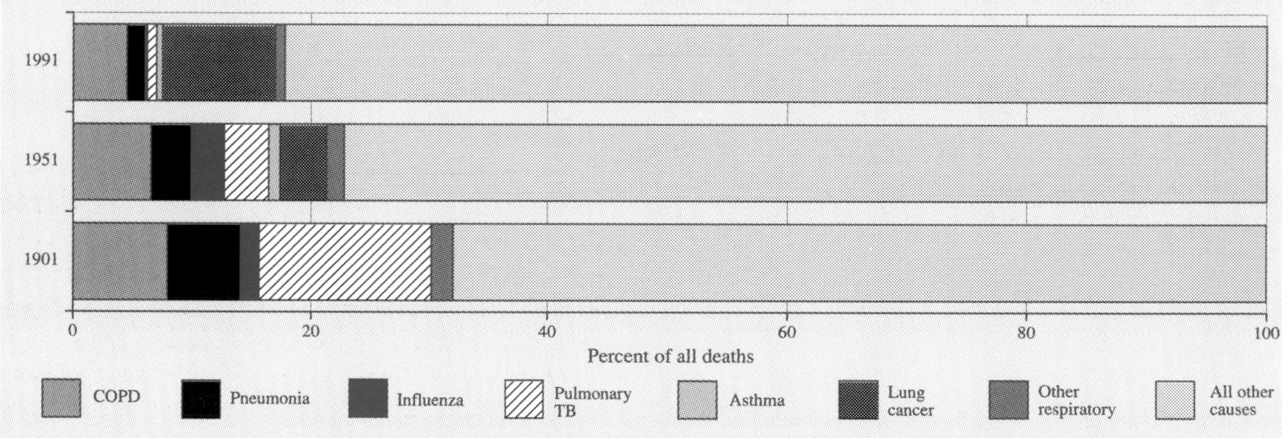

Figure 20.2

Major respiratory causes of mortality, ages 15-74, England and Wales

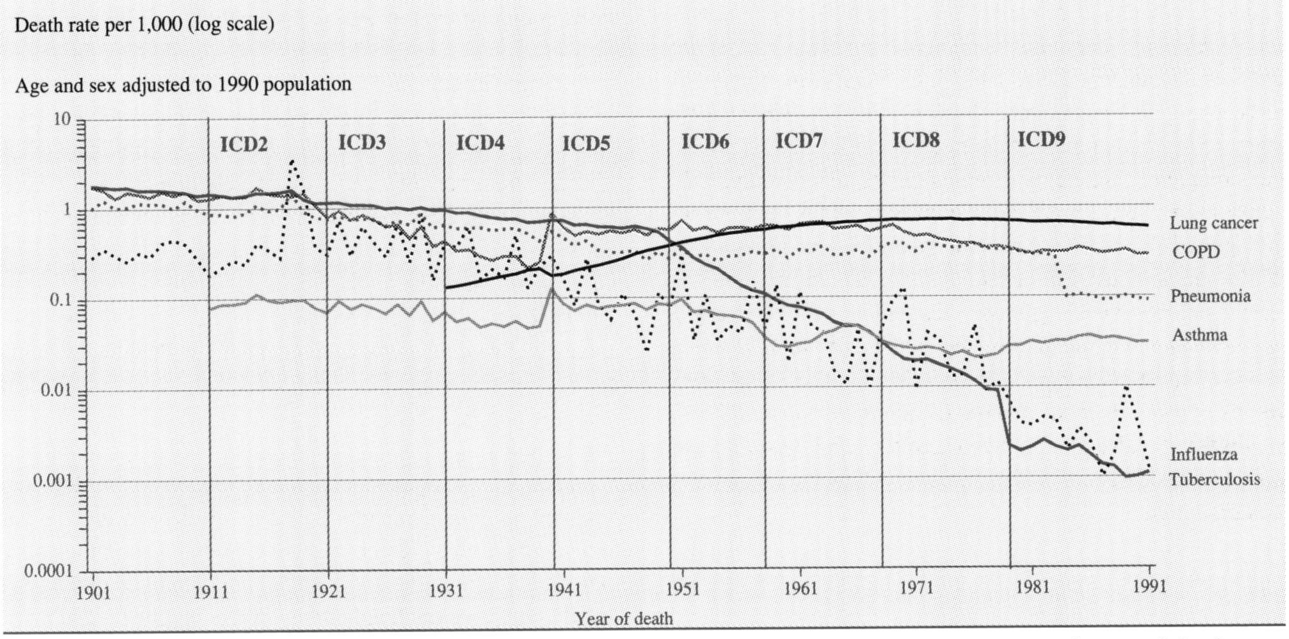

Death rate per 1,000 (log scale)

Age and sex adjusted to 1990 population

this can be difficult to detect on a log-scale plot if the alternative rate is an order of magnitude different, as is the case with COPD and asthma. Some changes in diagnoses on death certificates have been noted in published reports, such as the increasing trend in diagnosing terminal pneumonia as a primary cause of death, which ultimately led to the 1984 rule change described in Chapter 2.

Real changes in death resulting from a disease may be due to changes in the prevalence of the disease or changes in the case-fatality rate. Changes in disease severity or treatment may influence the latter.

For acute infections, recent or contemporary events are usually most important, whereas chronic diseases may have been initiated many years before the time of death. In trying to isolate these features, use is made of analyses attempting to separate the effects of age, the period of death and conditions in the lifetimes of different generations (cohort effects). Such age-period-cohort' analyses are described in Chapter 2.

Factors operating around the time of death, which may be consistent with observed period trends, include changes in the incidence of acute serious infectious diseases and changes in life-saving treatments. Examples of cohort risk factors that are influential in the early stages of the development of chronic respiratory illnesses are smoking and, possibly, allergen exposure. The interpretation of these period and cohort plots depends on the availability of data on temporal changes in hypothesised risk factors and changes in the therapeutic practices.

20.2 Data and methods

The ONS historical mortality and population datasets, described in detail elsewhere, were used for all these analyses.

Data for diagnosis, age-group, sex and year of death were available for the entire mortality dataset. Additional data on month of death were available for deaths occurring since 1959, and for month and year of birth for deaths occurring since 1969.

Both these mortality and population datasets contain data for the civilian population only. For the years 1915–20 and 1940–47, the selective recruitment of fit men into the armed forces caused an apparent increase in the mortality rate in the remaining civilians. To overcome this artefact, available data for non-civilian population and mortality were added to the dataset: for men aged 15–54 for the years 1915–20; for men aged 15–59 for the year 1940; and for men aged 15–59 and women aged 15–49 for the years 1941–47.

The mortality rates were adjusted for numerically important changes in the ICD code or ONS instructions to coders. Conversion factors (old to new) were calculated from published samples of deaths, coded according to both the outgoing and the incoming versions of the ICD. These were applied in a multiplicative manner to make data from each preceding version of the ICD comparable with the subsequent data. These adjusted data were used for all plots and analyses.

20.2.1 Period plots

Data were grouped into six 10-year age-bands from 15–74 years (an additional 5–14 year age-band was included for asthma). For each disease, the total number of deaths within each age-band was calculated separately for men and women for each year and divided by the estimated total mid-year population for that age-band to yield an age- and sex-specific mortality rate. These data were plotted on a logarithmic scale. The introduction of each new version of the ICD is identified by a vertical dotted line on the graphs.

20.2.2 Cohort plots

Five-year periods were defined commencing with 1911–15 and ending with 1986–90. Each age/sex/period-specific mortality rate was assigned to a cohort whose midpoint was identified by subtracting the midpoint for the 5-year age-group from the 5-year period midpoint. The resulting cohorts, which were identified by their midpoints, covered 10-year birth periods, each overlapping 5 years with the preceding cohort and 5 years with the subsequent cohort. Data were again grouped into the same six age-bands (seven for asthma) used in the period plots. For each of these age-bands the first cohort did not contain data for the younger half of the age-band and the last cohort did not contain data for the older half of the age-band. To avoid potential bias, the first and last cohorts of each age-band were not plotted. Hence, the cohort or year-of-birth midpoints range from 1846 to 1966. The data were plotted on a logarithmic scale.

20.2.3 Age-period-cohort analysis

Any linear trend over time (drift) could be due to a combination of cohort and period effects, but as birth cohort dates are derived arithmetically from age and year of death, it is not possible to determine the relative importance of cohort and period effects (Clayton and Schifflers, 1987). Such linear trends are termed 'drift'. An analysis was conducted to test whether the additional non-linear variation in mortality rates over time could best be explained by effects related to birth cohorts or periods of death, or both.

Sex-specific mortality rates for 5-year periods, overlapping 10-year cohorts, and 5-year age-groups were calculated for deaths occurring between 1911 and 1990. For COPD and pneumonia, data for ages 15–74 were used, whereas, for asthma, analyses were conducted using data for ages 5–54 years. In all cases separate models were fitted for men and women.

The models were fitted in GLIM3.77 using the iteratively re-weighted least squares regression method to allow for over-dispersion of residuals (Pocock *et al.*, 1981). The significance of effects was tested against the F distribution. A full model containing factors for age-groups, periods and cohorts (age-period-cohort model) was fitted initially to establish the appropriate weighting. Subsequently, a model containing factors for age-groups and a linear term for drift (i.e. a constant rate of change over the period of observation) was fitted. This model was then compared, separately, with one model containing factors for age-groups and periods, and another model containing factors for age-groups and cohorts, to establish whether period or cohort terms for non-linear temporal variation fitted the data significantly better than the linear trend. Finally, if significant non-drift period and/or cohort effects were identified, the age-period and the age-cohort models were compared with the initially fitted age-period-cohort model to test whether non-drift period and cohort effects were both required.

20.2.4 Sickness and invalidity data

The total number of spells of medically certified sickness or invalidity during the period 1962/63 to 1989/90 in each year and the proportion attributed to either influenza or COPD was plotted (DHSS, 1963–94). The composition of the COPD category varied during the period of observation. From 1962/63 to 1967/68 all bronchitis cases (ICD7 codes 500–502) were included. From 1968/69 to 1978/79 only non-acute bronchitis was included (ICD8 codes 490 and 491). From 1979/80 to 1989/90 emphysema and asthma were included along with non-acute bronchitis (ICD9 codes 490–493). The data were substantially influenced by the introduction of Statutory Sick Pay in 1983. This greatly reduced the total number of claims for sickness and invalidity benefit and had a disproportionate effect on the number of claims for short spells, for example, for influenza (DHSS, 1984). The number of women claimants dropped substantially after 1987, when women were no longer able to pay reduced rate National Insurance and still claim benefits (DSS, 1994).

20.2.5 Hospital In-patient Enquiry (HIPE)

These data are described in detail in Chapter 5. Data for month and year of admission (1968–85), age and sex for all records in which asthma was the principal diagnosis have been used to examine trends in admissions by age, sex, period and cohort. We have also assessed seasonal variation in admission rates using the method described below.

20.2.6 Seasonal variation

For the period 1959–91 the odds, for each disease, of death in any month compared with the odds of death in January were estimated by logistic regression. The logarithms of the odds were displayed graphically to detect seasonal trends. Separate models were constructed, together with confidence intervals, for each of three broad age-groups. Models were adjusted for effects of year of death, sex and, where necessary, the interaction between these. In models characterised by extra-random dispersion of the residuals, the reweighted least squares regression method was used (Pocock *et al.*, 1981).

The hypothesis that month-to-month variation in rates followed a seasonal pattern was tested by fitting a sinusoidal curved regression line to the data and testing whether the amplitude was significantly different from zero (Woodhouse *et al.*, 1994). The model was fitted by logistic regression with adjustment for year-to-year variation in rates. It was also used to test for difference in seasonal trends between men and women and between age-groups. Finally, the model was used to quantify the ratio of the seasonal maximum to the seasonal minimum (seasonal ratio).

This method was also used to describe and test monthly variation in hospital admission rates for asthma from 1968–85, as well as variation in mortality according to the subject's month of birth, for deaths occurring between 1969 and 1991.

20.3 Chronic obstructive pulmonary disease

COPD is defined as the group of pathologically distinct but clinically overlapping diseases: chronic bronchitis, emphysema, bronchiectasis, bronchial catarrh and other non-specific obstructive airway diseases. The classification and nomenclature for these have changed over the century, and hence separate analysis of these entities is not possible and the group as a whole is considered. For the most part, asthma has been separately identified and is not included within this category. In Chapter 9, Doll *et al.* have used a slightly different definition of COPD, called by the synonym 'chronic obstructive lung disease' (COLD).

20.3.1 Coding

In ICD1 (1901–10), asthma and emphysema were included in one category. Bronchitis was a separate category. From ICD2 onwards, asthma was classified as a separate entity. Acute bronchitis, which was listed separately from ICD3 onwards, and bronchiolitis, listed separately in ICD8 and ICD9, have not been included in these graphs. In ICD1 and ICD2 (1901–20), acute bronchitis was not separately identified (see below). In 1940, at the introduction of ICD5, coders were instructed to select the primary cause inferred by the certifier when more than one cause of death was listed. Previously, rules of precedence were operative. At the same time, 'subacute bronchitis' was reclassified from 'chronic' to 'acute bronchitis'. Occupational causes of bronchitis were classified separately from this time.

A major re-organisation among the categories of obstructive airway diseases occurred with the introduction of ICD6 in 1950, and a separate classification for bronchiectasis was introduced for the first time. In ICD7 (1958–67), some cases previously assigned to asthma were now assigned to bronchitis, if both causes were mentioned and the asthma was not specified as allergic. A further major reorganisation of bronchitis, bronchiectasis and emphysema occurred with ICD8 (1968–78).

The separate coding of acute bronchitis from 1921 onwards and the change in the rules of precedence in 1940 were the only numerically significant changes. Examination of the bridge-coding data for the introduction of ICD6, 7, 8 and 9 shows that the net change was less than 6 per cent in all cases. Dual coding of deaths occurring in 1939 allowed the calculation of accurate age- and sex-specific conversion factors to apply to rates before 1940.

There is no detailed bridge-coding information accompanying the introduction of ICD3 in 1921. Approximate age- and sex-specific conversion factors for deaths before that date have been estimated by calculating the proportion of all bronchitis and emphysema deaths in the period 1921–25 which were attributed to chronic or unspecified bronchitis or emphysema (i.e. not attributed to acute bronchitis). The data used in the graphs and analysis presented below have been adjusted by these conversion factors before 1940 and before 1921 (see Table 20.1).

20.3.2 Trends in mortality

Age-period-cohort analysis
Table 20.2 shows the comparison of models constructed according to the method of Clayton and Schifflers (1987) using data for men aged 15–74 dying from COPD. After adjustment for age, fluctuations in mortality rates over time beyond those explained by a linear trend (drift) are influenced to a significant extent by both period of death and cohort of birth. The conclusions for women are the same (data not shown).

Period effects (Figure 20.3)
Mortality caused by COPD changed little in the first two decades of this century but then declined during the period 1921–

Table 20.1

Conversion factors used to adjust rates for COPD prior to changes in 1921 and 1940

Year	ICD2 to 3 1921 to 1925*		ICD4 to 5 1939	
Sex/Age	M	F	M	F
15-24	0.75	0.66	1.33	1.51
25-34	0.76	0.66	1.54	1.71
35-44	0.81	0.67	1.78	1.85
45-54	0.83	0.73	2.03	2.18
55-64	0.83	0.74	2.31	2.71
65-74	0.83	0.75	2.42	2.68

* Based on proportion of all bronchitis deaths in the period 1921 to 1925 which were attributed to chronic or unspecified bronchitis.

Table 20.2

Age-period-cohort analysis of deaths occurring between 1911 and 1991 among men, aged 15 to 74, which were attributed to COPD

Model	Deviance	Degrees of freedom
1. Age + Drift	768.6	179
2. Age + Cohort	292.2	154
3. Age + Period	639.2	165
4. Age + Cohort + Period	187.8	140

Model comparisons	Change in deviance	Degrees of freedom
2. and 1. (cohort)	476.4	25**
3. and 1. (period)	129.4	14**
4. and 2. (period)	104.4	14**
4. and 3. (cohort)	451.4	25**
4. and 1.	580.8	39**

** $P<0.001$

40. From that time, mortality rates levelled off or increased slightly above age 54 until 1968, since when they have declined in men but not in women. Below age 54, mortality has been falling since 1940. There was an increase in mortality in younger age-groups between 1915 and 1919, and in all age-groups in 1940 (the latter likely to be the result of the revision of the ICD and rules for the selection of underlying cause).

Cohort effects (Figure 20.4)

Mortality rates decreased for cohorts born between 1841 and 1871. In men in the 55–74 year age-group, rates then increased to a maximum in those born around 1900. There has been a steady decrease in risk in men in all age-groups born since

that date. In women there has been a steady decline in mortality in those aged below 55 born after 1916, but a rise among those older than 54.

Age and sex effects

The markedly increased risk of death with advancing age is seen in both period and cohort plots. This effect of age has increased over time because deaths at young ages have decreased most. Since COPD is a group of diseases with different causes, this may not be surprising (see Chapters 9 and 12 on the contribution of smoking and atmospheric pollution). Mortality in men is higher than that in women in all ages, periods, and cohorts, although the difference is small in 15–34-year-olds.

Figure 20.3

Chronic obstructive pulmonary disease death rate by year of death

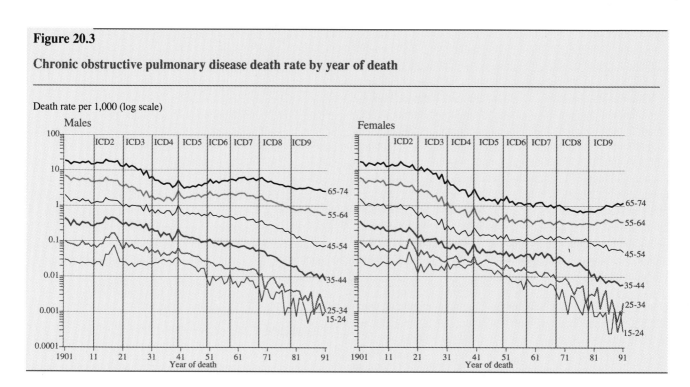

Figure 20.4

Chronic obstructive pulmonary disease death rate by year of birth

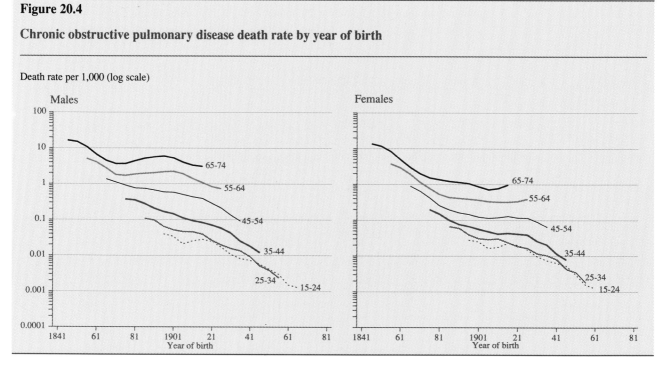

Seasonal trends (Figure 20.5)

There is a strong seasonal trend in risk of death from COPD, the risk being highest in January in all age-groups. There was a small but significant seasonal variation in the risk of death associated with month of birth (not shown). Subjects born in April were 6 per cent more likely to die from COPD than those born in September.

20.3.3 Trends in incapacity

Since 1962–63 there has been a downward trend in the proportion of spells of incapacity resulting from sickness and invalidity which are attributed to chronic bronchitis (see Figure 20.6). This trend is more marked for men than for women, and the excess of male incapacity from chronic bronchitis over that of women has diminished over this period. This may relate to the removal in 1987 of the provision for women to opt out of full National Insurance contributions (DSS, 1994).

20.3.4 Interpretation

Age and gender differences, cohort and period trends

The marked increase in morbidity and mortality from COPD with increasing age is consistent with Fletcher's model of COPD being due to an acceleration of the normal decline in lung function with age (Fletcher *et al.*, 1976). The higher mortality rates in men than in women may result from higher rates of exposure to two of the important risk factors for this disease: smoking and occupational dust and fumes, which differ with respect to birth cohort and period.

Smoking

The most clearly established risk factor for the development of COPD is smoking, which increases the rate of decline in lung function (Fletcher *et al.*, 1976; Fletcher and Peto, 1977; Lebowitz, 1981; Burrows *et al.*, 1987; 1988; Camilli *et al.*, 1987; Lebowitz *et al.*, 1987; Dockery *et al.*, 1988; Parker *et al.*, 1990), and induces an earlier onset of decline (Tager *et*

al., 1988). The increased rate of decline in lung function seen in current smokers quickly reverts to a normal rate of decline on quitting smoking (Camilli *et al.*, 1987). The risks of symptoms (Lebowitz, 1981; Barbee *et al.*, 1991) and mortality (Doll and Peto, 1976; Doll *et al.*, 1980; Kuller *et al.*, 1989) resulting from COPD are strongly related to smoking.

For men, the observed rise in risk of death from COPD between the ages of 55 and 74, among those born between 1871 and 1901, is at least partially attributable to the acceleration in the uptake of smoking during the second decade of the twentieth century (see Chapter 9). The influence of the later smoking epidemic among women is less clear. It may be too early to see the cohort effect on COPD mortality as a result of smoking in women.

The decline in risk of death caused by COPD in 55–74-year-old men, but not women, since 1968, coincides with the decreased prevalence of smoking among men since that time. This trend would be consistent with the known benefits of smoking cessation.

Figure 20.6

Spells of certified incapacity due to sickness or invalidity, males

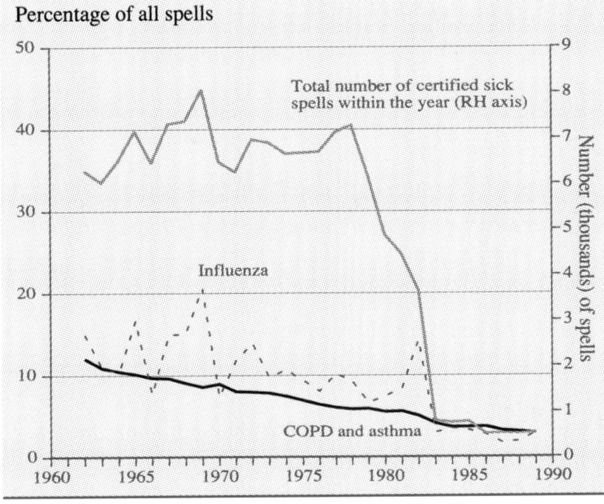

Percentage of all spells

Figure 20.5

Deaths due to COPD: 1958–91

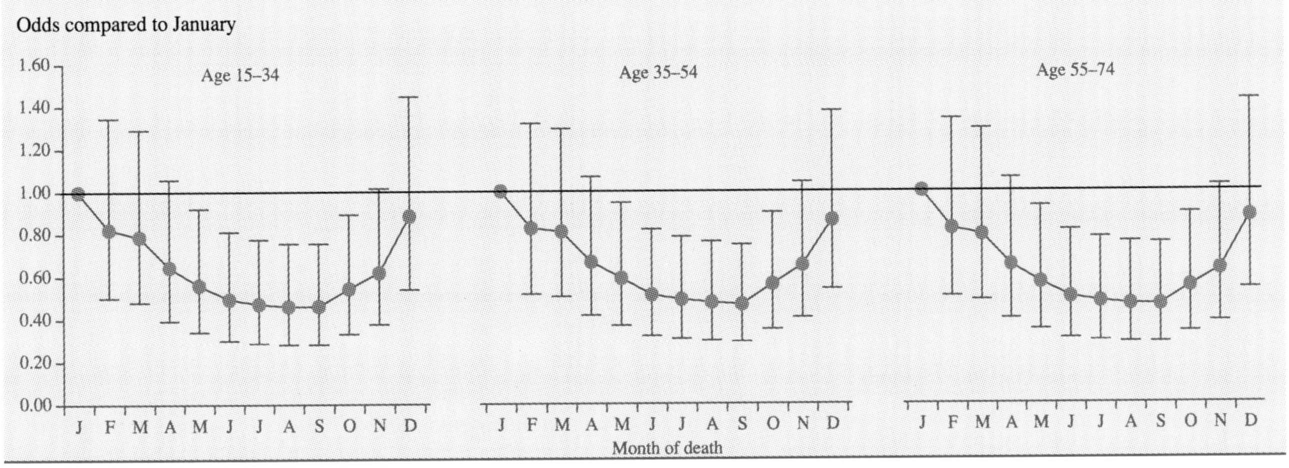

Odds compared to January

Month of death

The rise in risk of death in over-55-year-olds among men born between 1871 and 1901 is superimposed on a downward trend before and after those years. This trend is not consistent with changes in smoking and other explanations must be sought, including changes in the incidence of serious childhood infections, levels of air pollution, conditions for growth, and occupational exposure to dust and fumes.

Serious childhood infections

Early respiratory infections have long been thought to play a role in the development of subsequent respiratory illness. A history of childhood respiratory illness is frequently associated with adult respiratory symptoms (Colley *et al.*, 1973; Lebowitz, 1981), reduced lung function in adult life (Yamaguchi *et al.*, 1988; Barker *et al.*, 1991; Shaheen *et al.*, 1994) and mortality caused by chronic bronchitis (Barker and Osmond, 1986; Barker *et al.*, 1988, 1989). They also predict respiratory illnesses later in childhood (Holland *et al.*, 1969; Loughlin and Taussig, 1979; Voter *et al.*, 1988; Gold *et al.*, 1989; Strope *et al.*, 1991).

Unfortunately, there are many factors that make these studies difficult to interpret (Samet *et al.*, 1983). Many studies had problems of recall bias (Holland *et al.*, 1969; Lebowitz, 1981; Yamaguchi *et al.*, 1988) or selection bias (Loughlin and Taussig, 1979; Voter *et al.*, 1988; Gold *et al.*, 1989; Strope *et al.*, 1991) and others were ecological studies (Barker and Osmond, 1986; Barker *et al.*, 1989). In some instances, early respiratory illness is the first manifestation of subsequent chronic respiratory illness rather than a cause of it (Martinez *et al.*, 1988).

The incidence of fatal measles and whooping cough in children less than 5 years old was high and changed little between 1847 and 1900 (see Figure 20.7). In the first 20 years of this century there was a gradual decline, and after 1920 the rate of early childhood mortality caused by both these illnesses declined rapidly. The pattern of temporal variation of influenza mortality in children under 5 years of age is unusual, but mortality was high during the first two decades of this century (see Figure 20.7). Impressive though the reductions in serious childhood infections since the 1920s are, they cannot explain the decline in risk of death caused by COPD in successive cohorts born during the nineteenth century.

Air pollution

During the 1950s and early 1960s in London, severe foggy winters were associated with substantial excess mortality (Logan, 1949, 1953, 1956; Bradley *et al.*, 1958; Martin and Bradley, 1960; Martin, 1961, 1964). Deaths occurred mainly in elderly subjects with chronic cardiorespiratory illness. It was thought that excess mortality only occurred when particulate or sulphur dioxide (SO_2) pollution levels were very high (Holland *et al.*, 1979; Ware *et al.*, 1981). However, this concept of a threshold has been challenged in recent studies. Examination of the relationship between daily suspended particulate levels and daily mortality using data collected in London and several American cities (Ozkaynak and Spengler, 1985; Schwartz and Marcus, 1990; Schwartz, 1991; Pope *et al.*, 1992; Schwartz and Dockery, 1992a, b; Schwartz *et al.*, 1993) have revealed a dose-response relationship which exists throughout the range of exposure. These studies all show a significant effect of this form of pollution on cardiovascular and respiratory mortality. The effect is strongest among people aged over 65 (Schwartz and Dockery, 1992a).

The evidence for an association between long-term exposure to air pollution and mortality is conflicting. An index of pollution based on fuel consumption in 95 London and county boroughs between 1969 and 1973 showed no relationship to respiratory mortality in people aged 45–74 (Chinn *et al.*, 1981). This was in contrast to similar studies conducted over the preceding two decades (when pollution levels were higher) which had shown an association between this index and mortality. In a cross-sectional analysis of data from 98 districts across the USA there was a significant association between long-term particulate exposure and mortality rates (Ozkaynak and Spengler, 1985). Recent longitudinal data from the Six Cities Study in the USA have shown an increased risk for cardiopulmonary and lung cancer mortality, although not all cause mortality among subjects living in more polluted cities (Dockery *et al.*, 1993).

Although there is no continuous record of air monitoring back to the nineteenth century, it seems likely that air pollution was worse in the latter part of that century than during this century (Brimblecombe, 1987). Brimblecombe has combined data from several sources to show that the frequency of foggy days in London increased between 1750 and 1890 and declined rapidly after the turn of the twentieth century (Brimblecombe, 1987, p. 114). Furthermore, measures of smoke in London air during the 1880s revealed mean levels higher than those recorded in winters during the 1950s (Brimblecombe, 1987, p. 153). The major source of respirable air pollutants before the 1960s was the burning of coal, which yields particulate matter (black smoke) and SO_2. Total coal output increased from 104.5 mega-tonnes in 1868 to a peak of 287.4 mega-tonnes in 1913 and has declined since

---

Figure 20.7

Mortality due to measles, influenza and whooping cough in children aged below 5 years

Death rate per 1,000 (log scale)

Years with no deaths are shown with rate = 0.0001

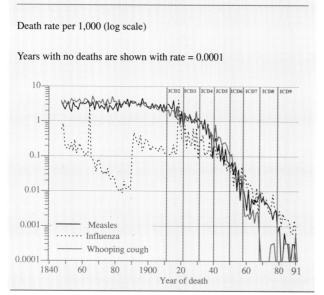

— Measles
····· Influenza
— Whooping cough

Year of death

Figure 20.8

Pollutant emissions in the United Kingdom 1950–90

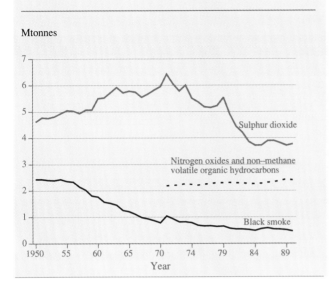

Mtonnes

then to 91.1 mega-tonnes in 1991–92 (Anon, 1964; British Coal Corporation, 1992), providing further evidence of a long-term decline in exposure to this form of air pollution. Since 1950, an annual emissions inventory has been published (Warren Spring Laboratory, 1972; Gillham et al., 1992) giving a national perspective on trends in air pollutants. Particulate emissions declined steeply after 1956 (see Figure 20.8), resulting from the introduction of the Clean Air Act in that year. The decline continued until the early 1970s but has flattened out since then. Total emissions of black smoke pollution are now less than one fifth of their level in 1950. Similar trends were observed for the output of SO_2 (Warren Spring Laboratory, 1972; Gillham et al., 1992).

Although the data are not conclusive, as mentioned in the previous paragraph it seems likely that particulate and SO_2 pollution in urban areas were at their worst in the latter part of the last century and the first 20 years of this century. The subsequent decline in this form of pollution is consistent with the cohort trend in COPD mortality. The steepest decline in particulate pollution occurred during the early 1960s. This precedes the decrease in mortality in men, which started from 1968, and hence acute effects of particulate pollution cannot explain the observed period trend.

Occupational exposures

Subjects exposed to dust, gases or chemical fumes at work have an increased risk of respiratory symptoms and, at least in the case of dust exposure, reduced lung function (Kauffmann et al., 1982; Krzyzanowski and Kauffmann, 1988; Viegi et al., 1991; Xu et al., 1992). Coal miners in the USA and the United Kingdom and gold miners in South Africa also exhibit a decrease in lung function, which is correlated with the extent of exposure to the mining seam (Love and Miller, 1982; Attfield, 1985; Hnizdo, 1992; Soutar et al., 1993).

Changes in occupational dust and fume exposure during the past 150 years are difficult to quantify. Census data on occupational groups are available from 1841–1981. However,

changes in the system of classification make the assessment of a continuous time series very difficult. Figure 6.10 of Chapter 6 shows that the proportion of the workforce engaged in mining reached a peak in 1911, when 9 per cent of economically active men were engaged in this occupation. In 1981 only 1 per cent of workers were miners, and the proportion has declined further since then. This decline has been accompanied, in the past 20–30 years, by an improvement in work practices, resulting in a decrease in their dust exposure. Employment in manufacturing industries increased between 1841 and 1951 and has reached a plateau since then. However, the nature of manufacturing and of work practices has changed markedly over the past 150 years.

It is likely that cumulative exposure to harmful agents at work has reduced, which may, in part, explain the cohort trend for decreasing mortality as a result of COPD.

Birth-weight, growth and development

The influence of antenatal factors in the development of COPD was established by the long-term follow-up of boys born in Hertfordshire in the period 1911–30 (Barker et al., 1991). Adult lung function was found to be significantly correlated with birth-weight: a 1 standard deviation difference in birth-weight predicting a 70 ml difference in FEV_1 (forced expiration volume in one second) in adult life. This relation suggests that in utero differences in lung growth have a life-long effect. Although the number of airways is fixed at birth, the number of alveoli increases until the age of 8 years and the size of alveoli and airways increases until growth of the chest wall is complete (Hogg, 1971). Hence, final lung function may be influenced by factors operating at any time during growth and development.

Data on trends in growth and development are described in Chapter 7. There has been a steady increase in the average height of working-class 15-year-old boys from 146 cm in 1850 to 169 cm in 1950 (Floud et al., 1990, p. 185). Cameron reviewed data on heights of schoolchildren collected during six London County Council surveys conducted in 1905, 1938, 1949, 1954, 1959 and 1966 (Cameron, 1979), and showed a progressive increase in height-for-age in both sexes throughout this period. However, this increase may not be accompanied by a proportional increase in the size of the thorax. The substantial increase in height of Japanese children and adults between 1957 and 1977 was entirely confined to an increase in leg length (Tanner et al., 1982).

It is plausible, but speculative, that the increase in height of schoolchildren during this century was accompanied by enhanced thoracic size, and hence lung size. As the proportional rate of decline in lung function after the cessation of growth is independent of the absolute value of FEV_1 (Fletcher et al., 1976), the absolute magnitude of FEV_1 at age 25 must be proportional to its absolute magnitude towards the end of life. Assuming the risk of death due to COPD is related to both the absolute and the percentage predicted FEV_1, improvements in lung growth would be expected to reduce the risk of death resulting from COPD. This would be consistent with Barker's data concerning in utero influences on adult lung function (Barker et al., 1991) but may also relate to postnatal influences on growth, including improvements in childhood nutrition.

Diagnosis and therapeutics

In spite of the changes in the ICD, the conditions chronic bronchitis, bronchiectasis and emphysema have been recognised in essentially the same form throughout this century and have probably been diagnosed as such (Osler, 1892; Allchin, 1902; Price, 1922; Beaumont, 1932). The overlap between chronic asthma and emphysema is discussed in section 20.4.

Although diagnostic advances, including the use of chest radiographs and the measurement of vital capacity (Price, 1922, p. 994), have increased the sensitivity and specificity of early diagnosis of COPD, they have probably not greatly altered the rate of death certificate diagnosis of this disease.

In the USA the false-positive rate for attributing death to chronic airway disease is less than 5 per cent (Mitchell *et al.*, 1971; Camilli *et al.*, 1991); but in Colorado during the 1960s the false-negative rate was 24 per cent (Mitchell *et al.*, 1971). The false-negative rate was lower in older subjects. Whether comparable figures apply to Britain is unknown, but there is evidence, within Britain and Europe, that doctors differ in their propensity to attribute chronic bronchitis, emphysema and asthma as causes of death (Gau and Diehl, 1982; Farebrother *et al.*, 1985; Burney, 1989). However, this is more likely to influence mortality rates for asthma than for COPD.

Therapeutic recommendations for chronic bronchitis and emphysema in the early part of this century included spending winter in warmer climates and the use of various inhaled therapies (Osler, 1892, pp. 494–5; Allchin, 1902, pp. 164–6; Price, 1922, p. 962; Beaumont, 1932, pp. 121–2). Inhaled bronchodilators became available in the 1920s (see section 20.4) and their introduction may be related to the decrease in mortality observed at that time. On the other hand, the subsequent advent of antibiotics from the late 1930s was not associated with any important change in mortality attributable to COPD. Home oxygen therapy for patients with hypoxaemia caused by COPD was introduced around 1968, but seems

unlikely to have had a major impact on mortality because, although male mortality declined, female mortality did not.

20.3.5 Conclusion

Examination of trends suggests that the separate epidemics of smoking in men and women have had important effects on mortality resulting from COPD during this century. However, the trends attributable to smoking are superimposed on a declining cohort trend for this disease. Decreasing particulate and SO_2 air pollution, reduction in occupational exposure to dust and fumes, and improvements in antenatal and postnatal growth may each have played a beneficial role.

20.4 Asthma

20.4.1 Coding

In ICD1 (1901–10), asthma and emphysema were coded as a single category. With the introduction of ICD4 (1931), 'summer bronchitis' and 'hayfever' were added to asthma as previously defined. During the currency of ICD5 (1940–50) many deaths were classified as asthma complicated by myocardial disease. These cases are not included in the graphs presented here. Also in 1940 the instructions to coders were changed so that, when more than one cause was specified, the primary cause was to be inferred from the certifier's statement rather than by applying rules of precedence. With ICD6 (1951) asthma was placed in the chapter for allergic diseases. The ICD5 changes were partially reversed with the introduction of ICD7 in 1958. If the certificate mentioned bronchitis as well as asthma, and the asthma was not specified as allergic, the case was assigned to bronchitis. Previously it would have been assigned to asthma. With ICD8 (1968) asthma was removed from the allergic diseases chapter to the respiratory diseases chapter. With ICD9 (1979) the precedence for bronchitis was removed. The main impact of this change was in deaths over the age of 44 (Stewart and Nunn, 1985). The effect of the 1984 ONS coding instruction on asthma mortality rates in people under 75 was less than 4 per cent.

Table 20.3

Conversion factors used to adjust rates for asthma prior to each change in the ICD

Age	ICD5 1939 M	F	ICD6 1949 M	F	ICD7 1957* M	F	ICD8 1967 M	F	ICD9 1978** M	F
5–14	1.00	1.00	1.11	1.00	1.00	0.86	0.98	1.00	1.30	1.30
15–24	1.00	1.04	1.19	1.03	0.91	0.96	0.95	0.97	1.06	1.06
25–34	1.03	1.04	1.08	1.23	0.82	0.84	0.94	0.95	1.06	1.06
35–44	1.09	1.06	1.38	1.16	0.89	0.81	0.94	0.97	1.06	1.06
45–54	1.09	1.11	1.46	1.30	0.65	0.84	0.90	0.97	1.33	1.33
55–64	1.06	1.12	1.58	1.61	0.67	0.75	0.87	0.97	1.33	1.33
65–74	1.06	1.16	1.69	1.54	0.62	0.62	0.87	0.96	1.34	1.34

*   Based on dual coding of deaths occurring from July to December, 1957.
** Based on dual coding of a 25 per cent sample of deaths occurring in 1978 (Stewart, 1985).
Estimates based on broad age-ranges (not sex-specific): 1–14 years, 15–44 years, 45–64 years and 65 years and over.

The age- and sex-specific conversion factors for each change in the ICD since 1940 are shown in Table 20.3, based on published analyses of dual coded certificates. Detailed age- and sex-specific rates are not available from the 1978 dual coding sample. Conversion factors for broad age-ranges (for both sexes combined) have been used as an approximation (Stewart and Nunn, 1985). These conversion factors were used in constructing the graphs and for the age-period-cohort analysis. No conversion factors are available for changes that occurred before 1939.

20.4.2   Trends in mortality

Age-period-cohort analysis

Table 20.4 shows the comparison of models constructed according to the method of Clayton and Schifflers (1987) using data for males aged 5–54 dying from asthma. After adjustment for age, fluctuations in mortality rates beyond those explained by a linear drift or trend are influenced to a significant extent by both period of death and cohort of birth. Among women the non-drift cohort effects were not quite significant but the non-drift period effects were (data not shown).

Period effects (Figure 20.9)

The most prominent feature of the pattern of asthma mortality during this century is the epidemic of the 1960s. The rise in asthma deaths started between 1959 and 1961, peaked in 1965 and 1966, and returned to pre-epidemic levels by 1970. It affected younger age-groups more than older. Short-term and less marked increases in asthma mortality occurred in 1915–19, 1940 (major change in coding) and 1981–87.

There has been no overall trend in mortality in younger age-groups over the course of this century. However, in men aged 35 and over and in women aged 55 and over, there was a gradual decline in mortality between 1901 and 1960. These

Table 20.4

Age-period-cohort analysis of deaths occurring between 1911 and 1991 among men, aged 5–54, which were attributed to asthma

Model	Deviance	Degrees of freedom
1. Age + Drift	699.5	149
2. Age + Cohort	356.9	126
3. Age + Period	613.2	135
4. Age + Cohort + Period	169.2	112

Model comparisons	Change in deviance	Degrees of freedom
2. and 1. (cohort)	342.6	23**
3. and 1. (period)	86.3	14**
4. and 2. (period)	187.7	14**
4. and 3. (cohort)	444.0	23**
4. and 1.	530.3	37**

**	P<0.001

are the age-groups in which the diagnosis of asthma is least specific and most likely to change over time; hence these trends need to be interpreted with caution.

Cohort effects (Figure 20.10)

In women there was a rising generational trend in the first half of the century in the risk of subsequent death resulting from asthma between ages 5 and 24. This was also apparent for men dying between ages 15 and 24. Among older age-groups the downward trend seen in the period graph was also apparent when mortality was plotted by year of birth.

Figure 20.9

Asthma death rate by year of death 1901–91

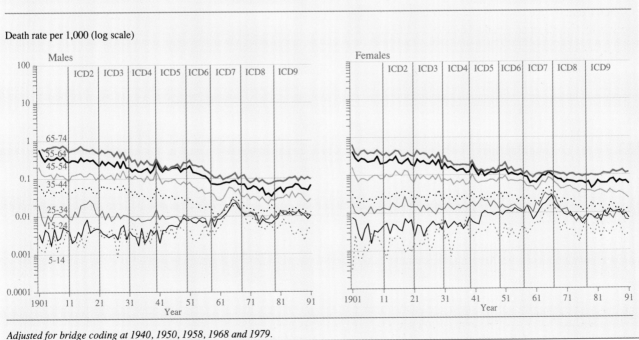

Death rate per 1,000 (log scale)

Adjusted for bridge coding at 1940, 1950, 1958, 1968 and 1979.

Age and sex effects

The increased risk of death with advancing age is apparent in both the period and the cohort plots. The epidemics of 1915–19 and the 1960s affected the younger age-groups disproportionately.

Before 1960, mortality in 35–74-year-olds was higher in men than in women. This sex distribution has reversed since 1960. In 15–34-year-olds there was little difference between the sexes before 1930. From then until 1968, mortality was higher in women, and since 1968, mortality has been higher in men in this age-group.

Women born before 1946 were more likely than men to die from asthma between the ages of 15 and 34, but since then, there is little difference between the sexes.

Seasonal trends (Figure 20.11)

There was significant seasonality in asthma mortality in all age-groups. However, there were important differences between age-groups in the direction and magnitude of this seasonal variation. Risk of death resulting from asthma among 5–34-year-olds reached a peak in August and a nadir in February. The seasonal ratio (August to February) was 2.00 for men and 1.50 for women in this age range. Among 55–74 year olds, a reverse trend was apparent, although it was less marked. The peak in mortality in this age-group was in January and the nadir in September. The seasonal ratio estimated from the sinusoidal model was 1.27 (February to August). In the intermediate age-group, the seasonal trend ratio (July to January) was much smaller (1.08).

There was also a significant seasonal variation in the risk of death resulting from asthma according to month of birth among 5–34-year-old males, but not females in this age-group.

The highest risk was for boys born in September (seasonal ratio 1.24). Less variation was seen in the older age-groups, with maximum seasonal ratios less than 1.2.

20.4.3 Trends in morbidity

Secular trend in hospital admissions (Figure 20.12)

There has been a progressive rise in hospital admissions for asthma from when these data were first collected in 1958 until the end of the HIPE data collection in 1985 (Burney, 1993). Recent Hospital Episodes Statistics (HES) data from 1989–92 show that this increase has flattened out and in some cases reversed.

The cross-sectional (period) data show an age-dependent variation in admission rate trends, the steepest increase being seen in the youngest age-groups. However, the data for men by year of birth (see Figure 20.13) demonstrate a uniform increase in admission rates in all age-groups up to 44 years. A similar pattern is seen among women, although admission rates in 15–44-year-olds are higher than in younger girls and lower than in older women. One interpretation of the data would be that the increase in admission rates is predominantly a cohort effect.

Seasonal trends in hospital admissions (Figure 20.14)

In the period 1968–85, the risk of admission to hospital for 5–34-year-olds reached a peak in September and October and was lowest in February. The seasonal ratio among 5–34-years olds was 1.97 for males and 1.57 for females (both September to March). There was no significant seasonal trend among 35–54-year-olds, and the trend among 55–74-year-olds was weak, peaking in February and March with a seasonal ratio of 1.13.

Figure 20.10

Asthma death rate by year of birth

Death rate per 1,000 (log scale)

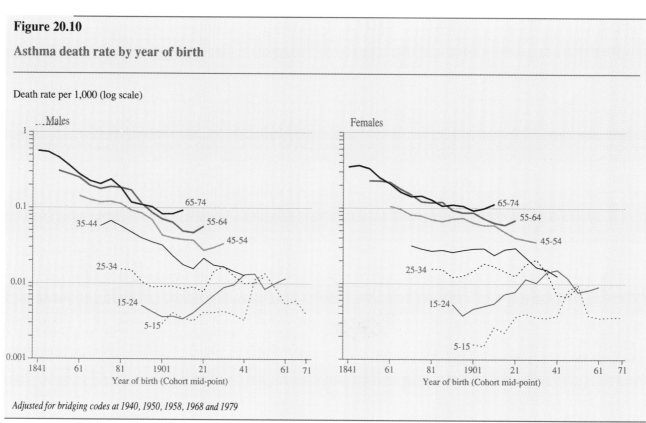

Adjusted for bridging codes at 1940, 1950, 1958, 1968 and 1979

Figure 20.11

Deaths due to asthma, 1958–91

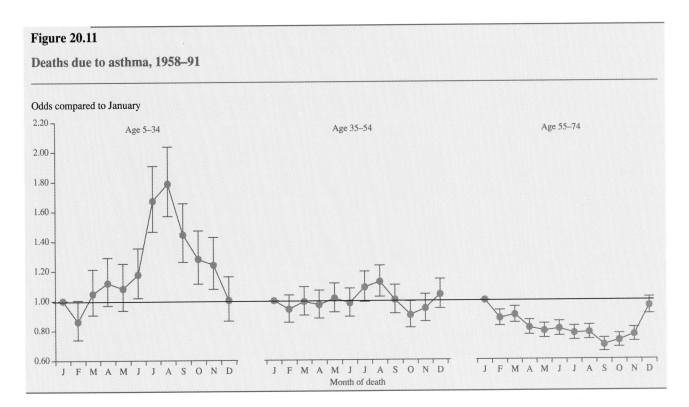

Odds compared to January

Age 5–34   Age 35–54   Age 55–74

Month of death

Figure 20.12

Admissions for asthma, 1957–85

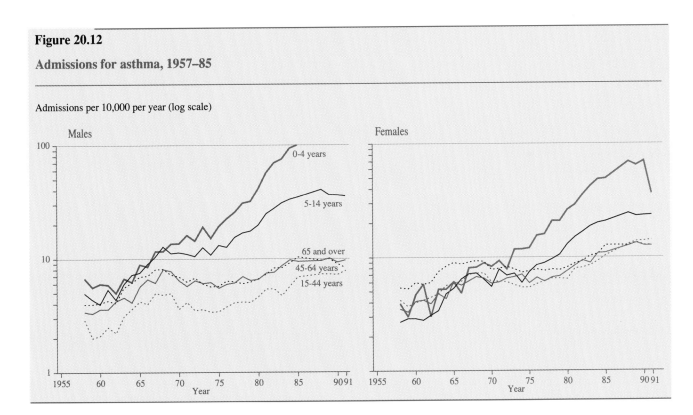

Admissions per 10,000 per year (log scale)

Males   Females

20.4.4 Interpretation

Time trends

Important changes in diagnostic fashion, especially in older age-groups, and changes in the ICD and in instructions to coders, mean that long-term time trends are subject to considerable error and must be interpreted with caution.

Hospital admission and mortality data show different patterns for the period for which they overlap. Sharply rising admission rates in all age-groups up to 44 years are not accompanied by any substantial similar trend in mortality in these age-groups over the same period. There are several possible explanations. Admissions may rise if there is a change in policy that favours earlier hospitalisation for patients experiencing exacerbations of asthma. This shift in policy may sig-

Figure 20.13

Admissions for asthma, 1957–85 by year of birth

Admission per 10,000 per year (log scale)

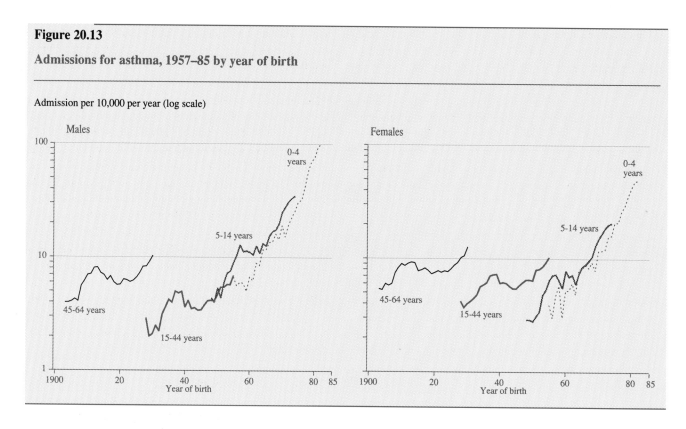

Figure 20.14

Hospital admissions due to asthma: 1968–85

Odds compared to January

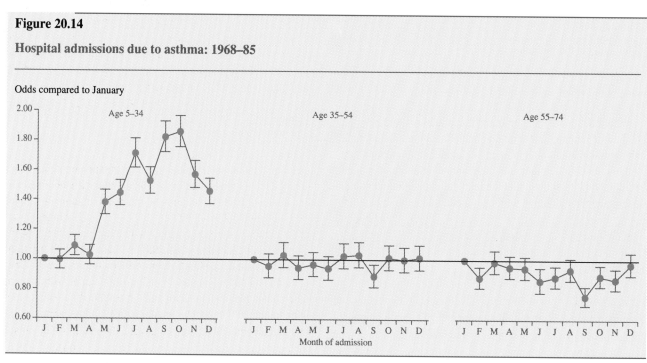

nify improved management of severe asthma, and decrease the risk of death resulting from asthma.

Differences in the way changes in diagnostic fashion influence hospital admission and mortality statistics are feasible. For example, the sensitivity of the diagnosis of asthma in a young adult or child who dies of this disease may be higher than the sensitivity of this diagnosis among those admitted to hospital, some of whom may be labelled as having bronchitis. Part of the increase in hospital admission rates for asthma may be the result of an increasing tendency to apply this diagnosis on admission to hospital, a trend that need not have been accompanied by a similar trend in death certification.

It seems likely that the propensity to attribute deaths to asthma in middle-aged or elderly patients is greater now than it would have been in the first half of this century. Attacks of acute asthma were well recognised at the beginning of the century (Osler, 1892, p. 499; Allchin, 1902, p. 177). However, chronic asthma was not clearly distinguished from emphysema. The prognosis for repeated attacks of asthma was thought to be the development of chronic emphysema (Osler, 1892, p. 500; Price, 1922, p. 972). Death attributable to asthma was rare. In fact, Osler states: 'We have no knowledge of the morbid anatomy of true asthma. Death during attacks is unknown' (Osler, 1892, p. 500). For this reason, we can assume that some patients whose death would now be attributed to chronic asthma would then have been certified as dying from emphysema. This diagnostic trend is at odds with the apparently higher mortality rate from asthma, especially in older age-groups, at that time.

There are reasons to believe that neither hospital admissions nor mortality accurately reflects changes in the prevalence of the disease. As noted above, long-term time trends are difficult to interpret. Furthermore, factors that influence the outcome of asthma for better or worse are not all the same as those that influence the likelihood of acquiring the disease. The epidemic of mortality and hospital admissions in the 1960s was almost certainly attributable to the use of high-dose, non-β_2-selective aerosols (Inman and Adelstein, 1969; Stolley and Schinnar, 1978).

Several studies have shown an increase in the prevalence of reported symptoms of asthma and reported diagnoses of asthma over the past 20–30 years in Britain (Morrison Smith, 1976; Burr et al., 1989; Burney et al., 1990; Ninan and Russell, 1992; Whincup et al., 1993). These data deal with change over a relatively recent period and there are problems with their interpretation. All except one rely on questionnaire data and, in the one that did use an objective test – the exercise challenge test (Burr et al., 1989) – the change in the prevalence of airway hyper-responsiveness to exercise was only apparent at the severe end of the range. The remaining studies could be influenced by changes in diagnostic fashion, although the measurement of symptoms is less subject to this confounder than the measurement of diagnosed asthma. Three studies involve only two measurements at widely spaced intervals (Burr et al., 1989; Ninan and Russell, 1992; Whincup et al., 1993) and at least one was conducted in a geographically constrained area in which migration has substantially changed the ethnic mix of the local population (Morrison Smith, 1976). Nevertheless, taken as a group, these studies do support the evidence from the hospital admission data that there has been an increase in the prevalence of asthma, at least in younger age-groups, over the past 20–30 years.

Risk factors

Risk factors operating around the time of the development of asthma are probably at least partly responsible for the rise in the prevalence in asthma. The presence of a significant cohort effect, which is especially pronounced in the data for hospital admissions, supports this hypothesis, but cannot distinguish whether the risk factors are pre- or postnatal, or both.

Little is known about the long-term time trends in most of the important risk factors for atopy, asthma and poor outcomes of asthma. Allergen exposure is relevant to all of these (Korsgaard, 1983; Sotomayor et al., 1984; Madonini et al., 1987; Platts-Mills et al., 1987; Green et al., 1989; Karjalainen et al., 1989; Lau et al., 1989; Crimi et al., 1990; Price et al., 1990; Sporik et al., 1990; Charpin et al., 1991; O'Halloran et al., 1991; Arshad et al., 1992; Bellomo et al., 1992). However, measurement of allergen exposure in a reproducible fashion has only been attempted in recent years and there are no data about changes in allergen exposure. Occupational asthma (Chan-Yeung and Lam, 1986; Blanc, 1987) is relatively rare

and is attributed to highly specific exposures. Data on this are lacking and clearly cannot explain the observed trends in childhood asthma.

It has been suggested that household size is inversely related to the clinical manifestations of atopy (Lebowitz et al., 1987; Strachan, 1989; Williams et al., 1992) and, more specifically, that the number of older siblings is inversely related to the risk of having allergic diseases (Strachan, 1989). This is not universally agreed, however, and one study has found the reverse: an increased prevalence of atopy in children from large families (Davis and Bulpitt, 1981). Furthermore, the observed mortality trends for asthma do not reflect the hypothesised relationship of family size, birth order and risk of atopy. Since 1938 there have been only small changes in the proportion of first, second, third or higher order births (OPCS, 1987). The proportion of children who were the first in a family declined to a nadir in 1960 but has increased since then. There have been no accompanying consistent cohort trends in the risk of death caused by asthma.

The Department of Health Committee on the Medical Effects of Air Pollutants examined the available evidence of possible links between outdoor air pollution and asthma (COMEAP, 1995). They concluded that while there is some epidemiological evidence that air pollution may provoke acute asthmatic attacks or aggravate existing chronic asthma, the effect is likely to be small and unimportant when compared with other factors, such as infections and allergens, which are known to provoke attacks. The increase in asthma over the past thirty years is unlikely to be the result of changes in air pollution.

Therapeutics

The major therapeutic advances in the management of asthma during this century started in the 1920s when the use of adrenaline by injection or inhalation was recommended (Osler and McCrea, 1920; Price, 1922, p. 972). Although strong coffee was long recognised as helpful in acute attacks, aminophylline was not recommended until the late 1940s (Christian, 1947; Beaumont, 1948; Young and Beaumont, 1950). Oral corticosteroids in the treatment of severe chronic asthma were first recommended in Beaumont's textbook in the 1950s (Beaumont, 1953; Young et al., 1956). Subsequent refinements since the 1950s have included the introduction of selective ß-agonists (Inman and Adelstein, 1969), selective β_2-agonists (Choo-Kang et al., 1969; Pride, 1969), cromoglycate (Howell and Altounyan, 1967; Anon, 1971; Silverman et al., 1972) and inhaled corticosteroids (Anon, 1972; Clark, 1972; Morrow Brown et al., 1972; Gaddie et al., 1973). The epidemic in the 1960s coincided closely with the rise and fall in sales of isoprenaline aerosol bronchodilators (Inman and Adelstein, 1969). However, there are no other sudden changes in mortality or admission rates which coincide with the other important therapeutic milestones for this disease.

Seasonal trends

There is a strong seasonal trend, peaking in late summer and early autumn, in hospital admissions and deaths attributed to asthma among subjects less than 35 years of age. The peak is slightly earlier for deaths than for hospital admissions. A reverse trend, peaking in January, is seen for deaths, and possibly admissions, in the oldest age-groups. This marked difference in trend in older subjects implies that different factors are responsible for exacerbations of asthma in these age-groups.

A seasonal peak in asthma admissions for children and young adults during autumn has been noted in several other studies in Europe and North America (Storr and Lenney, 1989; Bates et al., 1990; Mao et al., 1990; Weiss, 1990; Priftis et al., 1993). Bates et al. (1990) noted that the seasonal trend was not present in adults over 60 years. Similar to the data reported here, Weiss (1990) found a different and less marked seasonal pattern among people aged 35 and over in the USA. In this age-group, the highest admission rates were in winter. Weiss also found that the seasonal trend in asthma mortality differed between younger and older subjects. The peak in mortality in 5–34-year-olds was in July, 2 months earlier than the peak in admission rates. Storr and Lenney (1989) examined admissions to a children's hospital in Brighton and found several peaks in admission rates. The highest peak was in September but lesser peaks occurred at intervals throughout the year – particularly after school holidays.

The explanation for the seasonal pattern, and for the interaction with age, is not clear. Present evidence suggests that viral infections, in particular with rhinovirus, may be an important trigger for exacerbations of asthma in childhood (Johnston et al., 1995). Storr and Lenney (1989) hypothesised that the post-school holiday peak in hospital admissions with asthma might be attributable to increased transmission of respiratory tract viruses in the school environment. On the other hand, the known epidemiology of respiratory viral and mycoplasma diseases does not conform to the pattern observed for asthma admissions. In the United Kingdom, respiratory syncytial virus infections and influenza both occur as annual winter epidemics (Chakraverty et al., 1986; Winter and Inglis, 1987). Parainfluenza type 3 is a summer infection (Easton and Elgin, 1989) and mycoplasma pneumonia is endemic, with occasional epidemics peaking in winter (Noah, 1974). There are conflicting data on the seasonal pattern for rhinovirus infections. Using data collected over an 11-year period from several sources, Roebuck (1976) found the highest incidence of rhinovirus infections was in the months September to January. This pattern does partially overlap with the seasonal pattern in asthma admissions. However, more recent data from the PHLS laboratories (1978–87) show a very different pattern, with the highest reported identification of rhinovirus infection in the second quarter of the year. In both cases there is a year-round incidence with only modest seasonality. The epidemiological evidence linking the observed early autumn peak in asthma admissions to viral infections must be regarded as inconclusive.

Asthma becomes more severe during the pollen season in pollen-allergic patients (Sotomayor et al., 1984; Karjalainen et al., 1989; Crimi et al., 1990). This may be relevant to the lesser peak in admissions seen in July, but would not explain the large peak seen in autumn. Other outdoor allergens, such as moulds, may play a role. In 40 houses in Manchester, levels of house-dust mite allergen were higher in October than in other seasons; however, the variation was of a relatively small magnitude (Kalra et al., 1992) and probably does not explain the observed seasonal variation.

Some meteorological variables may be directly or indirectly responsible, however. A direct effect of temperature seems unlikely because it is relatively moderate in the month when admissions are at a maximum. Air pollution follows a seasonal cycle but particulates, which have been implicated the most in exacerbations of asthma (Forsberg et al., 1993), peak in winter and this, therefore, does not explain the observed pattern. SO_2 levels are now low in England and Wales and do not show marked seasonality (Air Monitoring Group, 1994). Ozone levels are higher in the summer months (Air Monitoring Group, 1994) but levels seen in the United Kingdom are low (Broughton, 1987) compared with international standards and are unlikely to cause many exacerbations of asthma. Oxides of nitrogen have recently been implicated in enhanced allergen responsiveness in people with asthma (Devalia et al., 1994). Levels of this pollutant have increased over the last decade (Gillham et al., 1992) but show no marked seasonal pattern (Air Monitoring Group, 1994). Seasonal variation in air pollutants is unlikely to explain the observed periodicity of asthma admissions.

It is perhaps not surprising that we found only a weak association between risk of death resulting from asthma and month of birth. The explanation for the observed association is unknown. It is unlikely to be attributable to seasonal variation in exposure to pollens because there is little association between month of birth and grass sensitivity (Burney, 1992).

20.4.5 Conclusion

Asthma has increased over the past 20–30 years under the influence of unidentified factors operating from early in life. At least one important epidemic in asthma mortality in the 1960s can be attributed to the adverse effects of treatment for this disease. The evolution of treatment does not seem to have had any other important effect on the pattern of mortality, although it may have prevented an increase in mortality accompanying the increase in prevalence. The role of allergen exposure, which has been proposed as a key risk factor for atopy, asthma or poor outcomes of asthma, cannot be satisfactorily investigated in this historical context because of the lack of knowledge of time trends in allergen exposure. In young adults the frequency of exacerbations of asthma requiring hospitalisation and the frequency of death resulting from asthma is highest in late summer and early autumn. This seasonal pattern is also unexplained.

20.5 Pneumonia

This section deals with all deaths attributed to non-tuberculous pneumonia and, separately, with the subset of deaths attributed to lobar and pneumococcal pneumonia.

20.5.1 Coding

Until the introduction of ICD8 in 1968, pneumonia was classified, primarily on anatomical grounds, as 'lobar pneumonia, bronchopneumonia and other, unspecified pneumonia'. In ICD8 a microbiological classification was introduced, which included 'viral', 'pneumococcal', 'other bacterial' and various less specific categories.

The most important change in coding practice was the reinterpretation by OPCS of WHO Coding Rule 3 in 1984. This meant that, where 'bronchopneumonia, unspecified' (code 485.0) or 'pneumonia, unspecified' (code 486.0), among others, was the only entry in Part I of the death certificate, and a major disease was listed in Part II, the disease mentioned in Part II was to be coded as the primary cause of death. The conversion factor to compare 1984 mortality with 1983 was 2.22 for 485.0 and 1.85 for 486.0. The effect was most marked among deaths in elderly people.

The reinterpretation of Rule 3 reversed a trend over the preceding 30 years, which could not be adjusted for; so the 1984 rule change was also not adjusted for in the graphs or the analysis.

The introduction of ICD5 in 1940 resulted in the removal of 'suffocative bronchitis' and 'necrotic pneumonia' and the addition of 'terminal pneumonia' and 'active and acute congestion of the lungs'. This had little impact on reported mortality rates for pneumonia: the net conversion factor, old to new, was 1.040.

20.5.2 Trends in mortality

Age-period-cohort analysis
Table 20.5 shows the comparison of models constructed according to the method of Clayton and Schifflers (1987), using data for men aged 15–74 dying as a result of lobar or pneumococcal pneumonia. After adjustment for age, fluctuations in mortality rates over time, beyond those explained by a linear drift or trend, are influenced to a significant extent by both period of death and cohort of birth. The conclusions are the same for women and when deaths attributable to all forms of pneumonia are examined (data not shown).

Period effects (Figures 20.15 and 20.16)
There was a sharp peak in total mortality resulting from pneumonia in 1918–19 especially in younger people. This was associated with the influenza pandemic at that time and affected mortality caused by lobar pneumonia as well as all

Table 20.5

Age-period-cohort analysis of deaths occurring between 1911 and 1991 among men, aged 15–74, which were attributed to lobar or pneumococcal pneumonia

Model	Deviance	Degrees of freedom
1. Age + Drift	2,511.3	179
2. Age + Cohort	1,053.0	154
3. Age + Period	1,809.1	165
4. Age + Cohort + Period	174.0	140

Model comparisons	Change in deviance	Degrees of freedom
2. and 1. (cohort)	1,458.3	25**
3. and 1. (period)	702.2	14**
4. and 2. (period)	879.0	14**
4. and 3. (cohort)	1,635.1	25**
4. and 1.	2,337.3	39**

**   *P<0.001*

pneumonia. There has been a gradual decline in pneumonia mortality throughout the century. The decline is most apparent in the 15–54-year-olds and was steepest soon after the advent of widely available antibiotics in the 1940s.

There was an increase in mortality reported as the result of lobar pneumonia from 1901, followed by a plateau in the 1920s, a small decrease during the 1930s and a steep decline with the advent of antibiotics.

There was a sudden large reduction in total pneumonia mortality in all age-groups in 1984 with the reinterpretation by OPCS of WHO Rule 3. For 30 years before this there had been little change for 35–54-year-olds and a small increase in 55–74-year-olds. In this oldest age-group a straight line can be drawn linking the steady decline before 1950 with the continued decline after 1984. The area above this line corresponds to excess deaths, which may be the result of the increasing trend before 1984 to identify terminal pneumonia as a cause of death. This rule change mainly affected bronchopneumonia, unspecified and pneumonia, unspecified, and did not affect coding of lobar or pneumococcal pneumonia.

Since 1983 there has been an increase in mortality attributed to pneumonia (but not pneumococcal pneumonia) among those aged 25–44, particularly in men. These will include deaths resulting from the pulmonary manifestations of AIDS.

Cohort effects (Figures 20.17 and 20.18)
There was a steady decline between 1856 and 1956 in the risk, at birth, of subsequently dying from pneumonia during adult life. This is apparent for all pneumonia and for lobar and pneumococcal pneumonia. The plateau and then the re-

Figure 20.15

Pneumonia death rate by year of death

Death rate per 1,000 (log scale)

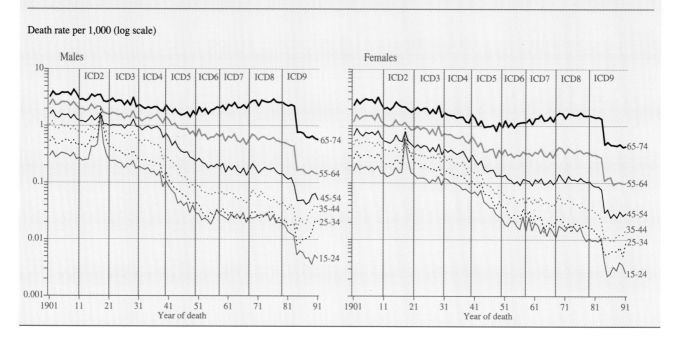

Figure 20.16

Lobar and pneumococcal pneumonia death rate by year of death

Death rate per 1,000 (log scale)

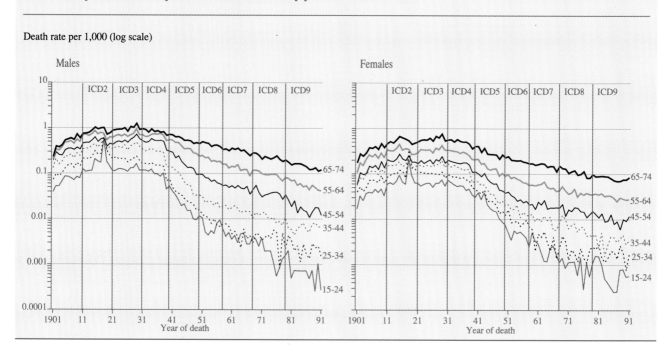

cent steep fall for all pneumonia in the older age-groups is the result of the increasing tendency to list bronchopneumonia as the underlying cause of death in the presence of other serious disease, and correction of this by the reinterpretation of WHO rule 3.

Age and sex effects

The period plots all show increasing risk of death with increasing age at death. However, the cohort plots show that the risk of death from lobar and pneumococcal pneumonia, for a given year of birth, is much less obviously influenced by age. There are two possible explanations: either there is a true interaction between age and period resulting in overlying cohort plots, or the risk is largely independent of age and the main determinant of risk of death from pneumonia, is when the person was born.

Over all periods, cohorts and adult age-groups, the mortality rate for pneumonia has been greater in men than women, although there was little difference in 15–34-year-olds in the period between 1940 and 1960.

Figure 20.17

Pneumonia death rates by year of birth

Death rate per 1,000 (log scale)

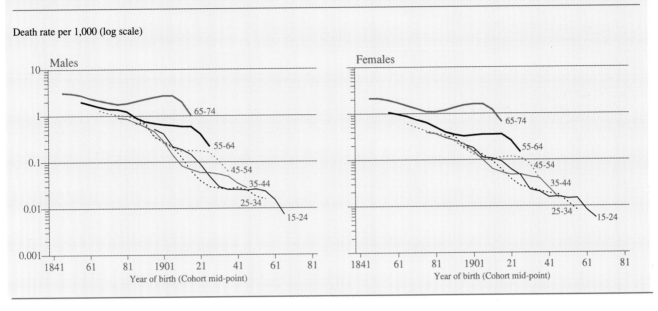

Figure 20.18

Lobar and pneumococcal pneumonia death rates by year of birth

Death rate per 1,000 (log scale)

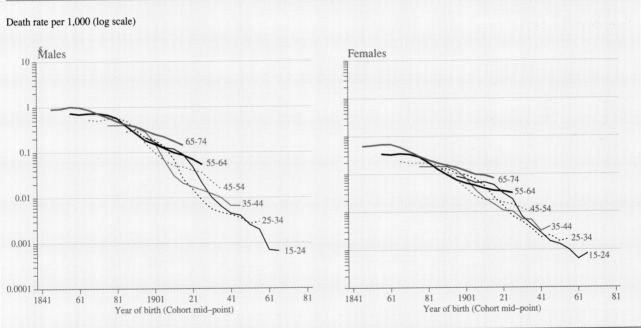

Seasonal trends (Figure 20.19)

There was a pronounced seasonal trend, in all age-groups in the risk of death resulting from pneumococcal pneumonia. Death rates were highest in January and lowest in August and September. The seasonal ratio (February–August) was 2.69 for men and 3.12 for women. There was no significant trend in any age-group in the risk of death according to month of birth.

20.5.3 Interpretation

Mortality and morbidity trends for all pneumonia and for lobar and pneumococcal pneumonia are broadly similar over the period of observation. The exception to this is the impact of OPCS reinterpretation of WHO Rule 3 and the changes in death certification practice over the preceding 30 years which did not affect certification of deaths caused by lobar or pneumococcal pneumonia.

Figure 20.19

Hospital admissions due to lobar and pneumococcal pneumonia: 1968–91

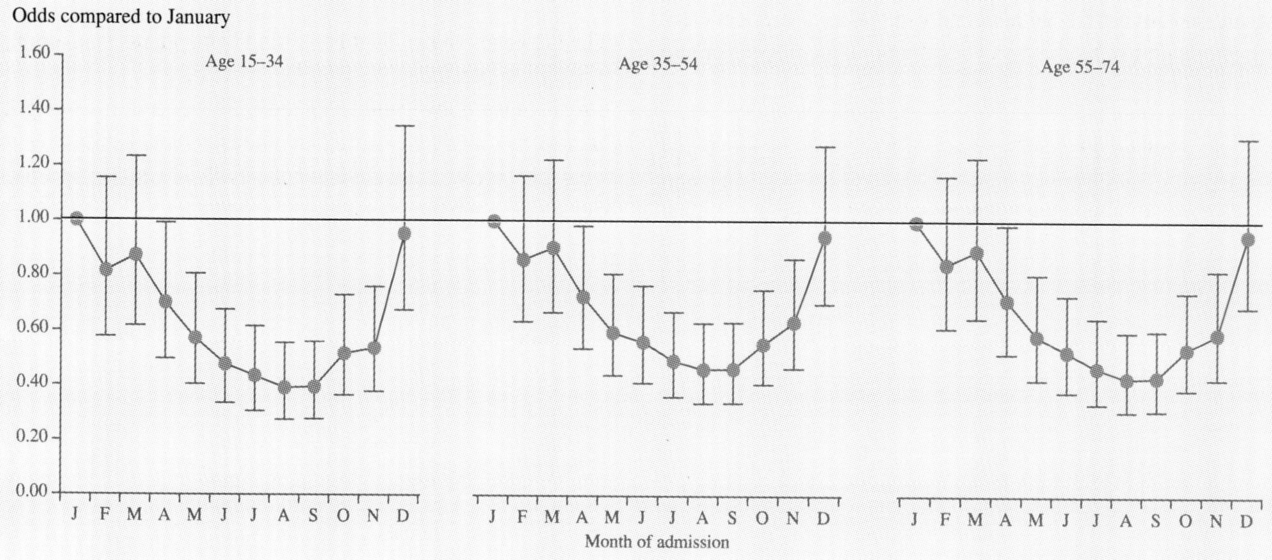

Odds compared to January

Month of admission

The most outstanding features of the time trend in pneumonia mortality are the decline in the death rate since the 1930s and the decline in mortality in all cohorts born since the middle of the last century.

Although the commencement of widespread use of sulphonamides in 1939 (Osler *et al.*, 1938, pp. 511–32; Young, 1941; Beaumont, 1942) resulted in an immediate, large reduction in mortality, this does not explain the subsequent continuing downward trend. Other important therapeutic developments, such as the availability of penicillin after 1946 (Florey, 1946; Christian, 1947) and the introduction of respiratory intensive care in the 1960s (Hilberman, 1975), did not have any perceptible effect on the time trend.

Influenza is a frequent precursor of pneumonia and there is evidence that this virus causes increased adherence of pneumococcal organisms to respiratory epithelium (Plotkowski *et al.*, 1986). Mortality from this disease has also declined steeply during this century (see Chapters 4 and 15). The last major influenza pandemic in 1918–19 resulted in a sharp rise in death resulting from pneumonia. However, it is not certain whether a reduction in the incidence of influenza has contributed to a reduction in pneumonia mortality. The reverse hypothesis, that improved survival from pneumonia has reduced mortality caused by influenza, is equally plausible.

The time trends for the prevalence of chronic diseases which may predispose to pneumonia (La Croix *et al.*, 1989), such as COPD, do not coincide with the time trends for pneumonia mortality.

Household crowding, which has been proposed as a risk factor for pneumonia, has decreased during this century (see

Chapter 10). The average number of people per room in a dwelling decreased from 0.95 in 1911 to 0.54 in 1981. This may have contributed to the continuing decline in pneumonia mortality.

Little is known about factors that may explain the observed cohort effect. The time trend for smoking (see Chapter 9), an important early aetiological factor in many respiratory diseases, is clearly not consistent with the cohort trend for pneumonia. Childhood mortality from measles and whooping cough is probably correlated with the incidence of severe cases of these childhood infections, which may predispose to later respiratory disease. Mortality from these decreased since 1900 but remained high throughout the second half of the nineteenth century, during which time cohorts with successively lower risk of pneumonia mortality were born (see Figure 20.7).

Increased age is commonly regarded as a risk factor for pneumonia mortality. However, the cohort plots suggest that this effect may not be as important as it seems when examined cross-sectionally. The age-period-cohort analysis demonstrates that there is, in fact, an independent effect of age, as well as period and cohort effects. This age effect may be partly masked by an interaction with period; that is, when effective chemotherapy was first available in limited quantities, it tended to be given preferentially to younger patients. This trend was noted at the time by the Registrar General (1947). The seasonal peak in mortality during winter and nadir during summer is explained, in part, by the seasonal increase in viral infections, especially influenza, during winter. Other possible, but not established, explanatory factors include the increased time spent indoors during winter and direct effects of cold weather on the risk of acquiring pneumonia.

20.5.4 Conclusion

The declining trend in mortality caused by pneumonia accelerated in the late 1930s, when antimicrobial chemotherapy became available for widespread use. Other therapeutic innovations do not seem to have had any major impact on the mortality trend.

The effect of antibiotics is followed by a continuing downward trend in mortality. Diminished household crowding, with consequent decrease in the risk of droplet infection, may partially explain this trend. Although the advent of the NHS in 1949 was not accompanied by any acceleration in the rate of decline in mortality, it is conceivable that the continuing downward trend is explained by improved access to medical care.

The increased risk of death resulting from pneumonia among elderly people today may be the manifestation of a cohort effect, those born in the early part of this century being at greater risk of death caused by pneumonia than those born later. The explanation for this cohort effect remains speculative.

Chapter 21

Renal diseases

By
Paul Roderick

Summary

- Over 100 different diseases affect the kidneys, many of which are self limiting, but severe disease may lead to end-stage renal failure (ESRF).

- Developments in understanding of the pathology of kidney disease were led in the nineteenth century by Bright in England and Rayer in Paris, and the first experimental haemodialysis was performed in humans in 1924. However, access problems limited its application to the treatment of acute renal failure. Kidney transplantation was introduced in the 1950s, but rejection was a major problem to be overcome in the 1960s and 1970s.

- Renal failure is often not recorded as the underlying cause of death on death certificates since it tends to be a complication of other diseases. The only sources of data on the incidence and prevalence of renal disease are the National Morbidity Surveys in General Practice. The EDTA provide data on the prevalence of patients on treatment and the incidence of patients onto renal replacement therapy (RRT).

- Mortality from genitourinary disease has declined since 1900, most dramatically in the period 1930–50, prior to the introduction of RRT.

- Mortality from renal disease is greater in people born in the Indian subcontinent or Afro-Caribbean Commonwealth.

- The number of transplants doubled in the 1980s and between 1989 and 1991 there were on average about 1,800 transplants per year. However, there appears to be a levelling off because of a shortage of donors, and waiting lists are growing. Graft survival has improved significantly over the last decade, with 10–year survival of 50 per cent.

- Provision of renal replacement therapy has risen sharply in the last decade. Current concerns are how to fund continued expansion of RRT, how to make this more accessible to the population, and how to maximise transplant supply, so reducing the need for more expensive dialysis facilities.

21.1 Introduction

This chapter largely describes the trends in mortality and morbidity from non-malignant chronic diseases of the kidney, and the utilisation of health care services for their treatment. Such diseases may lead to progressive chronic renal failure (CRF) and ultimately end-stage renal failure (ESRF). The last 30 years have seen the development and expansion of renal replacement therapy (RRT) by dialysis or kidney transplantation, which are both life-saving treatments for end-stage renal failure. Such treatments consume substantial health service resources (estimated at over 1 per cent) and this figure will rise as the prevalence of patients on treatment increases towards an equilibrium steady state-position. Acute renal failure is also an important cause of morbidity and mortality. Some other diseases of the genitourinary system are also significant causes of morbidity, particularly benign diseases of the prostate in older men, and renal calculi; these are not discussed in detail.

21.1.1 Types of kidney disease

Much renal disease is self-limiting but severe disease may lead to renal failure. Over 100 different diseases affect the kidneys. They may present with features such as pain, blood or protein in the urine, peripheral oedema or hypertension, or they may remain undiagnosed until the symptoms of renal failure develop.

Renal failure may be acute and reversible, or chronic and irreversible. Acute renal failure occurs in previously normal kidneys usually after major injury (e.g. major trauma, postoperative shock, shock due to hypotension or septicaemia). It can also be due to acute obstruction and to intrinsic renal disease. Such patients are often severely ill with failure of more than one organ system. Although renal support is only needed for days or weeks, mortality is high because of the severity of the primary causes.

More commonly, renal failure is chronic and irreversible, the kidneys being progressively damaged over months or years. In this form there are often few symptoms or signs and patients may present late in the disease with general symptoms such as tiredness, anaemia, breathlessness and oedema. There can be an acute deterioration of chronic renal failure. The later stages of chronic renal failure, at which there is loss of over 90 per cent of renal function (where the creatinine clearance, a marker of renal function, is below 5ml/min), is called end-stage renal failure (ESRF). Patients in this stage will die unless renal support is given. The reduced renal function in chronic renal failure leads to biochemical disorders with markedly raised serum creatinine and urea, and abnormalities of: red cell production leading to anaemia; salt water balance leading to hypertension; and calcium regulation leading to, for example, bone disorders, metastatic calcification and rarer complications.

Kidney diseases leading to ESRF have been categorised by the European Dialysis and Transplantation Association (EDTA). Most kidney diseases fall into the following categories:

Auto-immune disease
'Glomerulonephritis' describes diseases whereby glomeruli are destroyed by the body's immunological response.

Systemic disease
The most important cause is diabetes mellitus but renal failure also occurs in systemic lupus erythematosis, vasculitis, myelomatosis and amyloidosis.

High blood pressure
Severe and malignant hypertension damages the kidneys. Long-term follow-up of men recruited to the MRAT cardiovascular disease prevention study in the 1970s has shown that the risk of ESRF increases continuously with rising BP (Klag, 1996). Hypertension is a complication of chronic renal failure.

Obstruction
Any condition that blocks the outflow of urine can cause obstruction, the most common cause being benign prostatic hypertrophy.

Infection
Urinary infection in early childhood in the presence of vesico-ureteric reflux is the main cause of chronic pyelonephritis. Renal tuberculosis is now rare in the indigenous population but interstitial TB has recently been recognised as an important cause of chronic renal failure especially in immigrants from the Indian subcontinent.

Genetic
The autosomal dominant condition polycystic kidney disease is much the commonest. The many other genetic causes contribute less than 1 per cent of all cases of chronic renal failure.

The incidence of these causes of ESRF varies by age and ethnic group (see below).

21.1.2 Renal replacement therapy (RRT)

Renal replacement therapy describes treatment for ESRF in which the lost kidney functions are replaced by either dialysis or by transplantation. Dialysis can either be by haemodialysis, in which the patient's blood passes over filters and exchange of toxic products takes place, or by peritoneal dialysis, in which fluid is infused into the patient's peritoneal cavity (the most common form is continuous ambulatory peritoneal dialysis (CAPD)). Dialysis can be performed in a wide range of settings: hospital in-patient, outpatient, free standing (i.e. non-hospital unit) or at home. Renal transplants can come from live donors or, more commonly, from cadavers.

21.1.3 Historical context

Renal failure has probably been an important cause of death throughout the ages, although there is difficulty in obtaining data necessary to establish precisely its impact on mortality. Historically, even with the recognition of the value of autopsies, the kidneys were seldom examined (Richet, 1991). The assignment of the underlying cause of death on death certificates of patients with renal failure is inconsistent and overall it is under-recorded, as a cause of death.

Developments in understanding of the pathology of kidney disease were led in the nineteenth century by Bright in England and Rayer in Paris. The first experimental haemodialysis was performed in humans in 1924. However, access problems limited its application to the treatment of acute renal failure. The earliest medical management of patients with ESRF with any impact was that of high calorie–low protein diets introduced in the 1940s. However, it was the introduction of permanent vascular access by Scribner, and then Brescia with the AV fistula, that transformed the prognosis of ESRF (Kazuo, 1992). Kidney transplantation was introduced in the 1950s but rejection was a major problem. It was the work on immunosuppression that overcame this and which made transplantation the treatment of choice; of particular importance was the introduction of azathioprine in the 1960s and cyclosporin in the mid-1970s by Sir Roy Calne (Calne *et al.*, 1978). Although intermittent peritoneal dialysis was introduced in the late 1950s and a permanent indwelling catheter by Tenckhoff and Schechter in 1968, the development of continuous ambulatory peritoneal dialysis in 1976 led to rapid expansion of this modality (Gokal, 1992).

21.2 Methods of data analysis

21.2.1 Mortality

ONS mortality data from 1848 for England and Wales have been used. ICD coding has changed considerably over the period 1900 onwards to take account of scientific advances in the understanding of renal disease, as shown in the Appendix. This makes it difficult with certainty to trace 4-digit level ICD trends over the period, as it is unclear whether specific renal diseases are being recorded consistently over time. Hence groupings of ICD codes and the full genitourinary disease ICD chapter data are also presented here.

Another problem with death certification is that the cause of death is inconsistently recorded in patients with renal failure (Perneger *et al.*, 1995). This is partly because the cause of immediate death may be a complication, such as hypertensive stroke or heart failure superimposed on underlying CRF, and renal disease is then not often mentioned as the cause. This has been clearly demonstrated by a recent study using the Oxford Record Linkage Study data (ORLS) (Goldacre, 1993). For many years nearly all renal failure was termed 'Bright's disease', though as renal disease syndromes were described the diagnosis was split up.

Since 1990, renal failure standing alone on the death certificate, unqualified with respect to its cause, has been systematically referred to the Coroner.

ICD disease coding is not specific, so that, for example, within 'nephritis, nephrosis and nephrotic syndrome' (ICD9 580-9), there are the 4-digit categories 'acute renal failure', 'chronic renal failure' and 'renal failure not specified as acute or chronic'. There is, therefore, overlap in the ICD coding of acute and chronic renal failure despite the important clinical differences between them.

Five-yearly average age/sex-specific numbers and rates of renal disease are presented since 1911 or in some cases since later (where there were inconsistencies in coding). The age-bands used are 15–44, 45–54, 55–64, 65–74 and 75+. Directly age/sex-standardised rates using the standard European population as the standard are presented for 3-digit ICD analyses, as well as standardisation against the standard European population for the chapter level analysis. The codes used are shown in Appendix 21.1.

The relationship between social class and ethnicity and renal disease mortality are explored using data from the Decennial Occupational Supplement (OPCS, 1986). Both standardised mortality and proportional mortality ratios (SMR and PMR) have been shown for social and ethnic differences. For PMRs no knowledge of denominator populations is assumed. This is useful when there may be biases in deriving rates, as in the Decennial Supplement analyses. The actual number of deaths from renal disease is compared to the expected number derived from the proportions in the standard population and the total in the age/sex-band of the group of interest. It reflects an excess proportion, not an excess rate.

21.2.2 Morbidity

There are no routine data on the incidence and prevalence of renal disease except for the National Morbidity Surveys in General Practice. There have been ad hoc population-based studies, first in the 1970s. More recently there have been well designed studies of the incidence of acute and late stage chronic renal failure (Pendreigh *et al.*, 1972; McGeown, 1972, 1990; Feest *et al.*, 1990, 1993; Khan *et al.*, 1994) (see below).

21.2.3 Service provision and utilisation

Renal replacement therapy (RRT)
Data on the prevalence of patients on treatment (by type of RRT) and the incidence of acceptance onto RRT, and limited data on outcomes are available from the European Dialysis and Transplant Association (EDTA) Registry.

EDTA data are available from the United Kingdom and other Western countries from 1972 onwards. There are two questionnaires: centre-based and patient-based. The response rate in the United Kingdom has been high for the centre-based

Table 21.1

Completeness % of the EDTA patient- and centre-based questionnaire in the United Kingdom

Year	Patient	Centre
1984		91
1985		94
1986		93
1987		90
1988	68	85
1989	69	52
1990	45	100
1991	43	91
1992	55	95

Source: EDTA

one, but lower and falling for the more comprehensive patient questionnaire (see Table 21.1). This makes some of the analyses less robust, for example, age-specific rates. Moreover, geographical analysis is not possible on a population basis as patient data are collected by renal unit of treatment, not place of residence.

United Kingdom Transplant Support Service Authority (UKTSSA) has data on the kidney transplants performed in the United Kingdom and Eire, both live and cadaver, and on the transplant waiting list. The data pre-1978 are less reliable.

A recently completed survey of renal provision in all renal units in England was completed as part of a national review of renal services (unpublished Department of Health Review of Renal Services, 1994). The survey enabled population-based measures of acceptance (incidence of patients taken onto RRT) and stock (prevalence of patients on treatment) by age and sex, region, district, ethnic group and cause to be evaluated. Some data are presented here.

Causes of ESRF
This information has only been derived from the cause attributed to patients accepted onto RRT and collected by EDTA, and latterly by the National Renal Review. The accuracy of the coding by renal units is unknown. Moreover, doubts have been expressed about the validity of current coding systems (Perneger *et al.*, 1995).

Hospitalisation
Dialysis is largely an out-patient-based service unless there are complications which require admission to hospital, such as peritoneal infection in CAPD. Uncomplicated transplantation is similar; admission is only required routinely for the initial operation and establishment of graft function. Hospitalisation data are, therefore, less useful in assessing the impact of ESRF.

The main historical data source on hospitalisation is the Hospital In-patient Enquiry (HIPE) – a 10 per cent sample of all deaths and discharges available in computer-readable form from 1962 to 1985 (OPCS, 1987). Until 1981, the data were for England and Wales, after that for England only. The 10 per cent sample varied slightly per year so that there was not a constant multiplication factor. There is a problem in assessing more recent trends, as HIPE data were based on completed discharges and deaths, whereas more recent Hospital Episode Statistics (HES) are based on finished consultant episodes (FCE). There is scope for double-counting within HES data and they are probably only reliable from about 1990/91 onwards.

HIPE data have been analysed for the period 1968–85 for the following conditions:
  Nephritis, nephrosis and nephrotic syndrome
    (ICD 580-589)
  Infections of the kidney (ICD 590)
  Calculus of the kidney and ureter (ICD 592,594)
  Hyperplasia of the prostate (ICD 600)

Primary care
The Morbidity Statistics from General Practice (RCGP, 1992) provides data on episodes and consultations for certain renal diseases at primary care level-based on prospective ascertainment in a framework of spotter practices. Data are presented from the 1981 survey for the following College Codes:
  270 (ICD 580-83) acute and chronic glomerulonephritis
  271 (ICD 590.1,590.3,590.8,590.9) pyelonephritis
  272 (ICD 592,594) urinary calculus
  273 (ICD 593.6) orthostatic albuminuria
  276 (ICD 599.7) haematuria
  274 (ICD 595, 599.0) cystitis and urinary infection
  277 (remainder 590-99) other diseases of kidney, ureter
    and bladder
  278 (ICD 600) benign prostatic hypertrophy

21.3 Mortality trends

21.3.1 Causes of death

Chapter 4 describes the causes of death in England and Wales in 1992 by ICD chapter heading. Genitourinary disease deaths were relatively rare at just under 1 per cent of all deaths – there were 2,322 deaths in men and 2,984 in women. The most common cause was 'nephritis, nephrosis and nephrotic syndrome', with 39 per cent of all genitourinary deaths.

21.3.2 Genitourinary disease chapter level trend 1848–1994

Figures 21.1 and 21.2 show mean annual death rates by age and sex from all genitourinary diseases. These diseases have always been more common in men and in older ages, but in all groups there has been a decline in mortality since 1900, most marked in the older groups from 1930 onwards. There has been a slight rise in male rates over 65 in the 1970s. The trends for nephritis, nephrosis and nephrotic syndrome follow a very similar pattern over this period (see Figures

Figure 21.1

Genitourinary disease mortality rates in England and Wales, males, 1860–1990

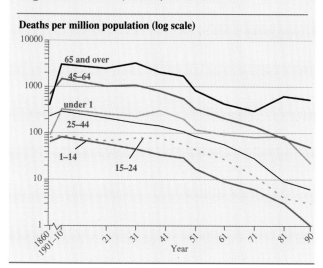

Figure 21.2

Genitourinary disease mortality rates in England and Wales, females, 1860–1990

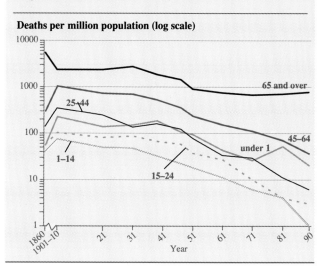

21.3 and 21.4). Overall rates have fallen dramatically in both sexes, particularly in the period 1930–50, prior to the introduction of Renal Replacement Therapy. Age-standardised mortality rates continued to fall since 1950 in all age-groups except above age 64, where there were increases from 1970 onwards, until the 1980s for ages 65–74 and until around 1990 for those aged 75 and over. RRT was widely available from the late 1970s (see Figure 21.4).

Mortality from infections of the kidney (see Figure 21.5) appeared to increase dramatically and then fall in the period 1930–50, to rise again 1950–65, and then to gradually fall. These patterns probably partly reflect a change in coding practices rather than true effects, as their magnitude was so large and precipitate (see below).

Genitourinary tuberculosis mortality rates rose in men, and to a lesser extent in women, during the wartime periods but then fell dramatically and have continued to do so, and genitourinary TB is now a rare cause of death (see Figure

21.6). However, there is emerging evidence that interstitial TB may be a significant cause of chronic renal failure in populations from the Indian subcontinent (Lightstone *et al.*, 1994).

Puerperal renal disease (see Figure 21.7) mortality rates fell sharply between 1930 and 1950, and have continued to fall since, reflecting improved maternal care in pregnancy and the puerperium, and mirroring the overall decline in maternal mortality. This would largely have been manifest as acute renal failure.

Data on deaths due to diabetes with renal complications and from hypertension with renal disease have only been available more recently. Diabetes mortality rates increased between the periods 1979–85 and 1986–91 in both sexes above age 54 (see Chapter 4). Some of this apparent rise may be due to ONS reinterpretation of WHO rule 3 from 1984 onwards (see Chapter 2). Hypertension rates fell steadily in both sexes from 1968 onwards.

Figure 21.3

Deaths from nephritis, nephrosis and nephrotic syndrome, males, standardised to European standard population, 1911–91

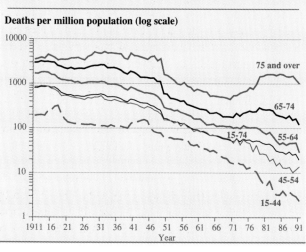

Figure 21.4

Deaths from nephritis, nephrosis and nephrotic syndrome, females, standardised to European standard population, 1911–91

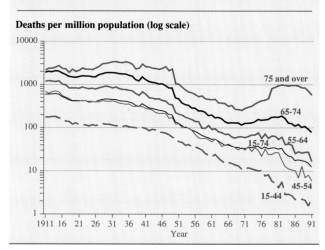

Figure 21.5

Deaths from kidney infection, standardised to European standard population, ages 15–74, 1940–91

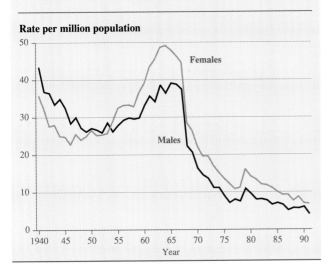

Rate per million population

Figure 21.6

Mortality from tuberculosis of the genitourinary system, standardised to European standard population, ages 15–74, 1911–91

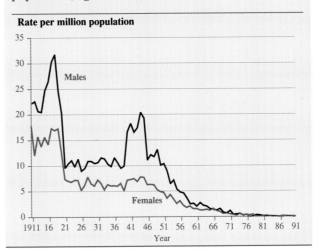

Rate per million population

Figure 21.7

Deaths from pregnancy-related renal disease, standardised to European standard population, ages 15–74, 1931–94

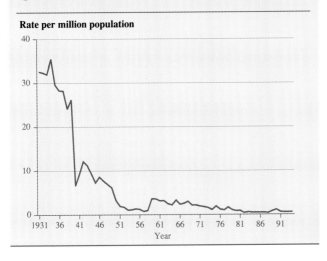

Rate per million population

perhaps be utilised to make a more valid assessment of the impact of renal disease on mortality.

21.3.4 Social class and mortality

The 1981 Occupational Decennial Supplement shows significant gradients in SMRs from both nephritis nephrosis and nephrotic syndrome and infections of the kidney. The gradients in PMRs are less marked. This suggests that mortality from kidney disease is increased along with many other chronic diseases such as cardiovascular disease in lower social groups, but the proportion does not vary by social group. Common determinants may underlie this excess mortality (e.g. hypertension, diabetes mellitus, nutritional and environmental factors; see Table 21.3).

21.4 Morbidity

21.4.1 Incidence of late stage chronic renal failure

It is important to determine the incidence of ESRF deemed suitable for RRT in order to be able to plan treatment provision. Initial studies largely used death certification to determine CRF incidence rates and hence were likely to under-ascertain the incidence. Population studies used general practitioner (GP) and hospital doctor surveys in defined populations in the 1970s. A study in Northern Ireland suggested an incidence rate of 48 per million population (pmp) in the age group 5–60; 38 pmp were thought to require dialysis (McGeown, 1972). A similar study in Scotland found an incidence rate under 65 of 109 pmp and a figure of 52 pmp requiring dialysis (Pendreigh *et al.*, 1972).

There have been more recent population-based studies of the incidence of late stage chronic renal failure as defined by serum creatinine levels of over 500 μmol/l, obtained from laboratory reports (Feest *et al.*, 1990; Khan *et al.*, 1994), or

21.3.3 Multi-cause analysis of cause of death

Data from the Oxford Record Linkage Study (Goldacre, 1993) showed that only a third of patients who had renal disease due to nephritis, nephrosis and nephrotic syndrome (ICD9 580-9) on discharge from hospital in Oxfordshire during 1979–86, and who died in the ensuing 4 weeks, had renal disease as the underlying cause on the death certificate. This disease coding was mentioned on 77.1 per cent of the death certificates of such patients. These figures are similar to those for diabetes mellitus (at 29.8 per cent and 68.6 per cent, respectively).

The figures vary by age; mention of renal disease is more likely in older age-groups (see Table 21.2).

As a result of this problem of under-ascertainment of renal disease as a cause of death, multi-cause coding could

Table 21.2

Deaths due to nephritis, nephrosis and nephrotic syndrome in Oxfordshire, 1979–86

	Total deaths of patients discharged with NNNS*	Underlying cause specified as NNNS underlying cause		NNNS on death certificate but not underlying cause	
		Number	(% of all causes in each age-band)		
<15	3	0		2	
15–64	205	34	(16.6)	106	(31.7)
65–74	290	95	(32.3)	126	(43.4)
75+	641	243	(37.9)	274	(42.7)
All	1139	372	(32.7)	506	(44.4)

Adapted from Goldacre (1993)
*Nephritis, nephrosis and nephrotic syndrome (ICD 580-9)

Table 21.3

Renal disease mortality by social class in England and Wales, 1979–83
Age-standardised mortality ratios (SMR) and proportional mortality ratios (PMRs) (E&W=100)

		Social Class (as defined by occupation)					
Males 16–74		I	II	IIINM	IIIM	IV	V
Nephritis, nephrosis,	SMR	45	72	103	100	117	180
nephrotic syndrome	PMR	86	105	108	94	101	101
Infection	SMR	30	63	90	75	104	248
	PMR	76	98	76	102	100	114
Females 16–59							
Nephritis, nephrosis,	SMR	56	62	88	92	111	204
nephrotic syndrome	PMR	81	80	101	93	101	152
Infection	SMR	7	43	72	95	113	188
	PMR	10	55	81	96	103	138

Source: OPCS Decennial Supplement

doctor survey (McGeown, 1990). These were undertaken in Devon, Blackburn, Grampian and Northern Ireland. All studies showed a marked rise in incidence with age. The incidence was greater in men but with no evidence of referral bias (personal communication). Studies of specific causes of chronic renal failure have largely found an excess in men (e.g. IgA nephropathy, membranous nephropathy) except for some causes of chronic pyelonephritis (Silbiger and Neugarten, 1995; see Table 2.14).

The fall in incidence with age in the Northern Ireland study suggests some under-ascertainment by the doctor notification method. The overall population rate in the Feest study was 148 pmp. These authors reviewed each case to see if they would have benefited from RRT (whether they were

treated or not) and concluded that there was an annual population need of 78 pmp per year under age 80 (the estimate had 95 per cent confidence limits of 68–93). There are some caveats with this figure: it does not take account of ethnicity; the clinical threshold may be too low; the over 80s do need to be considered; and it would be more appropriate to have an adult-only rate, as the denominator includes children, in whom ESRF is rare.

21.4.2 Incidence of acute renal failure (ARF)

The only population-based study was carried out in Devon by Feest, Round and Hammad (Feest *et al.*, 1993). Here, ARF was defined as a creatinine over 500 μmol/l which

Table 21.4

Incidence of late stage chronic renal failure in population based studies in the United Kingdom

Age-group	Feest Rate (pmp; number of cases = 210)	McGeown Rate (pmp; number of cases = 122)	Khan Rate (pmp; number of cases = 61)
0–19	6	24	15
20–39		37	
40–49		90	
20–49	58		36
50–59	160	197	159 for 50–69
60–69	282	220	ditto
70–79	503	167	472
80+	588	78	1153

subsequently fell below this level. The annual population incidence rate was 140 pmp. The age-related incidence rose from 17 pmp under age 50 to 949 pmp in over 80. Overall survival was poor at 34 per cent at 2 years; this did not differ markedly between age-groups above and below age 50. The incidence was greatest in men even after excluding prostatic disease (which was the most common cause in men). The dialysis rate was 18 pmp and the 'appropriate' referral rate to nephrologists estimated at 72 pmp. This estimate may be low, as first, the population studied had no cardiothoracic unit, and second, some patients with ARF may not have been suspected and therefore they may not have had a creatinine or urea level measured.

21.4.3 Ethnicity

Of particular interest is the impact of ethnicity on renal failure rates.

Mortality from renal disease is greater in people born in the Indian subcontinent or Afro-Caribbean Commonwealth; the numbers are rather small, especially for deaths due to kidney infection (Balarajan and Bulusu, 1990; see Table 21.5).

The relationship between ethnicity and ESRF was reviewed by the London Implementation Group Renal Services Review (London Implementation Group (LIG), 1993). People from the Indian subcontinent have a higher prevalence of NIDDM and higher mortality rates (Mather and Keen, 1985; Balarajan and Bulusu, 1990) and there is evidence of raised diabetic ESRF rates (Burden et al., 1992). Black people have an increased prevalence of both hypertension and NIDDM and higher mortality rates from cerebrovascular disease, hypertensive disease and diabetes (LIG, 1993). Systemic lupus erythematosus (SLE) is also more common in black people. Data from the US Renal Data System (USRDS) for 1988–90 have shown nearly fourfold increases in acceptance onto RRT in black people compared to white people. This increase is greatest for hypertensive ESRF (6.2) but also true for all other causes except polycystic kidney disease (USRDS, 1992). In the West Midlands, black people accepted onto RRT had a higher proportion of hypertensive/renovascular disease, diabetes and SLE than white people. In Asian people there were excess proportions of hypertension/renovascular disease but not of diabetes (Clark et al., 1993). In the Thames Regions in 1991–2 there were almost threefold increases in unadjusted acceptance rates onto RRT in both Asian and black people

Table 21.5

Mortality from renal disease in ethnic minorities in England and Wales, 1979–83 (E&W SMR/PMR =100)

Age 20–69		Nephritis, nephrosis, nephrotic syndrome (ICD 580-89)			Infection (ICD 590)		
		Deaths	SMR	PMR	Death	SMR	PMR
Place of birth							
Indian subcontinent	M	7	242	226	9	155	145
Indian subcontinent	F	76	372	350	14	164	157
Caribbean	M	36	199	247	3	93	117
Caribbean	F	26	228	217	2	209	189
African	M	16	270	245	2	163	155
African	F	10	263	224	4	240	206

Source: Balarajan and Bulusu (1990)

compared to white people (Roderick *et al.*, 1994). This was confirmed by the National Renal Review; age adjusted rates were 4.6 and 4.0 times higher, respectively. The relative rate increase rose with age; it was seven times higher in the over 65s, suggesting that there will be an increased demand for renal services as these populations age (Roderick, 1996). Rates were higher for diabetic ESRF and 'unknown cause' in Asians and for diabetes and hypertension in blacks. Their geographical distribution is clustered in certain areas, which will have substantially increased need and demand for RRT. It is not known to what extent the increased need and demand is due to a greater incidence of underlying causes, to reduced access to health care (e.g. for hypertension detection and control), to greater susceptibility to the underlying causes, or a combination of the three, or to what extent need is being met.

21.4.4 Provision of renal replacement therapy

EDTA acceptance and stock rates

In 1992 the stock of patients on renal replacement therapy (dialysis and transplantation) in the United Kingdom was over 20,000 with a population rate of 375 pmp. Of these, 52 per cent had a functioning graft, 19.4 per cent were on hospital haemodialysis, 23.2 per cent on CAPD and only 5.2 per cent on home HD. There was a steady rise in numbers during the 1970s and even greater rate of increase from the late 1970s onwards (see Figure 21. 8). This has been due to the increase in acceptance rates and to improvements in survival. For example, in South East Thames RHA the 1-, 4- and 8-year survivals for those accepted onto RRT in 1970–74 for 0–55-year-olds were 74 per cent, 52 per cent and 39 per cent; the 1980–84 figures were 90 per cent, 77 per cent and 65 per cent (EDTA). Key features of the modality mix were the predominance of transplantation as the single most common modality, the initial use of home HD but its decline since the mid-1980s, the steady but limited rise of hospital haemodialysis, and the expansion of CAPD in the 1980s.

Patients with serious comorbidity were initially largely excluded from RRT and Figure 21.9 shows, for example, that diabetics have only been accepted onto RRT in significant numbers during the 1980s. In 1975, diabetics were 1.4 per cent of the patients accepted in the United Kingdom. By 1984 this was 11.4 per cent, and in the National Review in England the percentage was 15 per cent. Nevertheless, some patients may still not be receiving treatment (Joint Working Party, 1989; Cameron and Challah, 1988).

The age distribution of RRT patients has changed. In the late 1960s and early 1970s patients were predominantly under 45; there was then an increase in the middle-age-group taken on. Until 1982 there were few patients over age 65 on dialysis but the elderly now form 16 per cent of those on dialysis (unpublished Department of Health Review of Renal Services, 1994). The age-distribution of new patients has also changed since the late 1970s with a greater proportion now being 65 or over (see Figure 21.10). In 1991–92, 37 per cent were over 65 compared with 1 per cent in 1976–78.

New patient 'acceptance' rates have increased steadily in the United Kingdom and are now in the mid-60s (see Figure 21.10). The national target which was set at 40 pmp in 1984 has been clearly exceeded. However, population need in the Caucasian population is estimated to be 80 per million per year under age 80 (Renal Association, 1991). Taking into account ethnic factors, a more liberal threshold, and treatment of over-80-year-olds, probably leaves the figure closer to 95–100 pmp. Some countries are reaching this (e.g. Wales, which has no major ethnic minority factor).

Geographical variation

As with most specialist services there is evidence of geographical inequality of utilisation and supply. This was first described for renal services (Dalziell and Garrett, 1987). The London Implementation Group's Review of Renal Services found marked variation in DHA acceptance rates in the Thames Regions in 1991 and 1992, reflecting both increased need due to ethnic minorities, but also reduced access to referral to the largely central London renal units and under-

Figure 21.8

Trends in the prevalence (stock) of patients on renal replacement therapy in the United Kingdom, by modality, 1975–1992

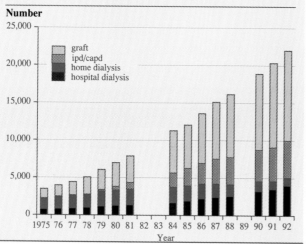

Figure 21.9

Trends in the prevalence (stock) of patients on renal replacement therapy in the United Kingdom, by diabetic status

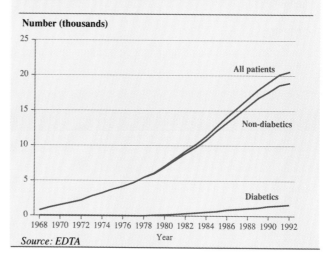

Source: EDTA

Figure 21.10

Acceptance rates onto renal replacement therapy in the United Kingdom, 1982–92

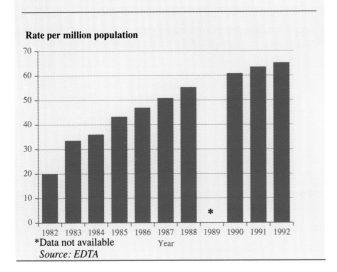

Rate per million population

*Data not available

Source: EDTA

referral (LIG, 1993). This variation has subsequently been found nationally in the National Renal Review. More equitable distribution of services is required to reduce geographical variation, although some areas (e.g. those with large ethnic minorities) have an increased need. An important determinant of acceptance is GP and physician referral patterns. A national survey by Challah in 1984 showed that there was incomplete knowledge among GPs and hospital physicians (compared to nephrologists) as to who would benefit from RRT (Challah *et al.*, 1984). It is not known if or how this pattern changed, but it is likely to be influenced by greater contact with nephrologists and more accessible local services.

EDTA data are not population-based as only the place of treatment is recorded. Some patients cross regional boundaries so that the data are not reliable estimates of regional rates. In 1991 EDTA-based regional rates varied from 138 (SW Thames) to 517 (NE Thames); the National Renal Review

found that the population based rates for these Regions were almost the same. Overall, there was significant inter-regional variation over the country (with rates ranging from 51 to 86 pmp).

European comparisons

Figure 21.12 shows the rise in RRT stock in several western European countries with United Kingdom catching up since 1985. In terms of modality, the United Kingdom relied heavily on the expansion of CAPD and transplantation, whereas France and West Germany concentrated on hospital HD and to a lesser degree on transplantation.

Although the United Kingdom has increased its acceptance rate it still lags behind other European countries (see Table 21.6). The highest rate worldwide was in the USA which had an acceptance rate 182 pmp in 1990 (USRDS, 1992).

Causes of ERSF

The only routine data on cause are derived from the EDTA Register of patients accepted onto RRT, available from the patient questionnaires. EDTA data, however, are incomplete in recent years. Data from the National Renal Review for non-Thames Regions in England showed that glomerulonephritis (20 per cent) and diabetes (17 per cent) were the most common causes, followed by pyelonephritis (13 per cent) and renovascular diseases, including hypertension (13 per cent) and polycystic kidney disease (8 per cent). However, 18 per cent of cases have 'unknown' cause, patients presenting in CRF or ESRF with small smooth kidneys which are not biopsied (see Table 21.7).

Transplantation

The UK kidney transplantation programme has been a great success. The numbers of transplants doubled in the 1980s and between 1989 and 1991 there were on average about 1,800 transplants per year (UKTSSA, 1993). However, there appears to be a levelling off because of shortage of donors (see Figure 21.13). This partly reflects welcome declines in the mortality from accidents and cerebrovascular disease. The

Figure 21.11

Percentage of new patients aged over 65 years accepted for renal replacement therapy in the United Kindom, 1967–91

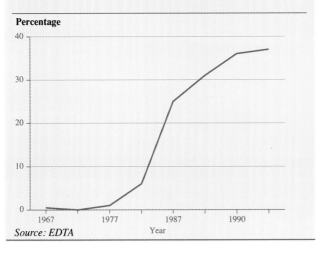

Percentage

Source: EDTA

Figure 21.12

Prevalence (stock) of patients on renal replacement therapy in selected Western European countries in 1980 and 1990

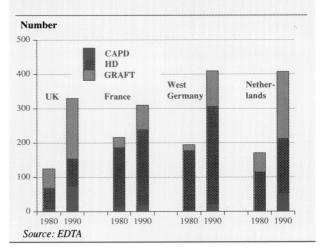

Number

CAPD
HD
GRAFT

Source: EDTA

Table 21.6

Western European acceptance rates onto renal replacement therapy

Per million population 1991

Austria	105
Sweden	97
Switzerland	96
West Germany	94
Belgium	87
Portugal	86
France	77
Norway	65
Netherlands	60
Spain	60
UK	**60**
Italy	54
Finland	54
Denmark	48

Source: EDTA

Table 21.7

European EDTA data for 1992 show the following breakdown by cause of all new acceptances in EDTA countries

Percentages

Glomerulonephritis	20
Unknown	18
Diabetes	17
Pyelonephritis	13
Renovascular (includes hypertension)	13
Polycystic kidney	8
Systemic	5
Drug	3
Hereditary, familial	1
Other	2

Source: EDTA

transplant waiting list has, therefore, grown markedly to nearly 5,000. Live transplant organs only make up a small percentage of total kidney transplants; between 1989 and 1991 there were 301 (5.2 per cent) out of 5,766 kidney transplants.

HLA matching (especially DR) improves the success of cadaveric transplantation; only 6 per cent have complete A, B and DR matching but 50 per cent are fully DR matched. The available kidneys have largely been given to younger patients, though as the age of patients on dialysis has changed, an increasing proportion are now being given to those over 55 (see Figure 21.14).

Figure 21.13

Cadaveric transplants performed and kidney transplant waiting lists, United Kingdom and Eire, 1972–93

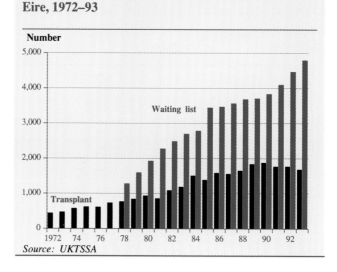

Source: UKTSSA

Survival on RRT

One- and 5-year survival for all forms of RRT in the United Kingdom between 1986 and 1991 were 85 and 60 per cent, respectively. This figure varies with age (see Table 21.8), with younger ages having 90 per cent 5-year survival (EDTA, 1992). Outcome is also influenced by comorbidity. Khan *et al.* (1993) showed that in two units in Scotland survival was also related to age and to the presence of other organ disease, whether cardiovascular, respiratory, liver, diabetes or to visceral malignancy. Others have found a similar picture; diabetics in particular have a poorer prognosis (Nicolucci *et al.*, 1992; McMillan *et al.*, 1990).

Comparison of modality survival is difficult because there are significant selection factors determining the treatment. Transplantation is the treatment of choice when available. Graft and, to a lesser extent, patient survival are influenced by many factors, including recipient and donor age and matching. Graft survival has improved significantly over the last

Figure 21.14

Cadaveric transplants performed in the United Kingdom and Eire, by recipient age, 1981–91

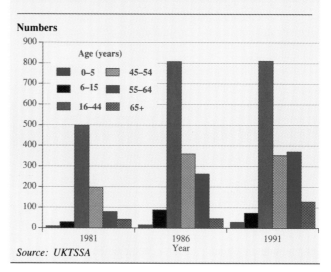

Source: UKTSSA

Table 21.8

Patient survival rates on all renal replacement therapy

All EDTA registry countries 1986-91

Age at start	1 year	5 years
15-24	96	89
25-34	97	89
35-44	94	77
45-54	90	69
55-64	82	48
65-74	73	32
75+	65	23
All	85	60

Source: EDTA

decade. Overall 1-, 5- and 10-year graft survivals were 78 per cent, 64 per cent and 50 per cent between 1981–91; the corresponding patient survival figures were 91 per cent, 73 per cent and 50 per cent (UKTSSA, 1993). Comparison of CAPD and haemodialysis in the Leicester unit 1975–84, with adjustment for case mix, showed that CAPD had a slightly lower mortality risk compared to haemodialysis (Burton and Walls, 1987) .

The most common cause of death on RRT is cardiovascular, followed by infection; these causes are both commoner in diabetics.

21.5 Health service utilisation data

21.5.1 Hospitalisation: HIPE data (Figure 21.15)

Nephritis, nephrosis and nephrotic syndrome (ICD 580-9)
Age-standardised rates increased slightly from 1968 until 1978 and then rose sharply to 1979, from when they rose steadily. This coincided with the change from ICD8 to ICD9. This was equivalent to a significant 8 per cent annual rise in both sexes. Rates for men were greater than for women but they have run in parallel. This probably reflects the trend to treat patients with ESRF by RRT rather than a true rise in incidence, because at the same time mortality from this cause was falling. The proportion of over 65s rose from 12 per cent to 37 per cent in men and from 12 per cent to 43 per cent in women.

Kidney infection (ICD 590)
In contrast to nephritis there was a significant decline in rates in both sexes of approximately 5 per cent per annum. Rates for women exceeded those for men in this category because both acute and chronic pyelonephritis are commoner in women. The reason for this fall is unclear but it is consistent with mortality trends.

Calculus (ICD 592, 594)
There was a just significant overall annual rise of 1 per cent in men largely due to changes in the 1980s.

Prostate (ICD 600)
Benign prostatic hypertrophy 'discharges' rose significantly by an average 1.3 per cent per year.

Figure 21.15

Trends in hospital discharges and death rates in England and Wales for selected renal diseases, males and females, 1968–85

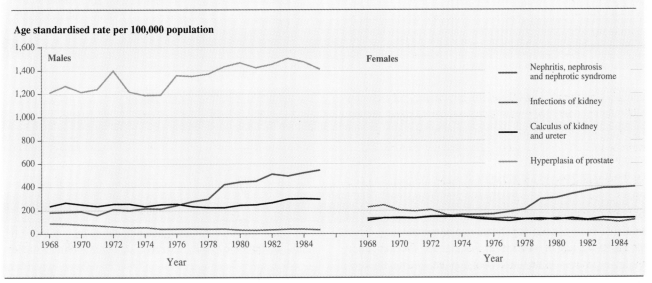

Age standardised rate per 100,000 population

Table 21.9

Genitourinary disease: rates for patient consulting their GPs in 1981

Patients consulting/1,000 at risk	Males	Females	All
Acute and chronic glomerulonephritis (ICD 580-83)	0.2	0.3	0.2
Pyelonephritis (ICD-590)	0.9	3.6	2.3
Urinary calculi (ICD 592, 594)	1.1	0.7	0.9
Orthostatic albuminuria (ICD 593.6)	0.1	0.1	0.1
Haematuria (ICD 599.7)	1.9	1.2	1.5
Cystitis and urinary infection (ICD 595, 599.0)	7.0	39.0	24.1
Other diseases of kidney, ureter and bladder (ICD remainder 580-99)	0.9	0.9	0.9
Benign prostatic hypertrophy (ICD 600)	3.7	n/a	—

Source: Morbidity Statistics from General Practice 1991/92

21.5.2 Renal disease in primary care.

Morbidity Statistics from General Practice 1991/2 shows that nephritis, nephrosis and nephrotic syndrome (ICD 580-89) was a rare cause of patient consultation, with 9 patients per ten thousand patient years at risk (Table 21.9); the associated referral rate was 1 per 10,000. The absolute numbers can be derived per GP by assuming an average list size of 2,000, i.e. less than two consultations for nephritis and less than one referral. Other diseases of the urinary system (ICD 590-99), however, were common, with 353 per 10,000 patient consulting and 21 per 10,000 referrals.

21.6 Discussion

Serious renal diseases are relatively uncommon but they are an important cause of mortality and morbidity, and their management requires substantial health care investment. Mortality rates have declined dramatically this century overall and for most underlying causes. The bulk of the change predates the introduction of renal replacement therapy. It is important to recognise that mortality statistics are an unreliable guide to true mortality because of the incompleteness of ascertainment and it is not known how this has varied over time. Moreover, separating mortality due to acute and chronic renal failure is difficult.

What explains these trends? Several authors analysed mortality rates in the 1950s and 1960s and found that there was a fall in nephritis and a rise in infection rates. Ascertainment effects were proposed by Waters as the explanation, given the greater interest in renal infection at the time (Waters, 1968). Kessner noted that the fall was greater in women, which would be consistent with this hypothesis (Kessner and Floer, 1967).

However, over the whole period the mortality falls probably reflect a true decline in the incidence of serious renal disease, although the reasons are largely speculative. For chronic renal failure it may be changes in other environmental and occupational exposures to nephrotoxins (e.g. lead) and to a change in the use of nephrotoxic drugs, such as analgesics. The fall in TB mortality mirrors wider falls and reflects improvements in socio-economic conditions, as most of the fall occurred before anti-TB drugs and BCG vaccination were widely available. Although post-streptococcal nephritis has declined, this would not have a major effect on mortality as both early and late mortality were low. Hypertension-related causes are falling recently, although whether this reflects improved management of malignant hypertension since the introduction of effective antihypertensive agents is not known. Of interest is the recent rise in diabetes-related mortality in the elderly. This could be due to ascertainment if more patients with NIDDM are being treated by RRT rather than to increases in the underlying incidence. One would not expect a marked change in congenital causes, because this is largely due to the autosomal dominant condition polycystic kidney disease, and the gene frequency will be relatively stable.

For acute renal failure (ARF) the distribution of causes has changed dramatically. For example, post-obstetric ARF has largely disappeared (as indicated by the decline in mortality from pregnancy-related renal disease), but ARF following major vascular surgery has increased, as such procedures are used more frequently. It is possible that ARF is more often coded now as the primary disease or procedure than as ARF.

End-stage renal failure is relatively uncommon, with an estimated 40–50 new cases a year requiring dialysis in the larger health districts with a population of 0.5 million. Nevertheless, it is an important disease for the NHS, as the costs of treatment are high. Provision of RRT for end-stage renal failure has increased steadily in the United Kingdom largely due to developments in transplantation and peritoneal dialysis. In contrast, other western European countries have relied more on hospital haemodialysis. There is still an unmet need for RRT and the prevalence of patients (stock) on RRT will rise even at current acceptance rates. Modelling work predicts a 50–100% increase in the next 10–15 years (NHS Executive: Renal Purchasing Guidelines 1996).

The elderly and those with serious comorbidity comprise an increasing proportion of patients being treated with RRT and so the marginal health gain is diminishing. An emerging problem is the need among ethnic minority populations for RRT. They have an increased incidence of underlying disease and a higher acceptance rate. As these populations age, need will increase sharply. In the 1991 UK Census, 2.7 per cent of the population were classified as Asian and 1.6 per cent as black. If the relative need of these populations for RRT is fourfold, the population rate in the United Kingdom would be 90.4 per million, or fivefold 93.8 pmp compared with the 80 pmp population need estimated in the white populations above.

Current concerns, then, are how to fund continued expansion of RRT, how to make this more accessible to the population and acceptable to the elderly population, and how to maximise transplant supply, thus reducing the need for more expensive dialysis facilities. Information available to purchasers and providers must improve. Mortality data on renal disease are not specific or complete, so it is an ineffective tool for monitoring and evaluating renal disease. Purchasers need to know about their acceptance and stock rate, the age and ethnic breakdown, modality split, and the outcomes in terms of mortality and major complications (Beech et al., 1993). A national renal register is proposed which could provide such information and facilitate provider audit against agreed process and outcome standards.

More emphasis is required on the prevention of end-stage renal failure. There are treatments available which can reduce or even prevent progression of chronic renal failure. These include better control of diabetes and more systematic detection and control of hypertension. This will involve greater collaboration between nephrologists and primary and secondary care. There is much less information on the prevalence of chronic renal failure in the population. Serious renal diseases are rare in primary care, with one new case of ESRF arising per year per 10,000 practices and with four to eight on RRT. However, there is a significant workload, at primary care level, of managing patients with symptoms of urinary tract disease, such as haematuria and urinary tract infection. Although only a minority will have serious kidney disease, improvements in the diagnosis and treatment of chronic renal failure could potentially reduce the incidence of ESRF.

Acknowledgements

We would like to thank Leo Cohn for computing support, Dr M Goldacre for advice on the Oxford Record Linkage Study and for providing HIPE data on behalf of ONS, Dr Elizabeth Jones for EDTA data, Dr Veena Soni Raleigh for her help on ethnic factors in need for renal replacement therapy, Professor Netar Mallick for assistance on the National Renal Review and the Department of Health for funding it, and finally Mrs Annette Hobbs for secretarial support.

Appendix 21.1 Disease codings for renal disease by ICD chapter

ICD revision, years covered:

1	1901–10
2	1911–20
3	1921–30
4	1931–39
5	1940–49
6	1950–57
7	1958–67
8	1968–78
9	1979–91

1.1 Nephritis nephrosis nephrotic syndrome

ICD	Codes
2	1190 1201 1202 1222 1223
3	1280 1290
4	1300 1310 1320
5	1300 1311 1312 1313 1320
6	590-4
7	590-4
8	580-4
9	580-7,589

1.2 Infection

ICD	Codes
5	1351 (cystitis) 1331 (pyelitis)
6	600 (infection) 605 (cystitis)
7	600 (infection) 605 (cystitis)
8	590 (pyelitis) 595 (cystitis)
9	590 (pyelitis) 595 (cystitis)

1.5 Tuberculosis

ICD	Codes	
1	0520	TB other
2	0343	TB other
3	0364	TB genitourinary
4	0300	TB genitourinary
5	0200	ditto
6	016	ditto
7	016	ditto
8	016	ditto
9	016	ditto

1.13 Pregnancy-related renal disease

ICD	Codes
4	1460
5	1401 1442 1471 1482
6	640 641 642.1 685
7	640 641 642 680 685
8	635 636 637 639.9
9	639.3 642.1 642.4–7 646.2 646.5 646.6 669.3

Chapter 22

Digestive disease

By
Jon Nguyen-Van-Tam and Richard Logan

Summary

- Almost 5 million people in Britain today consult their GP each year with a digestive complaint and over 25 per cent of these are considered serious.

- It is not possible to trace mortality patterns from digestive disease before 1900 because of the uncertainties of death certification for these conditions at this time. From 1900 until the early 1970s, however, there was a striking decline in death rates from digestive diseases.

- Long-term changes and trends in morbidity due to digestive disease are difficult to discern because data collection began only relatively recently, in the 1950s.

- The 1991–92 GP morbidity study shows a large increase since 1981–82 in the numbers of people consulting for non-ulcer dyspepsia. Consulting rates for other digestive diseases, including irritable bowel syndrome, have shown only small increases over the same period.

- Age-specific mortality from duodenal ulcer rose during the first half of this century but declined again from the 1950s until the early 1980s. Until the bacterium *Helicobacter pylori* was recognised, these trends were attributed traditionally to changes in smoking prevalence and the use of aspirin and other non-steroidal anti-inflammatory drugs.

- *Helicobacter pylori* is now known to play an essential role in the development of most peptic ulcers. Levels of *Helicobacter pylori* infection in Britain appear to be declining, as is peptic ulcer disease.

- For the first 20–30 years of this century mortality from appendicitis was very high. In younger age-groups mortality peaked in the early 1920s. Since 1940 mortality from appendicitis in both sexes and all age-groups has fallen dramatically.

- Decreases in hospital admission rates for appendicitis in young people in recent years are matched by increases in admission rates for abdominal pain. Some, if not all, of the apparent decline in appendicitis appears to be attributable to diagnostic reclassification.

22.1 Introduction: the nature of digestive complaints

By the time they reach adulthood, most people will have experienced one or more of a range of common digestive symptoms, such as abdominal pain, vomiting, and diarrhoea. In Britain during 1990–91, about 14 million days' work were lost owing to digestive problems (Department of Social Security, 1994). In fact, currently almost 5 million people in Britain consult their general practitioner (GP) each year with a digestive complaint and over 25 per cent of these are considered serious (McCormick *et al.*, 1995). Over 10 per cent of patients who consult their GP with a digestive problem are referred to a hospital (RCGP *et al.*, 1986). In 1985, the last year for which national hospital data are available from a consistent source (HIPE), over 400,000 admissions to hospital occurred because of a digestive disorder (DHSS and OPCS, 1987). In the same year, about 500,000 digestive tract operations or procedures (excluding those performed on teeth, gums or jaws) were performed in England and Wales, including many performed on people who were not admitted to hospital (DHSS and OPCS, 1987). Nevertheless, life-threatening digestive disease underlies only a small percentage of these symptoms; most are due to transient self-limiting gastrointestinal infections and to functional conditions, such as irritable bowel syndrome, that are associated with no known structural disturbance. Frequently it is not possible to distinguish functional gastrointestinal conditions from more serious diseases without use of special investigations or tests. Somewhat paradoxically, the increasing sophistication of gastrointestinal investigation has resulted in the recognition of milder forms of what would have been traditionally regarded as serious digestive disease. Some caution is therefore required when making comparisons of data collected over extended periods and it would be unwise to assume that the frequency of illness now diagnosed using sophisticated fibre-optic and video technology, is comparable to that recorded using only clinical signs and older techniques, such as barium contrast studies. This chapter will deal with non-malignant digestive disease by considering general trends in mortality and morbidity, before concentrating on two specific disease areas, peptic ulcer and appendicitis/abdominal pain, which together represent the commonest and most important causes of death from non-malignant gastrointestinal disease, and the most common reason for hospital admission.

22.2 Trends in mortality from digestive disease

Figure 4.15 of Chapter 4 illustrates the long term-trends in mortality from non-malignant digestive diseases among men

Table 22.1

Deaths from selected digestive disorders in England and Wales, 1901–91

	Men 1901	1931	1961	1991	Women 1901	1931	1961	1991
All causes (Number)	285,618	249,717	280,782	277,582	265,967	241,913	270,971	292,462
All gastrointestinal causes (Number)	16,297	10,805	7,546	7,923	16,059	8,806	7,011	10,585
All gastrointestinal as % of all causes	5.7	4.3	2.7	2.9	6.0	3.6	2.6	3.6
Major gastrointestinal causes of death	**Percentage of all gastrointestinal deaths**							
Duodenal ulcer-	-	10.7	20.7	13.5	-	1.9	7.4	10.5
Gastric ulcer/peptic ulcer (unspecified)	2.9	19.4	18.4	11.6	6.6	10.0	13.4	11.4
Chronic liver disease	14.6	9.7	9.8	22.0	12.0	6.4	9.0	12.8
Pancreatic disease	-	1.9	4.4	5.3	-	2.9	5.1	4.2
Cholelithiasis (gallstones)	8.2	6.9	5.7	4.7	9.5	19.0	13.7	5.3
Diverticular disease	-	1.7	5.3	5.1	-	1.8	10.5	10.5
Appendicitis	4.5	16.4	4.8	0.6	3.2	14.9	4.1	0.5
Inflammatory bowel disease	-	1.2	2.5	1.7	-	2.5	4.0	2.4
	Numbers of deaths							
Duodenal ulcer	-	1,158	1,564	1,071	-	164	516	1,113
Gastric ulcer/peptic ulcer (unspecified)	475	2,100	1,386	916	1,067	884	939	1,204
Chronic liver disease	2,375	1,050	737	1,747	1,933	560	633	1,355
Pancreatic disease	-	205	333	417	-	253	355	445
Cholelithiasis (gallstones)	1,335	741	430	370	1,532	1,671	959	561
Diverticular disease	-	183	401	408	-	159	739	1,107
Appendicitis	736	1,767	361	51	508	1,308	284	57
Inflammatory bowel disease	-	135	187	136	-	220	278	255

and women in Britain. In addition, Chapter 4 describes aggregate data for the earliest time periods (1848–72 and 1901–10). Given the uncertainties of death certification of digestive disease before the beginning of this century, mortality patterns prior to 1900 generally do not merit detailed consideration. From the beginning of this century until the early 1970s there was a striking decline in death rates from non-malignant digestive diseases. For both men and women mortality from digestive disease has been concentrated in the older age-groups, predominantly those aged 65 years and over. Within each age-band death rates in men and women have been of a similar magnitude in any given time period. Overall, these rates are low in comparison to non-gastrointestinal causes of death. For example, in 1921 among men aged 45–64 years, the age-standardised death rate from digestive diseases was 959 per million, while the death rate from diseases of the circulatory system was 4,348 per million – almost five times greater. In relative terms this difference has been increasing during the rest of this century (see Chapter 4). By 1990, among men aged 45–64 years, the death rate from digestive diseases had fallen by almost 70 per cent to 311 per million, while deaths from diseases of the circulatory system were recorded at 4,038 deaths per million – now more than 12 times greater than the level for digestive disease.

To gain a greater understanding of the historical pattern of digestive disease in Britain it is necessary to consider the broad distribution of deaths from specific disorders. Table 22.1 shows deaths from selected digestive disorders among men and women at four different points this century. The specific disorders in each table were selected because for each one there are representative data going back at least to 1931, and

because they are now the major contributors towards the overall burden of mortality from gastrointestinal disease. As most deaths from gastrointestinal disease occur in people older than age 60, and to take into account the increasing numbers of elderly in the population, the age-standardised mortality rates from the most important diseases shown in Table 22.1 are shown in Table 22.2. After standardisation it can be seen that overall the changes in mortality between the early and latter parts of this century are somewhat more pronounced than before. Table 22.1 shows the gradual decline in the contribution of gastrointestinal disease to all-cause mortality with gastrointestinal disease now accounting for 3 per cent of all deaths compared with about 6 per cent at the beginning of the century.

As the tables demonstrate, the single most important cause of death from digestive disease over the century has been peptic ulcer disease, which has accounted for 4,000–5,000 deaths per year since the end of the First World War; this topic is discussed in more detail later. Deaths due to liver disease rank second as a cause of death, and most (90 per cent) are due to chronic liver disease. The fluctuating numbers are mainly a reflection of changing levels of alcohol consumption in the United Kingdom; this is a subject of Chapter 8. The remainder are predominantly due to acute liver failure, secondary to either viral infection or poisoning by alcohol or drugs such as paracetamol.

Of the other major causes, deaths due to appendicitis show the greatest rise and fall and are discussed later. Deaths from gallstones also show a considerable decline during the century accounting for more than 2,800 deaths in 1901 and only

Table 22.2

Age-standardised mortality rates from selected gastrointestinal diseases among men and women aged 15-84 years in England and Wales, by selected quinquennia 1926–30 to 1986–90

Disease		1926–30	1946–50	1966–70	1986–90
Duodenal ulcer	Men	84.4	122.4	70.3	43.2
	Women	11.5	14.7	16.9	22.6
Gastric ulcer/peptic ulcer	Men	155.7	141.9	62.4	33.3
(unspecified)	Women	59.1	39.7	28.5	24.5
Chronic liver disease	Men	91.5	32.7	35.7	36.4
	Women	39.8	17.7	27.2	28.5
Pancreatic diseases	Men	15.3	9.4	15.1	18.1
	Women	15.9	10.4	12.3	12.6
Cholelithiasis (gallstones)	Men	30.2*	17.1	17.2	9.1
	Women	58.0*	32.7	19.0	8.4
Diverticular disease	Men	13.7*	16.1	19.0	12.8
	Women	10.4*	14.9	25.0	21.4

Death rate per million standardised to European Standard Population. * = *Mortality rate for 1931 only.*

around 900 today. For both conditions the decline in mortality undoubtedly reflects the dramatic advances in anaesthesia and surgery that have occurred this century, particularly since the incidence of both conditions was increasing during much of this period.

In contrast, deaths from diverticular disease and its complications (bleeding and perforation) have shown a steady increase, particularly in women, rising from fewer than 400 per year in 1931 to more than 1,500 in 1991. The increase is partly accounted for by an ageing population, as demonstrated by the less marked increase in the age-standardised rates (see Table 22.2). Also the prevalence of diverticular disease has almost certainly increased markedly, although most of the evidence for the increase is indirect. Deaths from pancreatic disease, which are predominantly due to acute pancreatitis, have almost doubled in the past 60 years, again this partly reflects an ageing population (see Table 22.2). However, the increasing age-standardised mortality in men is likely to be due to deaths from alcohol-induced pancreatitis. In contrast, deaths from the inflammatory bowel diseases ulcerative colitis and Crohn's disease are relatively few and are not increasing despite the increasing incidence of both diseases over the past 60 years (Srivastava *et al.*, 1995; Thomas *et al.*, 1995; Miller *et al.*, 1974).

The conditions listed in Table 22.1 account for almost two-thirds of digestive disease deaths. Other conditions of current importance but not shown in these figures because the data for earlier periods are less certain, include abdominal hernia, vascular insufficiency, unspecified gastrointestinal bleeding and non-malignant oesophageal disease. Abdominal hernia (716 deaths in 1991), as well as including deaths from inguinal and femoral hernias, included a quarter certified to diaphragmatic hiatal hernias where the underlying process is usually a peptic oesophagitis. The mortality rate from this condition and other non-malignant oesophageal disease (coded under ICD9 530) has more than doubled since 1968 (Panos *et al.*, 1995). Mesenteric vascular insufficiency (1,546 deaths in 1991), occurs acutely and reflects vascular disease elsewhere in the body. Similarly, many of the deaths coded to unspecified gastrointestinal bleeding (1,130 deaths in 1991) are due to generalised bleeding disorders and not to diseases with their origins in the digestive system.

22.3 Morbidity from digestive disease

Life-threatening disease represents only a small proportion of the total burden of gastrointestinal disease. It is important therefore to consider the data that exist to illustrate levels and patterns of morbidity, in particular, GP consultations and hospital discharge data. Before doing so, some further words of caution are appropriate. Concerns about the frailties of mortality data pale into insignificance when compared to the difficulties inherent in obtaining and interpreting changes and trends in morbidity data; virtually no data are available for the first half of the twentieth century, and aggregate data on national hospital admissions are consistently not available after 1985, after which major changes occurred to the data

collected. In order to set patterns of morbidity in perspective compared to mortality, Table 22.3 shows the 10 commonest reasons for GP consultation and hospital discharge among men and women, alongside their ten commonest causes of death from gastrointestinal disease in 1981–82. One of the most striking features is that irritable bowel, constipation and other functional digestive conditions, characterised by a disturbance in gastrointestinal motility and no known structural pathology, constitute the major burden of gastrointestinal disease in both men and women attending their general practitioner. Intestinal disease of presumed infective aetiology is the single most important digestive cause for GP consultation in both men and women; consultation rates for this condition are double those for any other single abdominal disorder. Food poisoning notifications including those where specific organisms have been isolated have shown a marked increase over the past 20 years and are likely to have contributed to increasing numbers with post-infective irritable bowel symptoms. Infective gastrointestinal disease is covered in Chapter 15 and is not discussed further in this chapter.

In the 1991/92 GP morbidity survey, 8.7 per cent of the population consulted their general practitioners that year with a digestive complaint (McCormick *et al.*, 1995). This was a 20 per cent increase from the 7.2 per cent consulting 10 years earlier but was not greatly different from the 8.2 per cent consulting in 1971/72 or the 10 per cent consulting in 1955/56 (RCGP *et al.*,1986). The increase was confined to adults, particularly those over 65 years in whom the increase was over 30 per cent. However, consulting rates for serious conditions such as peptic ulcer, inguinal hernia, appendicitis, liver and gall-bladder disease have not increased (McCormick, *et al.*, 1995; RCGP *et al.*, 1986). In contrast, the consulting rates for non-ulcer dyspepsia, which includes symptoms labelled as hiatus hernia, oesophagitis, gastritis and functional stomach disorders, have trebled in this 10-year period and account for almost a half of the consultations for non-infective conditions (McCormick *et al.*, 1995; RCGP *et al.*, 1986). Only a part of this increase can be attributed to more accurate endoscopic diagnosis of peptic ulcer.

The other major reason for consulting was symptoms ascribed to irritable bowel syndrome. Population surveys reveal that one or more of such symptoms are extremely common, being reported by 47 per cent of women and 27 per cent of men in a recent survey performed in Bristol (Heaton *et al.*, 1992). In this study 13 per cent of women and 5 per cent of men had sufficient symptoms (three or more) to make a diagnosis of irritable bowel syndrome according to standard criteria. Nevertheless, only half of these people had ever consulted a doctor about them, with the tendency to consult being related to the number of symptoms reported and the presence of abdominal pain. The GP morbidity surveys suggest that the numbers consulting have increased in recent years.

While so-called functional disorders are the main cause of people consulting general practitioners, conditions potentially needing surgical treatment either urgently or electively account for the majority of hospital discharges (see Table 22.3).

Table 22.3

Ten most common reasons for GP consultation, hospital discharge and death among men and women, 1981–82

GP consultation rate per 100,000 person-years		Hospital discharge rate per 100,000 population		Crude death rate per million population	
Men					
1 Intestinal disease presumed infective	4,200	1 Inguinal hernia	293	1 Duodenal ulcer	48.7
2 Functional disorder of stomach	1,990	2 Acute appendicitis	101	2 Chronic liver disease and cirrhosis	48.1
3 Irritable bowel syndrome	1,420	3 Duodenal ulcer	70	3 Gastric ulcer	28.1
4 Duodenal ulcer	1,400	4 Haemorrhoids	50	4 Vascular insufficiency of intestine	20.6
5= Inguinal hernia	1,050	5 Non-infective gastroenteritis/colitis	46	5 Intestinal obstruction	16.9
5= Haemorrhoids	1,050	6 Cholelithiasis (gallstones)	45	6 Diseases of the pancreas	16.4
7 Constipation	970	7 Other abdominal herniae	41	7 Diverticular diseases	13.7
8 Hiatus hernia	540	8 Diseases of the oesophagus	34	8 Gastrointestinal bleeding (unspecified)	11.3
9 Other disorders of stomach/duodenum	420	9 Other functional digestive disorders	33	9 Peptic ulcer (unspecified)	10.4
10 Anal fissure or fistula/perianal abcess	360	10 Gastrointestinal bleeding (unspecified)	32	10 Diseases of the oesophagus	8.5
Women					
1 Intestinal disease presumed infective	4,410	1 Cholelithiasis (gallstones)	95	1 Chronic liver disease and cirrhosis	41.3
2 Irritable bowel syndrome and other non-infective non-ulcerative disorders	2,210	2 Acute appendicitis	83	2 Duodenal ulcer	25.5
3 Functional disorders of stomach	1,950	3 Other disorders of the gallbladder	57	3 Gastric ulcer	38.7
4 Constipation	1,640	4 Other abdominal herniae	50	4 Diverticular disease	37.9
5 Haemorrhoids	1,190	5= Non infective gastroenteritis/colitis	42	5 Vacular insufficiency of intestine	33.2
6 Hiatus hernia	890	5= Diverticular disease	42	6 Intestinal obstruction	25.7
7 Cholecystitis/cholelithiasis	720	7 Other disorder of intestine	41	7 Diseases of the pancreas	16.6
8 Diverticulitis	680	8 Other functional digestive disorder	39	8 Gastrointestinal bleeding (unspecified)	16.0
9 Duodenal ulcer	570	9 Haemorrhoids	37	9 Peptic ulcer (unspecified)	12.8
10 Inflammatory bowel disease	380	10 Diseases of the oesophagus	33	10 Cholelithiasis (gallstones)	11.3

Emergency hospital admissions are generally the result of conditions producing acute abdominal pain and acute gastrointestinal bleeding. The latter is predominantly due to bleeding from the upper gastrointestinal tract (oesophagus, stomach and duodenum). In 1993 acute upper gastrointestinal bleeding was estimated to be the cause of 1,030 and 710 admissions per million in men and women respectively (Rockall *et al.*, 1995). Annual incidence rose sharply with age from 200 per million in people under 30 to over 4,000 per million in those aged over 75 years. Bleeding was ascribed to peptic ulceration in just over a third of cases and to peptic oesophagitis and acute erosive inflammation in 22 per cent, but in about a quarter no cause was clearly established, usually because active investigation of its cause was deemed inappropriate. Although crude mortality (case fatality rate) of acute upper gastrointestinal bleeding has stayed around 10 per cent for the past 50 years the age-adjusted mortality appears to have fallen by a third (Rockall *et al.*, 1995).

Numerous conditions can give rise to acute abdominal pain severe enough to result in hospitalisation. In people under 30 years, acute appendicitis and suspected appendicitis due to functional abdominal pain are the most common and are discussed below. Perforation of a peptic ulcer remains common, particularly in the elderly, although annual rates in those under 65 years are now less than 250 per million (see below) (Penston *et al.*, 1993). Remarkably little is known of the frequency of other conditions giving rise to acute severe pain, such as perforation or obstruction of the intestine, but they appear to be much less common. Acute pancreatitis has been estimated to affect 70 per million each year with a case fatality of 20 per cent (Corfield *et al.*, 1985).

Another important cause of hospitalisation is inflammatory bowel disease, namely, ulcerative colitis and Crohn's disease, which account for just under half of the hospital discharges, included under the label non-infective gastroenteritis/colitis. During the 1960s and 1970s, discharges for Crohn's disease increased steadily in both men and women to approximately 100 and 150 per million respectively (Sonnenberg, 1990); this occurred in parallel with an increase in incidence of Crohn's disease. Since then annual incidence in the United Kingdom appears to have plateaued at between 60 and 80 per million and tends to be higher in women than men

(Thomas *et al.*, 1995; Lee and Nguyen-Van-Tam, 1994; Fellows *et al.*, 1990). In contrast, hospital discharges for ulcerative colitis, initially higher in women than men, have declined in women to a level similar to that for men, which have shown little change, at around 100 per million. Incidence of ulcerative colitis is about twice that for Crohn's disease and has not increased significantly recently (Srivastava *et al.*, 1992; Sinclair *et al.*, 1983)

Discharges following elective surgery are dominated by those for cholecystectomy in women and inguinal hernia repair in men. Cholecystectomy rates in the United Kingdom were gradually declining until 10 years ago. No recent figures have been published for England but in Scotland and also in North America there has been an increase noted since the introduction of laparoscopic (key-hole) cholecystectomy, (Lam *et al.*, 1996). Gallstones are extremely common, being found in 12 per cent of men and 22 per cent of women over age 60 in a recent ultrasound survey in Bristol (Heaton *et al.*, 1991). In most people gallstones cause few or no symptoms and there is no evidence that the numbers with symptoms have increased lately. It seems likely, therefore, that the rise in cholecystectomy rates reflects a lower threshold for intervention rather than any increase in morbidity – a timely warning of the limitations of using procedure rates as a proxy measure of morbidity.

22.4 Specific conditions: peptic ulcer

As Table 22.3 shows, the most important causes of death from gastrointestinal disease in both men and women are chronic liver disease and peptic ulcer. Chronic liver disease is dealt with in Chapter 8, and this section focuses on peptic ulcer. Other reasons for examining peptic ulcer mortality in more detail are that, firstly, deaths from peptic ulcer are generally the result of either ulcer perforation or ulcer bleeding and

both are usually reliably diagnosed; and secondly, reasonably accurate figures are available for most of the twentieth century.

Figure 22.1 shows age-specific mortality from duodenal ulcer among men and women where the rise in mortality over the first half of the century can be seen in both sexes. A large proportion of this rise is commonly attributed to increases in the prevalence of smoking in the British population (see Chapter 9). It can also be seen that in all age-groups mortality from duodenal ulcer has been consistently and substantially higher in men than women. A decline in mortality is seen from the 1950s until the early 1980s, especially in men. These changes have been attributed to the decline in the prevalence of smoking, with the more substantial decline in men being consistent with the greater decline in prevalence of smoking among men (see Chapter 9). Somewhat surprisingly, duodenal ulcer mortality increased in women from the early 1970s until it began to plateau, or even decline, from 1981–85. Increases in mortality towards the mid-1980s have been noted previously (Walt *et al.*, 1986), and are thought, at least in part, to be the result of increased use of non-steroidal anti-inflammatory drugs (NSAIDs) for the alleviation of musculoskeletal pain. These drugs have been shown to cause both gastric and duodenal ulceration, including ulcer bleeding and perforation (Langman *et al.*, 1994; Henry *et al.*,1996) Prescribing of NSAIDs increased markedly during the 1970s and 1980s such that by 1990, 15–20 per cent of people over age 60 were taking a NSAID on a regular basis, (Langman *et al.*,1994). The recent small decline again after the mid-1980s may indicate increased awareness of the side-effects of NSAIDs and more selective prescribing of these drugs.

Figure 22.2 shows trends for gastric ulcer (which includes peptic ulcer with no site specified) for men and women. Under the age of 65 there have been declines in gastric ulcer mortality since 1945, greater at younger ages, but mortality among those aged 65 and over rose until the 1950s before declining.

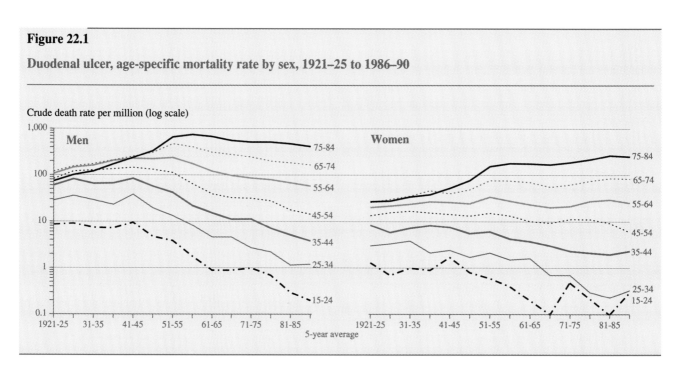

Figure 22.1

Duodenal ulcer, age-specific mortality rate by sex, 1921–25 to 1986–90

Crude death rate per million (log scale)

5-year average

Figure 22.2

Gastric ulcer/peptic ulcer age-specific mortality rate by sex, 1911–90

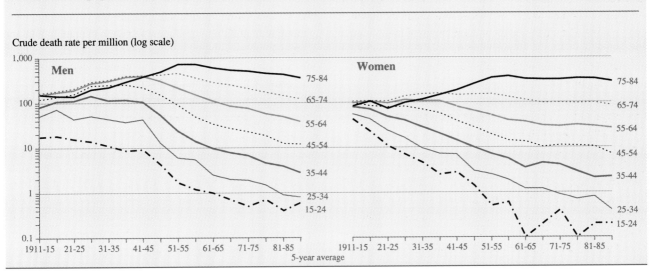

Crude death rate per million (log scale)

5-year average

What is also notable is that in the early part of this century the age-specific mortality rates for both duodenal and gastric ulcer in men and women showed less variation than currently. A similar pattern has now been observed in many countries in Europe as well as in the US and Japan (Susser, 1982; Sonnenberg, 1995). It is generally accepted that this pattern is indicative of a birth cohort effect whereby individuals born at a certain time were exposed to factors which preceding and succeeding birth cohorts were not exposed to. This can be demonstrated by plotting mortality rates for each age-band by the mid-year of birth of each cohort as has been done in Figures 22.3 and 22.4. What can be seen is that people born between 1870 and 1900 had the highest mortality rates and that the peak birth cohorts for duodenal ulcer mortality were 10–20 years later than those for gastric ulcer.

The environmental factor accounting for this cohort effect has not been definitely established. Recent attention has focused on the bacterium *Helicobacter pylori*, which is now

known to play an essential role in the development of most peptic ulcers. Helicobacter infection is equally common in men and women and is remarkably widespread, with a half or more of the United Kingdom population over age 50 being infected. It has been suggested that the crowded living conditions of the expanding cities at the beginning of the industrial revolution lead to a decline in hygiene and the spread and infection early in life with *Helicobacter pylori* (Sonnenberg, 1995). Infection with Helicobacter early in life is thought to result in more extensive gastric inflammation and a greater risk of gastric ulcer, while infection later in life, as might occur as living conditions and hygiene improve, results in inflammation confined to the gastric antrum and an increased risk of duodenal ulcer. Direct evidence in support of this hypothesis is lacking but no other factors have been identified that account adequately for the cohort effect. Moreover levels of *Helicobacter pylori* infection in the United Kingdom appear to be declining in parallel with the decline in peptic ulcer disease (Sonnenberg, 1995).

Figure 22.3

Age-specific mortality rate from duodenal ulcer by sex, 1841–1971

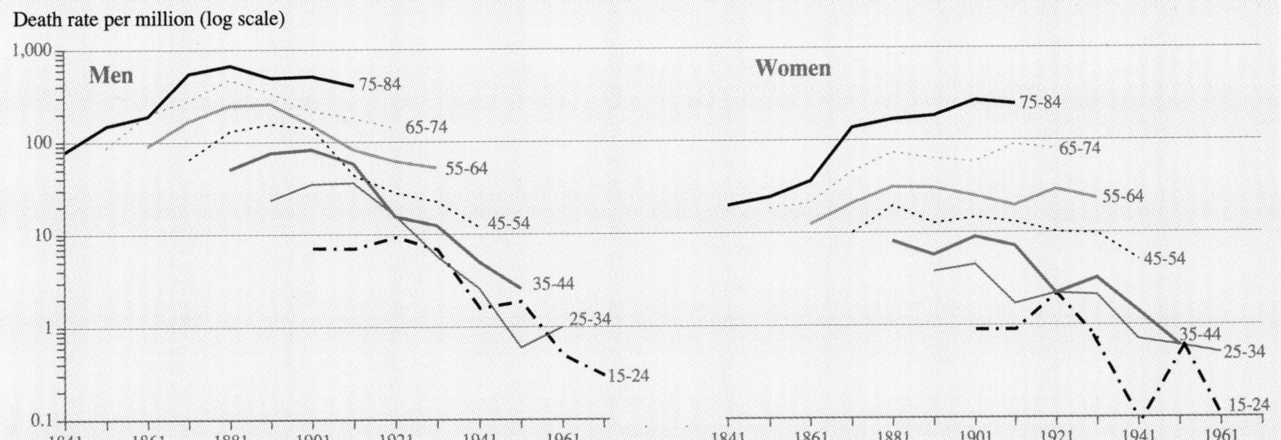

Death rate per million (log scale)

Year of birth

Figure 22.4

Age-specific mortality rate from gastric ulcer/peptic ulcer by sex, 1841–1971

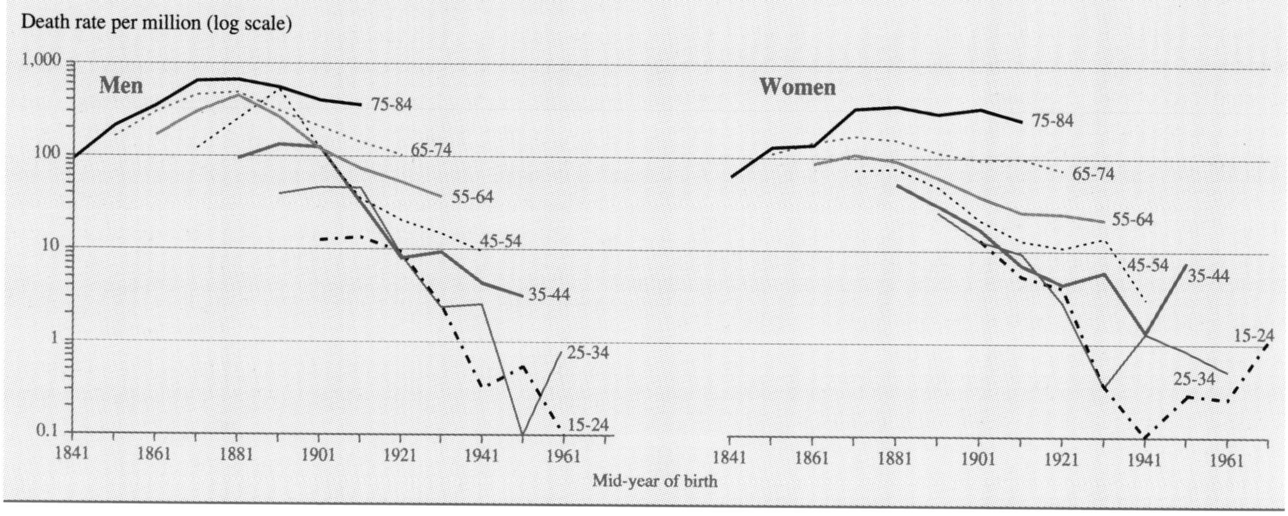

Death rate per million (log scale)

Mid-year of birth

22.5 Specific conditions: appendicitis and abdominal pain

Although some digestive disorders may produce little in the way of early symptoms (for example, stomach cancer), it is more often the case that the onset of digestive disease is associated with one or more of a wide variety of symptoms. People recognising these as abnormal, inconvenient, or distressing, may well decide, in the first instance, to consult with their general practitioner. The spectrum of digestive symptoms is extremely broad in terms of type, frequency and severity, and the commoner symptoms for which patients would be likely to seek medical advice naturally include abdominal pain; however, it is not always possible or practical to ascribe a definite diagnosis in every case. Data on abdominal symptoms for which general practitioners did not make specific diagnoses have been collected during the Royal College of General Practitioners National Morbidity Surveys (McCormick *et al.,* 1995; RCGP *et al.,* 1986). In each of these, the precise classification of symptoms has varied, which limits the extent to which the data from different periods are comparable. None the less, the results clearly demonstrate the range and frequency of digestive symptoms for which no diagnosis was made by general practitioners; detailed data for 1991/92 are shown in Table 22.4.

Table 22.4

Prevalence rates for abdominal symptoms 1991/92. Patients consulting their GP each year, per 10,000 person-years at risk

ICD9 code and symptom	0–4	5–15	16–24	25–44	45–64	65–74	75–84	85+
Men								
789.0 Unexplained abdominal pain	280	256	146	134	144	211	253	244
787.0 Nausea and vomiting	252	56	31	19	23	45	76	143
787.1 Heartburn	0	0	3	5	6	13	17	12
787.2 Dysphagia	2	1	2	4	13	30	42	53
787.6 Incontinence of faeces	8	8	0	0	1	1	18	42
Women								
789.0 Unexplained abdominal pain	259	348	471	365	247	272	269	327
787.0 Nausea and vomiting	241	59	105	63	54	80	118	162
787.1 Heartburn	1	0	20	22	12	23	18	8
787.2 Dysphagia	2	1	2	5	12	21	33	39
787.6 Incontinence of faeces	4	4	0	0	1	4	11	24

Source: OPCS Series MB5 No 3, 1995

It is perhaps unsurprising to discover that, of the digestive symptoms for which a definitive diagnosis is not readily evident, abdominal pain is by far the most common symptom that leads patients to consult their GP. The nature of abdominal pain is almost infinitely variable in terms of its quality, duration, timing and severity. Moreover, it is associated with a vast range of digestive and non-digestive disorders. As well as relatively minor disorders, such as constipation, many serious, treatable conditions, such as peritonitis, also begin with abdominal pain. Therefore, it is obviously important to discriminate between the two types of illness. In order to achieve this, sophisticated investigations (ranging from fibre-optic endoscopy to magnetic resonance imaging) may be needed; these are normally available only in hospitals, resulting in many patients being admitted. Even at this stage, a diagnosis is not always made; many patients admitted to hospital with abdominal pain are eventually discharged, after the pain has settled, without a definitive diagnosis ever having been made.

Between 1968 and 1981, in England and Wales, the hospital discharge rate for patients with undiagnosed abdominal pain rose appreciably from 1,230 per million in 1968 to 2,310 in 1981. The increase has been most pronounced in the younger age-groups, especially women aged 15–44 years. The hospital discharge rate in this group has continued to rise without abatement since the 1970s, almost doubling in just over 10 years (see Figure 22.5). About three times as many young women as young men are admitted to hospital each year with this condition.

Appendicitis was first distinguished in mortality statistics in 1901 (Donnan and Lambert, 1976); at that time, it gave the appearance of having suddenly appeared from nowhere. Figure 22.6 depicts mortality from appendicitis over the last century. The first remarkable feature is that in both sexes, and in all adult age-groups, mortality from appendicitis was initially very high and remained so, after the turn of the century, for the next 20–30 years; in the younger age-groups mortality peaked in the early 1920s, while among older adults this change took place about a decade later. These findings have been reported previously (Donnan and Lambert, 1976). However, it is interesting to note that mortality from appendicitis was increasing at the same time as surgical or operative mortality was undoubtedly decreasing. This suggests that in the early part of the century there was a genuine increase in the incidence of appendicitis. From the 1940s onwards, in both sexes and in all age-groups, the mortality from appendicitis has fallen dramatically. These changes coincide with substantial improvements in anaesthesia and surgical technique and probably a genuine decrease in incidence. However, death rates from appendicitis are now so low that they provide no meaningful indication of incidence. It should also be noted that, at all ages, mortality is consistently higher among men than women. Death rates are highest among the elderly, which undoubtedly reflects the hazards of abdominal surgery and general anaesthesia in elderly subjects.

Appendicitis is one condition that provides an example of the difficulties associated with accurate diagnosis of abdominal pain. In a great many patients presenting with lower abdominal pain, appendicitis should be considered high up in the differential diagnosis. Patients with appendicitis usually need surgery, and indeed the diagnosis cannot be confirmed without histological examination of the appendiceal stump. For this reason virtually every patient in whom appendicitis is seriously contemplated is nowadays admitted to hospital for observation, even though the presumptive diagnosis may not be subsequently confirmed. Because mortality from appendicitis is now extremely low, morbidity data are said to be the most reliable current indicator of incidence. Figure 22.7 illustrates that, in both sexes, hospital admission with

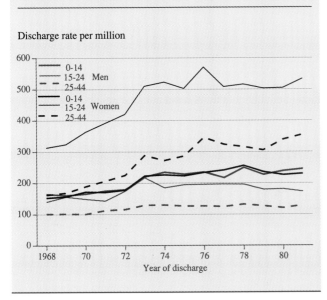

Figure 22.5

Hospital discharge rates with undiagnosed abdominal pain, 1968–85

Discharge rate per million

Year of discharge

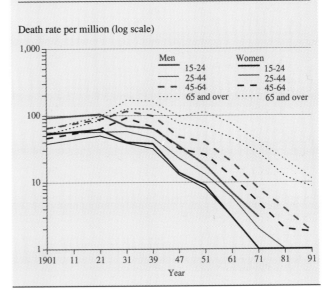

Figure 22.6

Mortality from appendicitis among adults in Britain, 1901–91

Death rate per million (log scale)

Year

Figure 22.7

Hospital discharge rates with main diagnosis of appendicitis, 1968–85

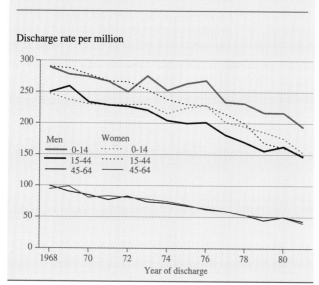

Discharge rate per million

appendicitis being confirmed at operation (negative appendicectomies) (Primatesta and Goldacre, 1994; Addiss *et al.*, 1990). Moreover, this situation is far more likely to occur in women than men (Primatesta and Goldacre, 1994; Addiss *et al.*, 1990), which undoubtedly reflects the particular difficulties in diagnosing abdominal pain among women of child-bearing age. Diagnostic sophistication has gradually increased through the use of tests such as ultrasound scans. In addition, the development of potent antibiotics and other improvements in surgical management have made perforation of the bowel less dangerous than it was; thus it has become safer to delay surgery. These changes may have resulted in progressively fewer episodes of abdominal pain being attributed to appendicitis (and therefore managed by early surgery), instead being assigned to abdominal pain of unknown origin and allowed more time to settle spontaneously. The evidence to support this possible explanation is explored below in greater detail.

Among men, declines in the admission rate for appendicitis are matched by corresponding rises in admission rates for abdominal pain; this is particularly easy to illustrate in boys and young men aged 15–44 years (see Figure 22.8). However, the decrease in admissions for appendicitis is not fully explained by diagnostic reclassification, and there may well have been some genuine reduction in incidence between the early 1970s and the early 1980s.

Among girls and women, the decrease in admission rates for appendicitis are probably more closely matched to increases in admission rates for abdominal pain; this 'mirror effect' is most easily seen among young women aged 15–44 years, although it is present to some extent in other age-groups (see Figure 22.9). In women it is perhaps less easy to conclude that there has been a genuine reduction in the incidence of appendicitis in the last decade.

appendicitis is commonest among children and young adults aged 15–44 years. However, since the late 1960s there has been a gradual decline across all age-groups in rates of admission for appendicitis among both men and women, with the rate of decline having been sharpest among young women. One previously suggested explanation for the decline in admissions for appendicitis and the rise in admissions for unspecified abdominal pain is diagnostic reclassification (Langman, 1979). In the past, a larger proportion of patients with acute abdominal pain were assigned a diagnosis of acute appendicitis, although this may not actually have been the case. Two epidemiological studies of appendicitis, one in the United States, one in Britain, both suggest that many emergency appendicectomies are performed without

Figure 22.8

Hospital discharge rates for unspecified abdominal pain and appendicitis in men, 1968–81

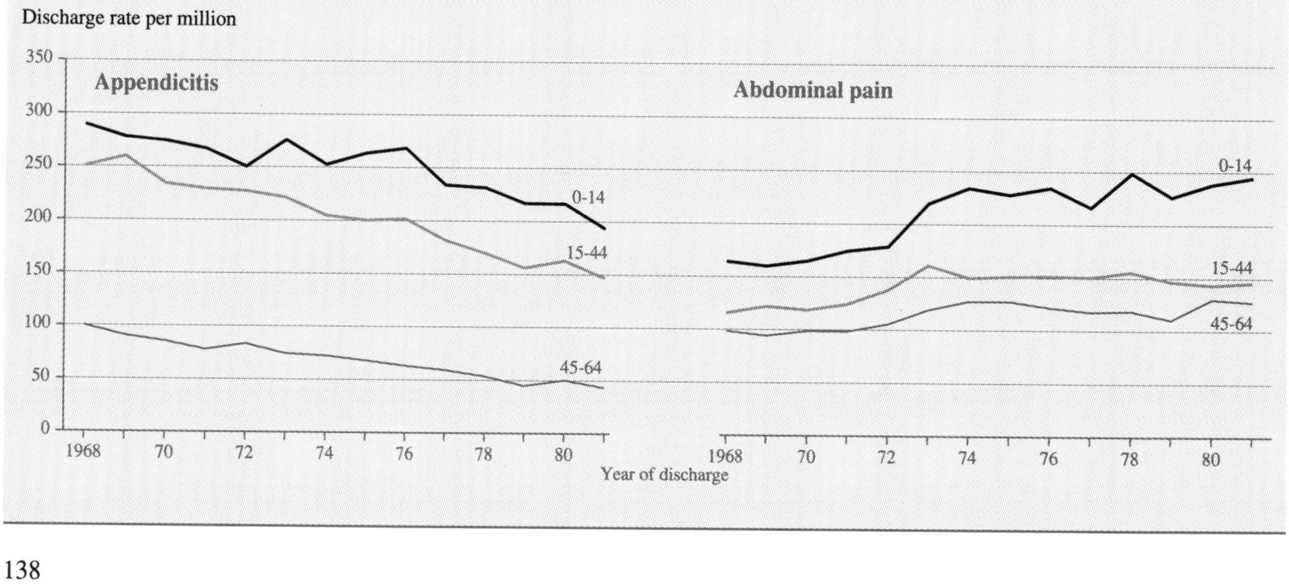

Discharge rate per million

Figure 22.9

Hospital discharge rates for unspecified abdominal pain and appendicitis in women, 1968–81

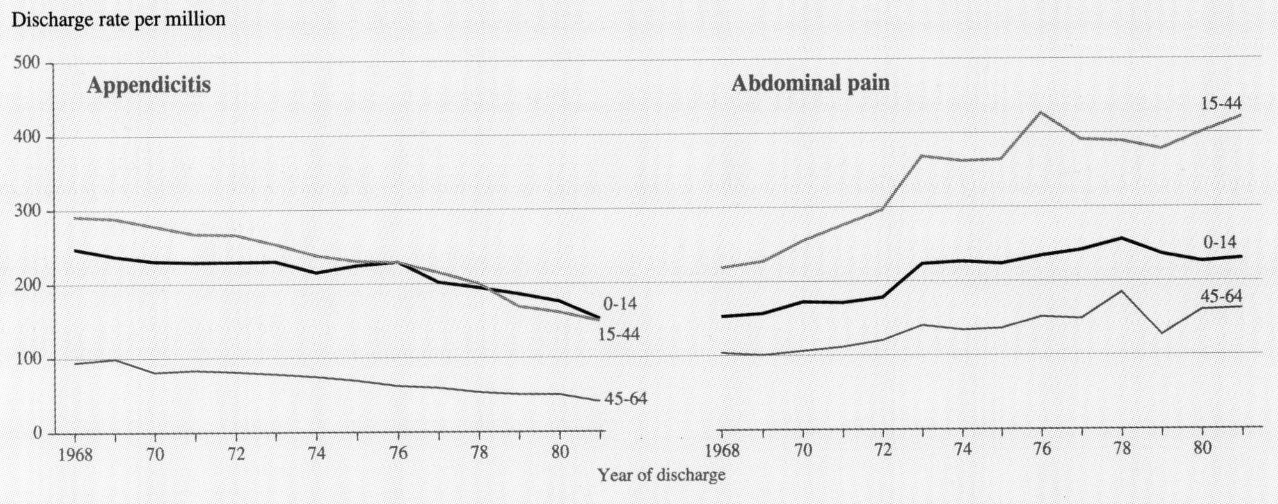

Discharge rate per million

22.6 Summary

This chapter has attempted a broad overview of the impact of digestive diseases on the health of adults in Britain. Firstly, trends in mortality have been discussed. Here, the evidence points to a substantial improvement in health over the last century; mortality from most serious or life-threatening digestive diseases has declined, with some notable exceptions, such as duodenal ulcer and diverticular disease in women, and pancreatic disease in men. These declines reflect, to a large extent, advances in medical treatment, especially surgery. From this perspective the impact of gastrointestinal disease in the twentieth century represents a medical success story.

Nevertheless, while the incidences of peptic ulcer and appendicitis have declined, others such as chronic liver disease, Crohn's disease and diverticular disease appear to have increased and are now a major burden on health services. Furthermore, for many conditions and complaints, consultations and hospital admission rates are increasing. These trends partly reflect increasing affluence, an ageing population and greater patient expectations – the penalty of successful treatment for other conditions. Thus, in spite of declining incidence of several major gastrointestinal diseases and generally falling mortality, the high prevalence of gastrointestinal symptoms and people's rising expectations from health care have ensured that gastrointestinal disease has been, and will continue to be, a major influence on the health of the nation for the foreseeable future.

Chapter 23

Musculoskeletal diseases

By
Deborah Symmons

Summary

- As the number of elderly people in the community has increased over the past 150 years, so the number of people with musculoskeletal conditions has also risen.

- In the last 100 years the application of immunology, biochemistry and radiology to the rheumatic diseases has assisted in identifying a number of distinct disease entities.

- Sources of data that have been used to investigate the epidemiology of the rheumatic diseases include mortality statistics, the RCGP morbidity studies, hospital in-patient statistics and several population surveys.

- There was a sharp growth in the incidence and prevalence of rheumatoid arthritis in the late ninteenth and early twentieth centuries. Since the 1950s it has declined, particularly among women. In very elderly people it is now more common in men than in women.

- Incidence of ankolysing spondylitis has been estimated at 6.6 cases per 100,000. Prevalence is estimated to be 1 per 1,000. Mortality data are difficult to interpret because many patients in the 1940s and 1950s were treated with spinal irradiation, which sometimes caused leukemia.

- The epidemiology of gout in Britain has changed dramatically in the last 150 years. This is due partly to altered dietary habits and partly to the introduction in 1963 of allopurinol, a drug that inhibits the formation of uric acid.

- Studies have shown that the prevalence of systemic lupus erythematosus is higher in black, Asian and Chinese communities than in white people. Prevalence is likely to be rising partly as a result of improved survival and partly because of increased recognition.

- The number of people with osteoarthritis is increasing. Knee osteoarthritis in particular is becoming more common. Cohort studies show that patients with osteoarthritis have an increased mortality.

- Joint replacement surgery has been widely practised in Britain for over 25 years. The main indication for operations is osteoarthritis.

- According to the RCGP morbidity studies the consultation rate for back pain has risen in the past 10 years. In Britain, work loss resulting from back disorders has doubled in the past 5 years.

- Studies from the Arthritis and Rheumatism Council's Epidemiology Research Unit estimate that lifetime prevalence of soft tissue rheumatism is close to 50 per cent of middle- and older age-groups.

- There has been a fourfold increase over the last 3 decades in mortality from osteoporosis in women, and the incidence of hip fractures has also increased.

23.1 Introduction

The term 'musculoskeletal diseases' encompasses a wide range of conditions affecting joints, bones, soft tissues and muscles. There are over 200 recognised disorders within this broad category. The present chapter covers only 10 of these conditions plus joint replacement (see Table 23.1) – chosen either because they are the most common or the most characteristic of their group.

The evolution of thought on the nomenclature and classification of the rheumatic diseases is reflected in their ICD (International Classification of Diseases; WHO, 1977) codes (see Table 23.1). Systemic lupus erythematosus (SLE) was coded as a disease of blood vessels in the seventh revision of the ICD (ICD7). Ankylosing spondylitis and juvenile chronic arthritis (JCA) were both classified as variants of rheumatoid arthritis until the ninth revision of the ICD (ICD9).

No age-group is spared, but the prevalence of musculoskeletal disorders rises with age. As the number of elderly people in the community has increased over the last 150 years (see Chapter 3), so the number of people with musculoskeletal conditions has also risen. At present 'arthritis and rheumatism' is the most frequent self-reported long-standing condition in Britain, with a rate of 80 per 1,000 adult women and 40 per 1,000 adult men (OPCS, 1989). Over half of the 6 million physically disabled adults in Britain are disabled by a musculoskeletal disease (Martin and White, 1988). Musculoskeletal disorders currently account for 18.7 per cent of all general practitioner (GP) consultations. This rose by 46 per cent between 1971 (RCGP, OPCS, 1979) and 1981 (RCGP, OPCS, 1988). Only 4 per cent of these patients are referred to hospital.

Some musculoskeletal disorders may affect other organ systems and be immediately life-threatening. However, the main burden of musculoskeletal disease is reflected not in mortality data, nor even in hospital in-patient statistics, but in morbidity data derived from general practice or community surveys.

23.2 Historical background and nomenclature

Rheumatic conditions have been recognised since the fourth century BC when Hippocrates described both gout and acute rheumatic fever. However, the emergence of distinct disease entities from the amorphous mass of rheumatic conditions has been a slow process. William Heberden commented on this at the end of the eighteenth century when he wrote, 'The rheumatism is a common name for many aches and pains, which have no peculiar appellation, though owing to very different causes'.

During the nineteenth century physicians tried to decipher and name different diseases, but by 1896 Gilbert Bannatyne remarked that 'Probably in no other department of medicine is there more hopeless confusion of nomenclature than in the so-called "rheumatic diseases" ' (Bannatyne et al., 1896). In the 100 years since then the application of immunology, biochemistry and radiology to the rheumatic diseases has enabled a number of distinct diseases to be defined. However,

Table 23.1

Musculoskeletal disorders included in this chapter, and their ICD codes

Grouping	Condition	ICD7	ICD8	ICD9
Inflammatory joint disease	Rheumatoid arthritis	722*	712.1 712.3	714 – 714.2
	Juvenile chronic arthritis	722*	712	714.3
	Ankylosing spondylitis	722.1	712.4	720.2 – 720.9
	Gout	288	274	712.0* 274.0
Joint failure	Osteoarthritis	723	713	715
Connective tissue disease	Systemic lupus erythematosus	456*	734.1	710
	Scleroderma	710	734	710.1
Bone disease	Osteoporosis	733*	723.0	733.0
	Fractured neck of femur	N820	N820	820
	Fractured vertebra	733*	723.9*	733.1
Soft tissue rheumatism	The shoulder syndromes, other bursitistendonitis, tenosynovitis, synovitis and peripheral enthesopathy			726 727 (exc. 727.1 and 727.4) 728, 729 (exc. 729.5 and 729.8)

Includes other conditions.

the situation remains in a state of flux and debates continue on, for example, the correct nomenclature for childhood arthritis and on whether rheumatoid arthritis is one disease or many.

Most of our current understanding evolved during the time period covered by this book. For many centuries the word 'gout' was used as non-specifically as 'arthritis' is today. In 1686 Thomas Sydenham distinguished acute rheumatic fever as a separate entity. However, it was not until 1848 that Sir Alfred Garrod, a physician at the West London Hospital, discovered an excess of uric acid in the blood of patients with gout. In 1859 he proposed the term 'rheumatoid arthritis' for those arthritic patients who did not have gout. The term 'osteoarthritis' was first introduced by John Kent Spender, a physician in Bath, in 1888. He believed that rheumatoid arthritis and osteoarthritis were forms of the same disease. The modern distinction between rheumatoid arthritis and osteoarthritis was drawn by Sir Archibald Garrod (son of Sir Alfred) in his contribution to the 1907 edition of Allbutt and Rolleston's System of Medicine (Copeman, 1964). The British Ministry of Health adopted the two terms in 1922. The characterisation of rheumatoid arthritis was further assisted by the discovery of rheumatoid factor, an autoantibody directed against immunoglobulin, independently by Erik Waaler in 1940 (Waaler, 1940) and Harry Rose in 1948 (Rose et al., 1948). Rheumatoid factor is an antibody against the person's own immunoglobins.

The first clear description of juvenile chronic arthritis (JCA) appeared in 1897. It was written by George Frederick Still while he was a medical registrar at Great Ormond Street Hospital (Still, 1897). For many years all forms of JCA bore his name, but the term 'Still's disease' is now confined to the form of JCA with a systemic onset.

The literature on ankylosing spondylitis (AS) begins with a pathological description by Bernard Connor, an Irishman, in his MD thesis presented to the University of Rheims in 1691. His description seems to have gone largely unnoticed until Adolf Strümpell (1884, Germany), Vladimir Bechterew (1897, Russia) and Pierre Marie (1898, France) focused on the clinical features of the condition. Ankylosing spondylitis has enjoyed a wide variety of names since then.

In the USA, it was believed to be a variant of rheumatoid arthritis and was called 'rheumatoid spondylitis' until 1963. However, it is now clear that AS has more in common with the other forms of seronegative (seronegative here means no rheumatoid factor) arthritis, such as psoriatic arthritis and Reiter's disease, than with rheumatoid arthritis. This is partly explained by the association of all the seronegative forms of arthritis with the HLA-B27 antigen. The close link between AS and HLA-B27 was described by Derek Brewerton and his group from the Westminster Hospital in 1973 (Brewerton et al., 1973).

The first description of systemic lupus erythematosus (SLE) is attributed to Biett in 1822. In 1851, Cazanave used the term 'lupus erythematosus' to describe the cutaneous mani-

festations of the disease. The earliest and classic descriptions of the visceral features of SLE were given by William Osler in 1904. When the LE cell test was first described in 1948 (Hargraves et al., 1949), it became clear that SLE, like rheumatoid arthritis, is an autoimmune disease. The phenomenon was attributed to antinuclear antibodies in 1950 (Haserick, 1950). Antinuclear antibodies arise when the body's defence mechanisms react to the body's own cell constituents, in this case cell nuclei. Methods to detect antinuclear antibodies have been available since 1958.

The term 'scleroderma', referring to a persistent hardening and contraction of the body's connective tissue, was first used by Fantonetti in 1836 and early descriptions of the disease appear between 1842 and 1847.

People have been troubled with back pain and sciatica throughout recorded history. The last 150 years have seen a number of changes in the way that back pain has been perceived. The first was the idea that back pain might be provoked by trauma. This was put forward by Erichsen in 1866, following a spate of accidents during the building of the railways (Allan and Waddell, 1991). The second was the discovery of the ruptured vertebral disc, which then explained the link between back pain and sciatica (Mixter and Barr, 1934).

There has been difficulty in knowing whether everyone was speaking about the same disease, even when the terms for individual rheumatic disorders have been agreed upon. Unfortunately, the great majority of rheumatic diseases do not have a unique identifying feature. Instead, they consist of a cluster of symptoms, signs and laboratory features. To facilitate comparisons between groups of patients, and as an aid to epidemiological surveys, various sets of diagnostic criteria have been proposed. The American Rheumatism Association (ARA) – now the American College of Rheumatology (ACR) – has led the way in developing such criteria. Even when such criteria exist, there can be difficulties in applying them in the population setting, because they often require either blood tests or radiology, which may not be available.

23.3 Sources of data

23.3.1 Mortality statistics

Mortality data from 1958 (ICD7-9) have been examined and are presented by disease. Annual mortality rates have been age-adjusted to the mid-1990 population for England and Wales by direct standardisation. The data are presented as 3-year moving averages in order to iron out fluctuations caused by small numbers. Although any trends observed are likely to be real, it is important to remember that attributing the cause of death can be difficult. Cohort studies of patients with inflammatory joint disease and connective tissue diseases have shown that these patients tend to die prematurely, most commonly from infection, renal disease or cardiovascular disease. The underlying musculoskeletal disorder is often not recorded on the death certificate. In a study from

Figure 23.1

England and Wales population: persons, 1901–91

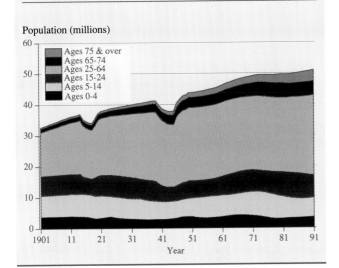

Population (millions)

Legend:
- Ages 75 & over
- Ages 65-74
- Ages 25-64
- Ages 15-24
- Ages 5-14
- Ages 0-4

Year

Birmingham of rheumatoid arthritis patients, rheumatoid arthritis was mentioned on only 36.2 per cent of death certificates (Prior *et al.*, 1984).

In 1984 there was a change in the OPCS 'Part II ruling'. This meant that diseases recorded in Part II of the death certificate as being a contributory condition could, at the discretion of the coder, be recorded as the underlying cause of death. This may account for the apparent increase in mortality for some of the rheumatic diseases from 1984 onwards, noted in this chapter.

23.3.2   GP morbidity studies

The four national morbidity studies of the Royal College of General Practitioners (RCGP) (Logan and Cushion, 1958; RCGP, 1979, 1988, 1995) provide the only national population-based data on the incidence and prevalence of musculoskeletal disease. There are no attempts to standardise diagnoses and so reliability for some of the less common disorders may be low.

23.3.3   Ad hoc epidemiological surveys and cohort studies

John Lawrence, the founder of the Arthritis and Rheumatism Council's Epidemiology Research Unit, carried out a number of population surveys in the 1950s and 1960s in Leigh, Wensleydale and Watford (Lawrence, 1977). These are still widely quoted. A number of epidemiological surveys, on a smaller scale, have been carried out since and are quoted in this chapter. In addition, cohort studies have been utilised which give information on natural history and cause of death.

23.3.4   General Household Survey

The General Household Survey (GHS) is an annual survey that started in 1971 (OPCS, 1989). It covers six domains:

population, housing, employment, education, health and social services. The sample size is around 14,000 households. The content of the structured interview changes in response to the information needs of government departments. All diagnoses are self-reported and most musculoskeletal complaints are grouped under 'arthritis and rheumatism' or 'back pain'. Questions about long-standing illness or disability are asked each year, but questions about the type of illness were only asked in 1988–89.

23.3.5   Health and Lifestyles Survey

The Health and Lifestyles Survey was conducted in 1985 (Blaxter, 1990); 9,003 adults aged over 18 who lived in private households in England, Wales and Scotland were interviewed. Health status was ascertained during two home visits by a trained observer. Diagnoses are self-reported.

23.3.6   Hospital in-patient statistics

Most patients with musculoskeletal disorders who are referred to hospital attend only as out-patients. Unfortunately, there are no national data on out-patient referrals and attendances. The number of in-patient beds and indeed the provision of rheumatology services varies widely around the country (Grahame *et al.*, 1986). The last 10 years have seen a considerable increase in the number of rheumatologists (Symmons *et al.*, 1991a). Any changes in in-patient admissions will reflect more these trends in personnel and service provision than underlying alterations in morbidity. This data source has therefore been used very little.

23.4   Review of specific diseases

23.4.1   Rheumatoid arthritis

Background

Rheumatoid arthritis is a symmetrical inflammatory polyarthritis. It usually begins in the small joints of the hands and feet. The inflamed synovium (lining of the joint cavity) erodes the articular cartilage and underlying bone and eventually causes joint deformity and progressive disability. It is more common in women than men and rarely occurs before puberty. Extra-articular features include nodules, pericarditis, pulmonary fibrosis and peripheral neuropathy.

Disease definition

It is clear that early studies of rheumatoid arthritis included patients with SLE and AS. Classification criteria for rheumatoid arthritis were first proposed by the American Rheumatism Association in 1958 (Ropes *et al.*, 1958). They comprised a list of 11 criteria. People with three or more criteria were classified as having probable, five or more as having definite and seven or more as having classical rheumatoid arthritis. A revised set of criteria was produced in 1987 (Arnett *et al.*, 1988), including only seven criteria and abandoning the concept of probable rheumatoid arthritis.

Figure 23.2

Time trends in incidence of rheumatoid arthritis: UK general practice, 1976-87

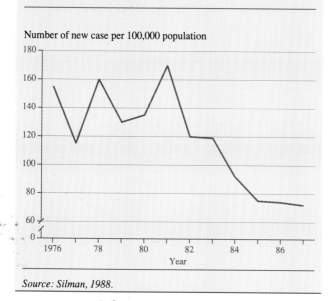

Source: Silman, 1988.

Incidence of rheumatoid arthritis

There have been three estimates of the incidence of rheumatoid arthritis in Britain. The first, of 1,200 per 100,000, was derived from two cross-sectional population studies in Leigh and Wensleydale, 5 years apart, in the 1950s (Lawrence, 1977). This is likely to be a considerable overestimate. The second used the weekly returns of the RCGP research practices to estimate the annual incidence of rheumatoid arthritis from 1976 to 1987 (Silman, 1988 see Figure 23.2). No diagnostic criteria are used; the figures are probably an overestimate and include cases of undifferentiated inflammatory arthritis. The sharp decline in incidence seen from 1981 onwards has also been seen in other countries (Dugowson et al., 1991) and has been attributed, by some, to a protective effect of the oral contraceptive pill (Vandenbroucke et al., 1982).

The latest and most rigorous assessment of rheumatoid arthritis incidence comes from the Norfolk Arthritis Register, which has been established in the Norwich Health Authority. Based on GP notifications it estimated an annual incidence in 1990 of 36 per 100,000 for women and 14 per 100,000 for men (Symmons et al., 1994, see Figure 23.3).

The prevalence of rheumatoid arthritis

Until recently the only study of the prevalence of rheumatoid arthritis was that of Lawrence (1961), which showed an overall prevalence of definite rheumatoid arthritis of 1.6 per cent in women and 0.5 per cent in men. Figure 23.4 shows the prevalence of probable plus definite rheumatoid arthritis.

With few exceptions, studies of the prevalence of rheumatoid arthritis in European populations have yielded a similar overall prevalence of definite rheumatoid arthritis of around 0.8 per cent. A recent study (conducted in 1990–91) of middle-aged women (aged 45–64) in Chingford yielded a prevalence of 1.2 per cent (Spector et al., 1993). This contrasts with Lawrence's finding of 2.5 per cent for the same group (Lawrence, 1961).

Mortality of rheumatoid arthritis

The age-adjusted annual mortality rates fell progressively in women from 1959 to around 1985 (see Figure 23.5). They then rose sharply and are now falling again. The same pattern was seen in men. This rise is probably an artefact caused by the change in the coding of Part II information noted in section 23.3.1. The age-specific mortality rates increase with age in both sexes, but rise more sharply in women (see Figure 23.6).

Cohort mortality studies of rheumatoid arthritis from Britain have all shown a reduced life expectancy for patients with rheumatoid arthritis (see Table 23.2). The study of Reilly et al. (1990) is the only one that follows patients from early in their disease. The most common causes of death were infection, circulatory and gastrointestinal deaths.

Figure 23.3

Incidence of rheumatoid arthritis in the Norwich Health Authority, 1990

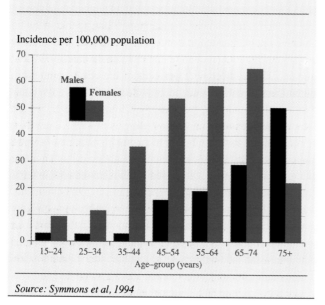

Source: Symmons et al, 1994

Figure 23.4

The prevalence of rheumatoid arthritis, 1958–60

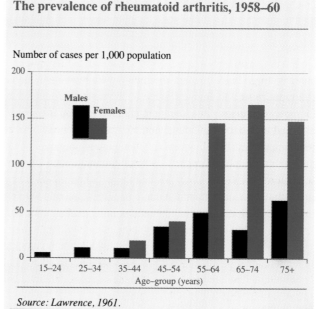

Source: Lawrence, 1961.

Figure 23.5

Annual mortality rate for rheumatoid arthritis (3-year moving average), 1959–90

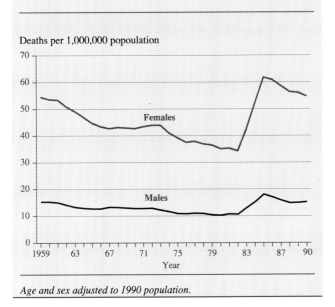

Deaths per 1,000,000 popoulation

Age and sex adjusted to 1990 population.

Figure 23.6

Age-specific mortality rates for rheumatoid arthritis, 1987–91

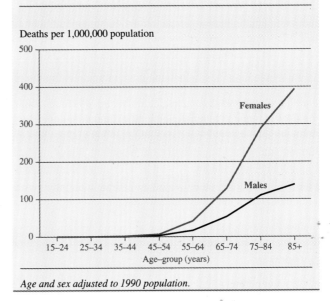

Deaths per 1,000,000 population

Age and sex adjusted to 1990 population.

Table 23.2

British studies of survival in rheumatoid arthritis

Author	Year of cohort inception	Mean follow-up (yrs)	Year of publication	SMR Males	SMR Females	Both
Duthie	1948–51	9	1964	225*	195*	
				155†	122†	
Lewis	1966–76	NS	1980			113
Prior	1964–78	11	1984	257	336	298
Reilly	1962	25	1990	144	137	140

NS Not stated.   *Age 50–59.   †Age 60 and over.

Trends

Once a rheumatic disease has been defined it has usually been possible to go back through the medical literature and skeletal remains and to find evidence of the disease going back for many centuries. Java man (a skeleton over 500,000 years old) had an osteoarthritic hip and Egyptian mummies have been found with AS. However, it has proved impossible to find unequivocal evidence of rheumatoid arthritis before the description in 1800 by Landré-Beauvais. This has led to speculation that rheumatoid arthritis may be a 'disease of civilisation', which first appeared during the industrial revolution. Recently, skeletal remains from 4,000 years ago have been found in Kentucky and Alabama (Rothschild and Woods, 1990) with erosive changes suggestive of rheumatoid arthritis, leading to the proposal that – like tobacco and the potato – rheumatoid arthritis may have been a gift from the New World to the Old!

Rheumatoid arthritis was first described in England in 1848. It seems likely that the incidence and prevalence rose sharply during the late nineteenth and early twentieth century, so that by the 1950s it affected 1 per cent of the adult population. Since then there is evidence of a decline in both the incidence and prevalence, particularly among women. In men the situation has not changed and there is now evidence that, in very elderly people, rheumatoid arthritis is more common in men than in women (see Figure 23.3). As well as a decline in incidence, there is a suggestion that rheumatoid arthritis may be becoming less severe (Silman *et al.*, 1983) with successive cohorts of patients (by year of birth) being less likely to be seropositive (i.e. rheumatoid factor present), erosive, or to have nodules. Nevertheless, rheumatoid arthritis remains a common and serious problem. It is still the most common form of inflammatory joint disease and has a high toll in terms of disability and mortality (Scott *et al.*, 1987).

23.4.2 Juvenile chronic arthritis

Juvenile chronic arthritis is defined as an inflammatory arthritis of more than 3 months' duration with an onset before the age of 16 (Wood, 1978). Its relevance to adult health relates to the late deaths and persistent disability that it may cause. The incidence of JCA is estimated to be 11 per 100,000 children in Britain. After 15 years of follow-up of 243 children with JCA admitted to hospital, 30 per cent had severe functional impairment, 3 per cent were chair or bed-bound and 7 per cent had died (Ansell and Wood, 1976). Most of the deaths occur as a consequence of infection or amyloidosis (a generalised deposit of amyloid protein in the liver, kidney, spleen and other body tissue, which interferes in their function and is a feature of a number of chronic inflammatory diseases).

23.4.3 Ankylosing spondylitis

Background
Ankylosing spondylitis is an inflammatory disorder of the spine. The inflammation starts in the sacroiliac joints and progresses up the spine. Unlike most other rheumatic diseases, it is more common in men than women. The condition is complicated by ankylosis, so that, untreated, the spine may become completely rigid. The peripheral joints may be affected and extra-articular features include iritis, upper lobe pulmonary fibrosis, aortic incompetence and cardiac conduction defects.

Disease definition
Classification criteria – known as the 'New York criteria' – were proposed in 1968 (Bennett and Wood, 1968). Radiological evidence of sacroiliitis is essential in order to satisfy the New York criteria. The principal symptom of AS is low back pain and, without radiological evidence of sacroiliitis, it is difficult to distinguish the minority of low-back pain sufferers who have AS, from the majority who do not.

Incidence of ankylosing spondylitis
The only true incidence study comes from Rochester, USA (Carbone *et al.*, 1992). It estimated an annual incidence rate of 6.6 cases per 100,000, with a male to female ratio of 3:1, and a peak age of onset in both sexes of 25–34. These figures remained constant over five decades (1935–89). A study of members of the National Ankylosing Spondylitis Society (a UK-based self-help group) suggested that the age of onset of AS is increasing (Calin *et al.*, 1988), but the methodology of this study has been criticised (Fries *et al.*, 1989).

Prevalence of ankylosing spondylitis
Lawrence (1963) estimated the prevalence of AS in Northern England to be 1 to 3 per 1,000 population. The Fourth National Morbidity Study shows a patient consultation rate for AS of 1 per 1,000 (RCGP, 1995).

Mortality due to ankylosing spondylitis
Studies of the mortality of AS are complicated by the fact that many patients were treated with spinal irradiation in the 1940s and 1950s. This treatment was sometimes complicated by the development of leukaemia and other cancers (Smith and Doll, 1982). Data from the USA suggest that non-irradiated patients have a normal life expectancy (Carbone *et al.*, 1992). Deaths from the late effects of irradiation may account for the slight rise in age-adjusted annual mortality rates in males since 1959 (see Figure 23.7). The age-specific mortality rates rise sharply with age in males (see Figure 23.8).

23.4.4 Gout

Background
The existence of gout can be traced back to the time of Hippocrates. The condition occurs as a result of precipitation of monosodium urate crystals from supersaturated solution in synovial fluid (joint lubricant). This produces one of the most painful forms of arthritis. A similar process may occur in other tissues leading to the formation of tophi and, in the

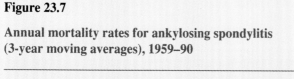

Figure 23.7

Annual mortality rates for ankylosing spondylitis (3-year moving averages), 1959–90

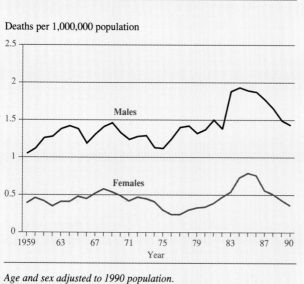

Age and sex adjusted to 1990 population.

Figure 23.8

Age-specific mortality rates for ankylosing spondylitis, 1987–91

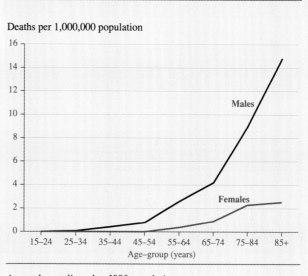

Age and sex adjusted to 1990 population.

kidneys, to gouty nephropathy. The epidemiology of gout in the UK has changed dramatically in the last 150 years – partly because of altered dietary habits and partly because of the introduction, after 1963, of allopurinol, a drug that inhibits the formation of uric acid. Changed diet has made gout more common, whereas allopurinol has made it unnecessary to suffer more than a couple of attacks.

Disease definition

Most patients with gout have raised serum uric acid concentrations but the correlation is far from perfect. Diagnostic criteria for gout were first proposed in 1968 (Bennett and Wood, 1968). A further two sets of criteria were proposed by the ARA in 1977 – one for the clinical setting and the other for survey work (Wallace *et al.*, 1977). In practice, most epidemiological studies use their own criteria.

Incidence of gout

Data from the Second and Third National Morbidity Studies (RCGP, 1979, 1988) (see Figure 23.9) show that there was an increase in the incidence of gout of around 30 per cent in both sexes and all ages between 1970 and 1982. Incident cases (based on the diagnostic opinion of the individual GP) were defined as those with a first-ever episode of gout.

Prevalence of gout

The prevalence of gout can be expressed in a number of ways. The numerator in the rate may be either all those who have ever had an attack of gout, or all those who experience an attack within a particular time frame (period prevalence). The denominator in the rate may be the whole population or the population at risk. The period prevalence of gout in 1981–82 was 2.7 per 1,000 persons at risk (RCGP, 1988) and in 1991–92 it was 4.0 per 1,000 persons at risk (RCGP, 1995; see Figure 23.10). These rates are similar to those obtained from a general practice survey which found a prevalence of 6.1 per 1,000 in men and 1.0 per 1,000 in women (Currie, 1979).

Mortality attributed to gout

Most deaths attributed to gout relate to the renal complications.

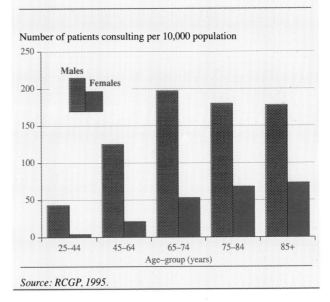

Figure 23.10

Period prevalence of gout from the Fourth National Morbidity Study, 1991–92

Number of patients consulting per 10,000 population

Source: RCGP, 1995.

Trends

The incidence of gout appears to be rising but, as a result of treatment, the prevalence of chronic tophaceous gout is falling. Data from the USA showed a progressive rise in serum urate levels from 1961 to 1978 (Glynn *et al.*, 1983). Predictors of increase were weight gain, alcohol consumption and triglyceride level.

23.4.5 Systemic lupus erythematosus (SLE)

Background

SLE is the most common of the diffuse connective tissue diseases. Its immunological hallmark is the presence of circulating antinuclear antibodies, which may be directed against a variety of nuclear components (see section 23.2). Most of the wide variety of clinical manifestations of SLE can be attributed to the deposition of immune complexes (i.e.

Figure 23.9

Annual incidence of gout from the Second, Third and Fourth National Morbidity Studies

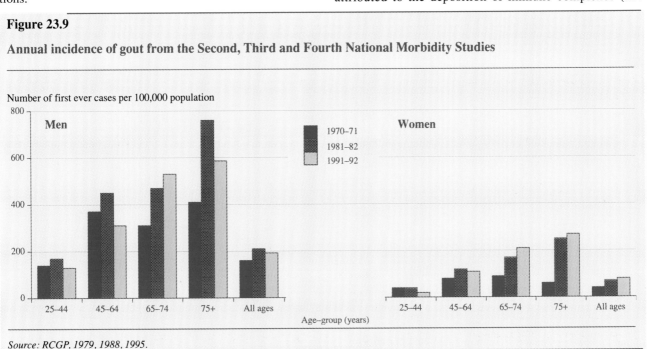

Source: RCGP, 1979, 1988, 1995.

aggregations of autoantibody and the cell components which are their targets, together with other proteins which are part of the body's defence mechanism). The most common organs to be involved are the skin, joints, kidneys, lungs and brain. Renal involvement, particularly in the past, was associated with a poor prognosis. There is a marked difference in the susceptibility and severity of SLE between ethnic groups. SLE has a high prevalence among black, Indian and Chinese people. Thus, with the immigration to Britain of people from the West Indies and the Indian subcontinent since the 1950s, SLE has become an increasingly common disease in some parts of Britain.

Disease definition

The visceral manifestations of SLE were first described in 1904 (Osler, 1904). The ARA proposed a preliminary set of classification criteria for SLE in 1971 (Cohen *et al.*, 1971), which were revised in 1982 (Tan *et al.*, 1982). They have gained widespread acceptance. Before 1972 all studies used their own independent diagnostic criteria.

Incidence of SLE

The only study of the incidence of SLE in the UK was conducted in 1989–90 (Hopkinson *et al.*, 1993; see Figure 23.11). The study attempted to ascertain new cases of SLE from multiple sources. It found a crude incidence rate of 3.7 per 100,000 population, with sex-specific incidence rates of 1.3 per 100,000 for men and 6.1 per 100,000 for women. The peak age of onset in both sexes was 50–59.

Prevalence of SLE

There have been three estimates of the prevalence of SLE. Hochberg used data from the Third National Morbidity Study (RCGP, 1988) to obtain an overall prevalence estimate of 6.5 per 100,000. The prevalence in women was 12.5 per 100,000 (Hochberg, 1987). This is thought to be an underestimate for a number of reasons. First, it included no male cases. Second, many mild cases may have remained undiagnosed or the patients may not have attended their GPs during the study

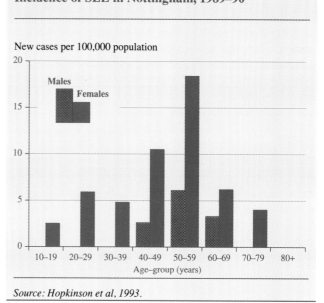

Figure 23.11

Incidence of SLE in Nottingham, 1989–90

Source: Hopkinson et al, 1993.

year.

The two other prevalence studies used similar methodologies of case ascertainment from multiple overlapping sources. The first study from Leicester identified hospital-diagnosed cases and found an overall prevalence of 20.2 per 100,000 for the white population and 50.4 per 100,000 for the Asian population (who came mainly from the Gujarat region of India) (Samanta *et al.*, 1992; see Figure 23.12). SLE is not only more common in Asians than in white people, but also has a worse prognosis (Samanta *et al.*, 1991). The second study from Greater Nottingham, where the population is 95.9 per cent white, found an overall prevalence of 24.0 per 100,000 (Hopkinson *et al.*, 1993). Both studies showed a marked female predominance. There are no studies of SLE in black populations in Britain. Studies from the West Indies show SLE to be a common disease there (Wilson and Hughes, 1979; Nossent, 1992).

Figure 23.12

Prevalence of SLE in Whites and Indian Asians in Leicester, 1989

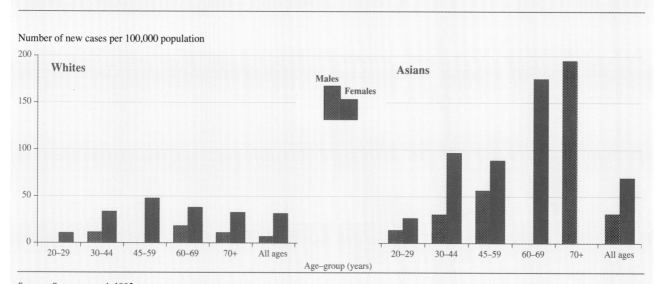

Source: Samanta et al, 1992.

Mortality attributed to SLE

Mortality data for SLE were not tabulated until the introduction of ICD8 in 1968. The age-adjusted annual mortality rate since then is shown in Figure 23.13. Since 1968 the age-adjusted mortality rate for SLE has fallen in both men and women. There has been no further fall since 1983. The age-specific mortality rates (see Figure 23.14) increase with age in both sexes up to age 75 and then fall. In 1983 the maximum rate in women was in those aged 55–74. The maximum rate is now in the 75–84 age-group in both sexes.

Trends

The peak age of onset of SLE in England is 50–59 (Hopkinson *et al.*, 1993). Twenty five years ago the peak age of onset in the USA was 15–44 (Siegel and Lee, 1973), and in 1977 it was 45–54 (Hochberg, 1985). The temporal trend is thus for an increasing age at onset. The prevalence of SLE is likely to be rising, partly as a result of improved survival, and partly because of the higher frequency of the disease in the black, Asian and Chinese communities. The mortality has fallen in both sexes – probably as a result of improved prognosis. However, the peak age-specific mortality rate has risen. This may be as a result of improved treatments (patients with SLE living longer) or there may be a cohort effect (patients develop SLE later in life and so die from the disease later).

23.4.6 Scleroderma

Background

Scleroderma is the least common disorder included in this chapter, but has the highest mortality. It is a multisystem disease characterised by obliterative microvascular lesions leading to atrophy and fibrosis of many organs. Apart from the skin, the organs most frequently involved are the lung, kidney, bowel and heart.

Disease definition

The ARA proposed criteria for the classification of scleroderma in 1980 (Masi *et al.*, 1980). These have not found universal acceptance.

Incidence of scleroderma

A single study of the incidence and prevalence of scleroderma has been conducted in the West Midlands Region (Silman *et al.*, 1988). Multiple overlapping sources, including consultants, GPs, patient self-help groups and in-patient statistics were used to identify all new and old cases of scleroderma resident in the region. The overall incidence of scleroderma was estimated as 1.1 per million for men and 6.2 per million for women. The peak age of onset was 45–54 for both sexes.

Prevalence of scleroderma

The same study (Silman *et al.*, 1988) yielded prevalence estimates of 31 per million. The female excess in prevalence is more marked before the menopause.

Mortality from scleroderma

Like SLE, scleroderma was not identified separately in mortality statistics until the introduction of ICD8 in 1968. Mortality data for scleroderma for England and Wales from 1968 to 1985 have been analysed by Silman (1991). The results showed overall mortality of 0.9 and 3.8 per million per year in men and women respectively. Taken with the incidence figures quoted (Silman *et al.*, 1988), these figures suggest that around 60 per cent of women, and an even greater proportion of men, with scleroderma die from their disease.

Trends

There was an average increase in mortality from scleroderma of around 3 per cent per year between 1968 and 1985 (Silman, 1991). As the prognosis of the disease is, if anything, improving, then this increased mortality probably reflects an increase in incidence – as has been reported from the USA (Steen *et al.*, 1988).

23.4.7 Joint failure – osteoarthritis

Background

Joint failure is the most common form of joint disorder in Britain. It is the final common pathway of many conditions,

Figure 23.13

Annual mortality rate for SLE (3-year moving averages)

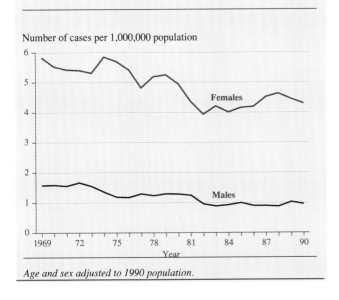

Number of cases per 1,000,000 population

Age and sex adjusted to 1990 population.

Figure 23.14

Age-specific mortality rates for SLE 1987–91

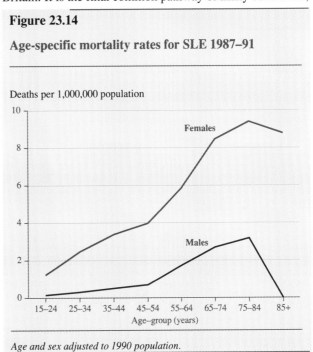

Deaths per 1,000,000 population

Age and sex adjusted to 1990 population.

including rheumatoid arthritis, trauma and gout. In addition, certain people have a genetic predisposition, manifest as primary generalised osteoarthritis, to develop joint failure. The predominant symptoms of primary and secondary osteoarthritis are pain, particularly on use, gelling after inactivity, and disability. The radiological manifestations of osteoarthritis are of new bone formation (osteophytes) and joint-space narrowing. Osteoarthritis may affect any joint and wherever it occurs the pathological and radiological changes are similar. However, the epidemiology of osteoarthritis differs considerably between joints. This is particularly so for osteoarthritis of the hip and knee.

Disease definition

As the radiological changes of osteoarthritis are more specific than the symptoms, early definitions were based on radiological findings (Kellgren *et al.*, 1963). However, symptomatic and radiological osteoarthritis do not always coincide. As a cause of morbidity, it is symptomatic osteoarthritis that is of relevance. The American College of Rheumatology has recently developed sets of clinical criteria for osteo-arthritis of the hip (Altman *et al.*, 1991) and knee (Altman *et al.*, 1986), but these have been criticised because they are based on distinguishing osteoarthritis from rheumatoid arthritis, rather than osteoarthritis from normality.

Incidence of osteoarthritis

The onset of joint pain and the appearance of diagnostic radiological features are both insidious. It is, therefore, very difficult to estimate the incidence of osteoarthritis. The RCGP morbidity studies (RCGP, 1979, 1988, 1994) record the number of people consulting for the first time with symptoms attributable to osteoarthritis (based on the opinion of the individual GP). Figure 23.15 shows the incidence by age-group in the 1981–82 study. The incidence is higher in women at all ages and almost double in very elderly people (75 and over).

Prevalence of osteoarthritis

Most community surveys of the prevalence of osteoarthritis are based on the radiological definition of Kellgren and Law-

rence (Kellgren *et al.*, 1963). Lawrence's surveys, carried out in Leigh and Wensleydale in the 1950s and 1960s (Lawrence, 1977), showed that the prevalence of moderate or severe osteoarthritis (grade 3 or 4) in one or more joints rises progressively with age (see Figure 23.16). Sixty per cent of those aged over 65 had moderate or severe osteoarthritis in at least one joint. Other studies show that the prevalence of radiological osteoarthritis continues to rise with age up to the age 90 and over. Osteoarthritis is slightly more common in men before the age of 45, but more common in older women (coinciding with the age of the menopause).

Studies that estimate the prevalence of symptomatic osteoarthritis are better measures of the community burden of disease. Various definitions of pain have been used, such as 'pain on most days of the prior month' (Hart *et al.*, 1991) and 'pain on most days of a month last year' (Guccione *et al.*, 1990). The age-specific prevalence of symptomatic osteoarthritis is increasing (see Figures 23.17 and 23.18). These data empha-

Figure 23.16

Prevalence of moderate or severe radiological OA in at least one joint, 1958–66

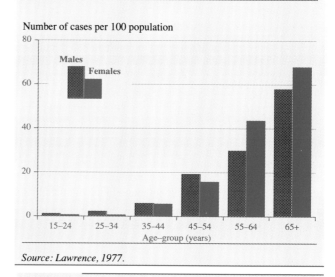

Number of cases per 100 population

Source: Lawrence, 1977.

Figure 23.15

The incidence of symptomatic OA in England and Wales, 1981–82

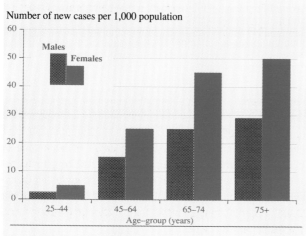

Number of new cases per 1,000 population

Source: RCGP, 1988.

Figure 23.17

Prevalence of symptomatic OA in England and Wales (age and sex adjusted to 1990 population)

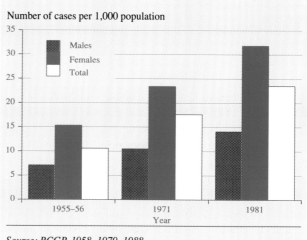

Number of cases per 1,000 population

Source: RCGP, 1958, 1979, 1988.

Figure 23.18

Prevalence of symptomatic OA in England and Wales

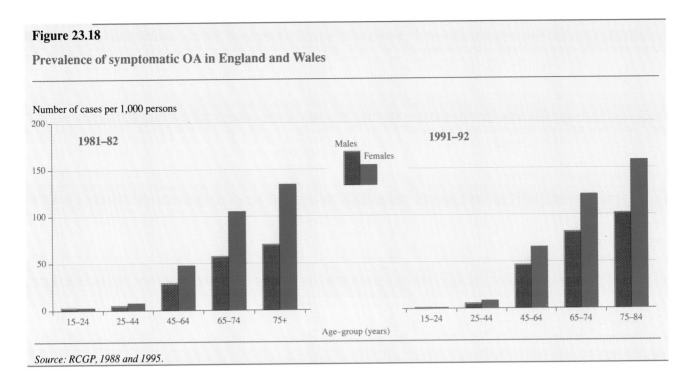

Number of cases per 1,000 persons

Age–group (years)

Source: RCGP, 1988 and 1995.

sise the marked increase in the prevalence of osteoarthritis with age. Not everyone is equally susceptible to osteoarthritis. Obesity is strongly associated with osteoarthritis of the knee especially in women, but not with osteoarthritis of the hip. Osteoarthritis of the hip is more common in farmers (Croft *et al.*, 1992) and osteoarthritis of the knee in occupations which involve lifting (Anderson and Felson, 1988). Osteoarthritis of the knee is three times more common than osteoarthritis of the hip. This ratio is rising.

Mortality

Cohort studies show that patients with osteoarthritis have an increased mortality (Monson and Hall, 1976; Lawrence *et al.*, 1987). However, osteoarthritis is seldom mentioned on the death certificate so no insight into the magnitude of the problem is given from national mortality data.

Trends

The number of people with symptomatic osteoarthritis is rising sharply as the proportion of elderly people in the community rises. Age-adjusted figures from the RCGP morbidity studies (see Figures 23.17 and 23.18) suggest that the prevalence may be rising even faster than demography would dictate. In particular, osteoarthritis of the knee is becoming more common.

23.4.8   Joint replacement surgery

Total hip replacement (THR) has been widely practised in Britain for over 25 years, and total knee replacement (TKR) for around 15 years. Trends in the numbers of operations performed in NHS hospitals are shown in Figure 23.19 (data from Williams *et al.*, 1992a, b). The numbers of TKR are rising sharply but in 1989–90 the number of TKRs was still only one third the number of THRs. The main indication for both operations is osteoarthritis – and osteoarthritis of the knee is 3 times more common than osteoarthritis of the hip.

Figure 23.19

Numbers of hip and knee replacements in NHS hospitals in England, 1967–90

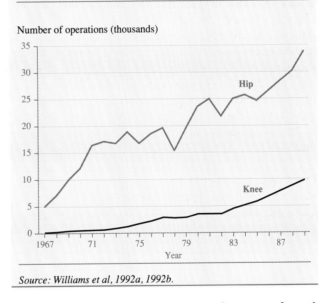

Number of operations (thousands)

Year

Source: Williams et al, 1992a, 1992b.

In the USA similar numbers of both operations are performed. Around 75 per cent of large joint replacements are performed in those aged over 65.

23.4.9   Back pain

Background

Back pain is a symptom not a disease. It may be triggered by a great variety of factors (see Table 23.3). In spite of this long list, it is impossible to establish the cause of back pain in most acute episodes (Dillane *et al.*, 1966) and in up to 50 per cent of chronic cases (Pope *et al.*, 1980). In population-based studies it is, therefore, probably best to regard back pain as a single symptom complex rather than to attempt to group those with back pain by cause.

Table 23.3

Causes of back pain

1. Mechanical causes	4. Infective causes	7. Referred pain
Ligament and tendon strain	Ostemyelitis	From:
Vertebral fractures	Discitis	Duodenal ulcer
Prolapsed inter-vertebral disc	Paravertebral abscess	Pancreas
Spondylolysis and spondylolisthesis	Brucellosis	Renal tract
Congenital abnormalities		Gynaecological disorders
		Lower bowel
2. Degenerative conditions	5. Neoplastic causes	
Degenerative disc disease	Primary benign tumours	
Lumbar spondylosis	Primary malignant tumours	
	Metastatic disease	
3. Inflammatory conditions	6. Metabolic bone disease	8. Psychogenic pain
HLA-B27 related spondarthropathies:	Osteoporosis	
Ankylosing spondylitis	Osteomalacia	
Reiter's disease	Paget's disease	
Psoriatic arthritis		
Inflammatory bowel associated		
arthritis		

Case definition

There is no standard definition of back pain. Confusion is found in both official statistics and ad hoc surveys. The ONS Hospital In-patient Enquiry diagnostic group D134 includes all ICD9 codes from 720.1 to 724.9. This includes cervical spine disorders but excludes AS. DHSS sickness figures for dorsopathies cover codes 720.0 to 724.9 and so include AS as well as neck problems. The Third and Fourth RCGP Morbidity Studies (1988, 1994) code neck problems; AS; and strains and sprains of the vertebral column separately from other causes of back pain. In ad hoc surveys, the definitions used have included 'back pain during the 2 weeks preceding interview' (Dunnel and Cartwright, 1972), 'back pain at the time of interview' (Symmons *et al.*, 1991b) and 'back pain on most days for at least 2 weeks' (Deyo and Tsui-Wu, 1987).

Incidence of back pain

Back pain tends to be episodic and most episodes settle within 6 weeks (Liang and Komaroff, 1982). However, back pain is also recurrent and one of the strongest predictors for back pain in the future is back pain in the past (Pedersen, 1981; Symmons *et al.*, 1991b). Thus, 'incidence of back pain' can mean either 'first ever attacks of back pain' or 'new attacks of back pain' during the given time frame. The lifetime incidence of back pain ranges up to 80 per cent (Wells, 1985). A number of studies have suggested that less than 20 per cent of back pain episodes are brought to medical attention (Frymoyer and Cats-Baril, 1991) – a figure that is borne out by the ratio of self-reported to consultation rates in England and Wales (see Table 23.4).

The Second and Third RCGP Morbidity Studies (RCGP, 1979, 1988) examined the number of new attacks of back pain during a 1-year period (see Figure 23.20). The 1981–82 figures show that incident back pain is more common in men aged 25–44, but more common in women at all other ages. Overall, 1 in 18 adults consults his or her GP each year with a new episode of back pain. This is equivalent to 2.3 million individuals in 1991.

Prevalence of back pain

A number of estimates of the prevalence of back pain are available for the British population (see Table 23.4). Walsh (Walsh *et al.*, 1992) suggests that the lifetime prevalence of back pain is consistently higher in men than in women and approaches 70 per cent by the age of 60. The 1-year prevalence is higher for men than for women except for the age-group 40–49. However, the sex ratio is reversed when it comes to consultations for back pain. The Health and Lifestyles Survey shows that back pain is a particularly common symptom in elderly women. Taken together, these figures suggest that short-lived episodes of back pain are more common in women, whereas chronic, persistent back pain is more common in men. This impression is born out by the consultation figures. On average, around 1 in 5 people with back pain appears to consult his or her GP. The consultation rate is now higher for women than for men. In the last 10 years the consultation rate has risen for all age-sex groups. During the same time there has been a sharp increase in sickness and invalidity benefit for back pain (see Figure 23.21). Whether this results from a true increase in the prevalence of back pain or from less willingness to tolerate it cannot be deciphered from these figures.

Hospital referral patterns

In a publication in 1985, the Office of Health Economics estimated that between 10 and 20 per cent of those who consulted their GPs with back pain were referred to hospital (Wells, 1985). They reported that there were 62,572 discharges (or deaths) from hospital with back pain diagnoses in England, Wales and Scotland in 1982. The single most important identifiable cause of hospitalisation (accounting for 24.7 per cent of cases) was intervertebral disc disorders. Most patients with disc problems were aged between 25 and 44.

Table 23.4

Estimates of the prevalence (percent) of back pain

Source	Sex	Age-band					
		15–24	25–44	25–64	65–74	75+	All ages
3rd RCGP Morbidity	M	4.1	7.5	8.2	6.4	5.9	6.8
(1981–82) (1 year)	F	4.2	7.1	8.6	7.1	6.8	6.9
	T	4.1	7.3	8.4	6.8	6.5	6.8
4th RCGP Morbidity	M	4.6	8.2	10.5	8.7	8.2	
(1991–92) (1 year)	F	5.8	9.6	12.6	10.6	9.9	
	T	5.2	8.9	11.6	9.8	9.2	
Health and Lifestyles	M		14.3	18.3	19.3	16.5	
Survey (1985) (1 month)	F		16.6	23.2	46.9	21.0	
	T		15.6	21.0	25.3	19.0	

		Age-band			
		16–44	45–64	65–74	75+
GHS (1989)	M	3.7	6.7	4.4	2.4
(long-standing illness)	F	3.3	4.6	2.8	3.7
	T	3.5	5.7	3.5	3.2

		Age-band			
		20–29	30–39	40–49	50–59
Walsh 1991	M	35.4	37.1	38.2	40.5
(1 year)	F	27.0	33.6	43.7	35.7
(lifetime)	M	52.0	60.4	64.2	70.5
	F	45.2	53.8	62.8	63.7

Figure 23.20

Consultation rates for new episodes of back pain in England and Wales

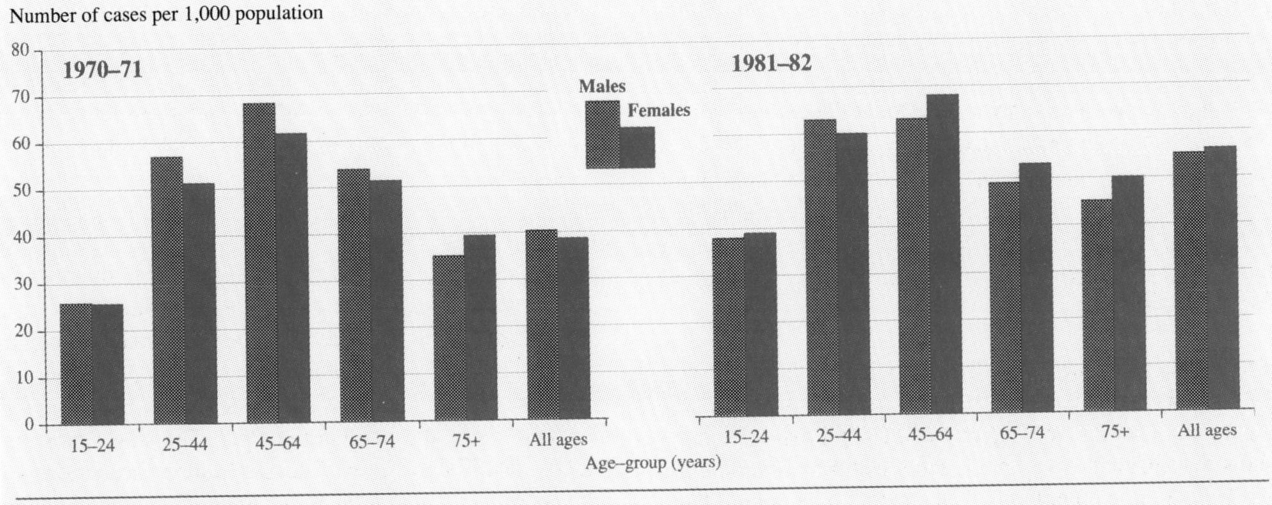

Source: RCGP, 1979, 1988.

Figure 23.21

Sickness and invalidity benefit claims for back pain

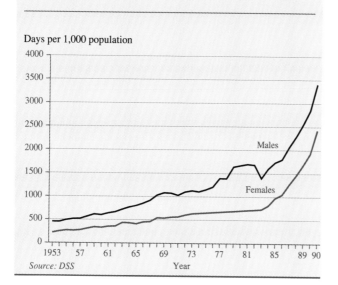

Days per 1,000 population

Source: DSS

Papageorgiou and Rigby (1991) have proposed a rule of 'fifths' when considering the epidemiology of back pain in Britain. One in five of the population are experiencing back pain at any particular time; 1 in 5 of these consult the GP; and 1 in 5 will be referred to hospital. One in five of those attending as out-patients will be admitted and, of these, 1 in 5 will undergo surgery.

Trends

Figure 23.20 shows that in the 10-year period between the Second and Third Morbidity Studies, consultation rates for new episodes of back pain had risen by an average of 1.5 per cent in men and 1.7 per cent in women. The rise was most marked in those aged under 45 and over 75. There was a further even greater rise in the next decade. In Britain, work loss resulting from back disorders has doubled in the last 5 years. Back troubles now account for one seventh of all sickness and invalidity benefits (see Figure 23.21). Back disability is increasing faster than any other form of disability

(Waddell, 1992). Frymoyer and Cats-Baril (1991) propose that the number of people with back pain is not increasing but the number of individuals who believe that they are disabled has exploded.

23.4.10 Soft tissue rheumatism

Background

Soft tissue problems originate in the non-articular part (non-bone or joint) of the musculoskeletal system. There are several soft tissue junctions at which minor injury and inflammation can occur causing pain. These include tenoperiosteal (tendon-to-bone), ligament-periosteal (ligament-to-bone), myofascial (bone-to-muscle) and costochondral (rib-to-cartilage) junctions. In addition, disorders may arise within the soft tissue structures of muscle, ligament, tendon and tendon sheath.

Case definition

Disorders of soft tissue can be classified by clinicopathological process (e.g. tendinitis), by anatomical region (e.g. shoulder pain) or by aetiology (e.g. repetitive strain injury). In practice, it is often difficult to discern the underlying process and so the more pragmatic approach of classifying by region is adopted. The most common sites for non-articular pain are the neck, shoulder, upper arm, elbow and wrist. The same problems are encountered in defining a 'case' of shoulder pain as a 'case' of back pain (see section 23.4.8).

Incidence of soft tissue rheumatism

There are no studies of the incidence of soft tissue rheumatism at the population level. The Second and Third RCGP Morbidity Studies (RCGP, 1979, 1988) provide estimates of the number of new episodes presenting to GPs (see Figure 23.22). The incidence of soft tissue rheumatism rises up to age 65 and then falls. The incidence rate is higher for women than for men at all ages except over age 75. Incidence rates are higher for both men and women in age-groups over 24 in the 1981–82 study than in the 1971–72 study.

Figure 23.22

Consultation rates for soft tissue rheumatism in England and Wales

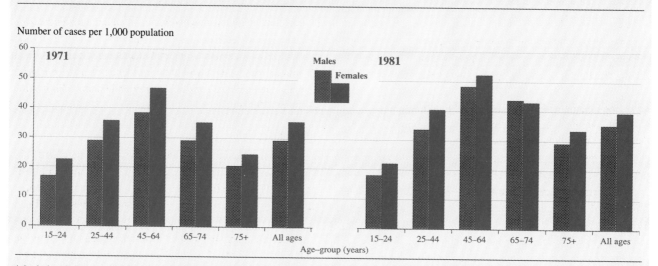

Number of cases per 1,000 population

Age–group (years)

* Includes shoulder pain, bursitis, tendinitis, tenosynvitis and other non-articular rheumatism.

Prevalence of soft tissue rheumatism

Studies from the ARC Epidemiology Research Unit suggest that up to 20 per cent of the middle and older age-groups may have experienced some soft tissue problem in the previous month. Lifetime prevalence is close to 50 per cent.

Trends

Figure 23.22 shows that consultation rates for new episodes of soft tissue rheumatism had risen in both sexes and for all age-groups between 1971 and 1981. Whether this represents a true increase in incidence or a lower tolerance of symptoms is not clear.

23.4.11 Osteoporosis

Background

Osteoporosis is defined as a reduction in bone mass. The public health importance of osteoporosis lies in its association with fractures of the hip, pelvis and distal radius. It is estimated that, at the age of 50, the lifetime risk of such fractures is 40 per cent in white women and 13 per cent in white men (Melton *et al.*, 1992). The risk in other ethnic groups is lower but not inconsiderable.

Incidence of hip fracture

Hip fracture is the most important consequence of osteoporosis, in terms of both morbidity and cost. Each year around 45,000 people in England and Wales fracture their proximal femurs. The annual age-specific incidence rates for various years is shown in Figure 23.23. These graphs, which are based on hospital admissions for fracture, show that the incidence of hip fracture rises sharply with age, especially after age 65. Over the age of 50 there is a female to male ratio of around 3:1. In addition, the Oxford data show that in the three decades up to 1983, the age-specific incidence rates had doubled for those aged over 65 (Boyce and Vessey, 1985). Similar secular trends have been observed in other European countries and in the USA (Melton *et al.*, 1987). The reason for this change in incidence is not known. Recent paleopathological data suggest that age-specific bone mass has fallen in women in the last two centuries (Lees *et al.*, 1993). One possible explanation for this change and the increased hip fracture rate is the lower amount of physical activity undertaken by present-day women. Hospital admission data for England and Wales (Spector *et al.*, 1990) and a recent paper from Leicester (Anderson *et al.*, 1993) suggest that the increase in age-specific hip fracture incidence may have stopped at around 1980.

Incidence and prevalence of vertebral fracture

Vertebral fractures occur at an earlier age than hip fractures. Many vertebral fractures are asymptomatic and so it is only possible to determine the incidence of the condition by conducting two cross-sectional radiological surveys and estimating the number of new fractures that have occurred. The definition of vertebral fracture is also difficult. A vertebral fracture can be defined either as a partial loss of height on the anterior edge or middle section of a vertebral body (wedge fracture) or as a collapse of the entire vertebral body (compression or crush fracture). Exact radiological definitions of

Figure 23.23

Annual age-specific incidence of hip fracture

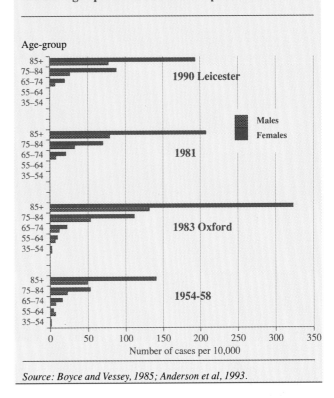

Source: Boyce and Vessey, 1985; Anderson et al, 1993.

wedge fractures vary and can make a substantial difference to estimates of prevalence (Cummings, 1991).

Prevalence rates have been estimated in female out-patient attenders in Leeds (Nordin *et al.*, 1980). Crush fracture prevalence rose from 2.5 per cent at age 60 to 7.5 per cent at age 80 years. Wedge fractures, however, were present in around 60 per cent of women aged over 75. Using data from the USA, Cooper and Melton (1992) have estimated that each year 34,000 women will present with clinically diagnosed vertebral fractures in Britain, 8,000 of whom will attend hospital.

Incidence of fractures of the distal radius (Colles' fractures)

Distal radius fractures are the most common fractures in women up to the age of 75; thereafter, hip fractures are more common. As with hip fractures, there is a winter peak in incidence. However, whereas most hip fractures follow a fall indoors, Colles' fractures are usually associated with an outdoor fall. In the United Kingdom, the incidence of distal radius fracture in women rises linearly between the ages of 45 and 65, and the plateaus. In men, the incidence remains constant between the ages of 20 and 80 (Miller and Evans, 1985; Winner *et al.*, 1989).

Mortality associated with osteoporosis

In spite of the rise in the incidence of hip fracture up to 1980, the annual mortality attributed to hip fracture has been falling since 1970 (see Figure 23.24). On the other hand, deaths attributed to osteoporosis or fractured vertebrae have been rising (see Figure 23.25). There has been a fourfold increase over the last three decades in women, which may now be flattening out. These figures almost certainly underestimate the mortality caused by osteoporosis. Thirty five per cent of

Figure 23.24

Annual mortality for hip fracture (3-year moving averages)

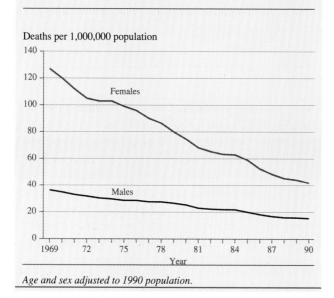

Deaths per 1,000,000 population

Age and sex adjusted to 1990 population.

Figure 25.25

Annual mortality rate for osteoporosis (3-year moving averages)

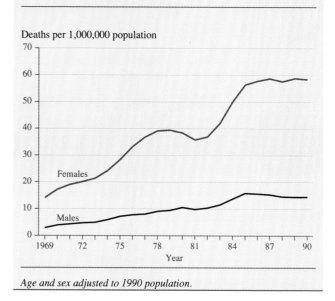

Deaths per 1,000,000 population

Age and sex adjusted to 1990 population.

patients admitted to hospital with fractured neck of femur die within the next 2 years (Donaldson *et al.*, 1989). The fracture is mentioned on the death certificate in less than 6 per cent of cases.

23.5 Prevalence of physical disability in the community

An alternative approach when trying to assess the burden of musculoskeletal disease in the community, is to disregard the underlying diagnosis – which may, in any case, be inaccurate – and concentrate on symptoms and functional impairment. The GHS in 1989 (OPCS, 1989) and the Health and Lifestyles Survey in 1984–85 (Blaxter, 1990) both included questions about the health of the respondents. Both rely on

self-reported diagnoses but give an insight into the prevalence of musculoskeletal symptoms at the population level (see Table 23.5). These data show that in any month about a fifth of the population have painful joints and about an eighth painful feet.

The 1986 OPCS Disability Survey (Martin and White, 1988) undertook home visits in order to assess disability in each of 13 functional areas. The prevalence of locomotion disability rose from 3.1 per cent in those aged under 60 to almost 50 per cent in those aged over 75. The survey showed that 6 million adults (14.2 per cent) in Britain have one or more disabilities. Musculoskeletal problems gave rise to 46 per cent of disabilities in private households and 37 per cent of disabilities in communal establishments. In the same year (1986) the ARC Epidemiology Research Unit undertook a survey of

Table 23.5

Prevalence (per cent) of musculoskeletal symptoms in the population

Source	Sex	Age-band			
		18–44	45–64	65+	All ages
Health and Lifestyle Survey (1985)					
Painful joints	M	12.2	26.9	30.5	20.0
	F	10.9	33.3	44.7	23.9
Painful feet	M	10.1	14.6	17.4	12.9
	F	10.3	21.3	27.9	16.9

		Age-band			
		16–44	45–64	65–74	75+
GHS (1989)					
Long-standing illness due to	M	1.4	7.2	10.8	17.1
arthritis and rheumatism	F	2.5	12.9	21.1	28.2

Figure 23.26

Prevalence of disablement due to rheumatic disorders in Calderdale, West Yorkshire, 1986

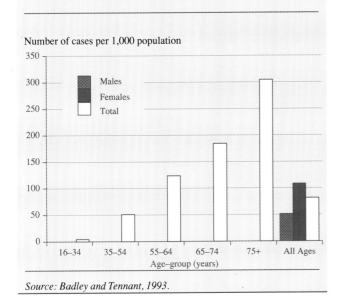

Number of cases per 1,000 population

Source: Badley and Tennant, 1993.

rheumatic disablement in Calderdale, West Yorkshire (Badley and Tennant, 1993). A two-stage screening procedure was used. In the first phase, a screening questionnaire was sent to 1 in 3 households. A stratified sample of those who screened positive (reported disability caused by a rheumatic disorder) was seen for an in-depth interview. The prevalence of rheumatic disablement rises steeply with age (see Figure 23.26).

Almost one third of those aged over 75 have a significant musculoskeletal problem. Of those with disability, 58 per cent had unspecified arthritis (mainly osteoarthritis), 9.3 per cent had rheumatoid arthritis, 31.5 per cent had back or neck disorders and 2.3 per cent had soft tissue rheumatism (based on a self-reported diagnosis).

23.6 Summary

This chapter summarises the epidemiological data on the incidence, prevalence and mortality of the most common musculoskeletal diseases in Britain, and on physical disability. Nearly all the musculoskeletal diseases increase in incidence with age, and so, with the increasing proportion of elderly people, the prevalence of these diseases has risen dramatically in the last 150 years. In addition, there is evidence that the age-specific incidence rates of osteoarthritis, gout, back pain and osteoporosis may be rising. Most musculoskeletal disorders are also more common in women than in men – and it is women who have enjoyed the greater increase in life expectancy. The prospect for the future, therefore, is for an increasing burden of rheumatic disease in an ageing population. Only rheumatoid arthritis appears to be on the decline. Rheumatoid arthritis, SLE and possibly AS all have an older age of onset now. Mortality data are difficult to interpret because musculoskeletal disorders are so often omitted from the death certificate. Nevertheless, it does appear that the mortality from SLE has declined, and that from osteoporosis, scleroderma and AS has risen.

Chapter 24

Accidents: trends in mortality and morbidity

By
John Nicholl and Patricia Coleman

Summary

- Since a peak in the 1930s there has been a consistent decline in the numbers and rates of deaths resulting from all accidental causes.

- The declining trend in the accidental death rates is greater for men than women, and for children aged 0–14 years than for adults.

- Of the causes specified, deaths from fire and drowning show the biggest percentage declines.

- Trends in non-fatal accidents are difficult to identify, but the available data sources indicate that during the last 20 years, patterns of consultation and service use have been increasing steadily.

On the roads:

- A decrease in the numbers of people killed or seriously injured across all modes of transport in road traffic accidents (RTAs) is evident, but the benefits are not distributed evenly across all road users.

- The proportion of people involved in serious RTAs who die has remained constant, and in some modes of transport appears to have increased.

- The data suggest that the reduced mortality is attributable to changing patterns of exposure and to successful primary and secondary accident prevention measures.

At home:

- The numbers of fatal home accidents have fallen to an extent similar to that observed in RTAs.

- Deaths from head injuries have remained relatively constant with most of the reduction resulting from declines in the numbers of deaths attributed to falls. Coding inconsistencies surrounding deaths from falls in the elderly population may be the largest factor contributing to the overall reduction.

At work:

- Reductions have occurred in the numbers and rates of fatal accidents to employees. These will be attributable in part to changes in exposure linked to the decline of hazardous industries, as well as to changes in the occupational stricture and patterns of employment.

At play:

- The patterns of death during sports and leisure activities are erratic and reflect three major incidents occurring in a 10-year period each of which resulted in the deaths of a large number of people.

24.1 Introduction

Accidents are the cause of only 2 per cent of all deaths occurring in England and Wales each year. However, they are the most common cause of deaths in people under 35 and account for 8.3 per cent of all potential years of life lost under age 75. Furthermore, accidental injuries account for 7 per cent of all episodes of care in NHS hospitals, and they are also estimated to be responsible for 7 per cent of all NHS expenditure (Department of Health, 1993a).

The significant contribution of accidents to death and illness might itself make accidents a primary target for national efforts to improve health. However, it is the fact that most accidents are considered avoidable, and consequently that much of this burden of ill health could be prevented, which has underlined the importance of accidents in the Health of the Nation (HoN) targets. The HoN targets are to reduce the death rates from accidents in children under 15 by at least 33 per cent, in young people aged 15–24 by at least 25 per cent and in older people aged 65 and over by at least 33 per cent, between 1990 and 2005. No targets exist for reducing morbidity from accidents. This is not because morbidity is considered less important but at the present time no integrated national system exists for measuring levels of accident-related morbidity in all settings.

Achievement of the HoN targets will depend on the extent to which accidental deaths are in fact preventable, as well as the efforts being made by the health and other services to develop prevention strategies. National and local strategies for primary prevention (i.e. preventing accidents), secondary prevention (i.e. preventing or reducing the severity of injuries in accidents that do occur) and tertiary prevention (i.e. minimising or preventing the health outcomes of injuries) via education, engineering, legislation, medical advances and many other initiatives have all been pursued to a greater or lesser extent in the past. The long- and short-term historical trends in accidental deaths and morbidity have been examined in order to help assess the possibilities for the prevention of accidents, and to set the changes which are occurring with the development of HoN strategies in their historical context.

This chapter first assesses changes since the beginning of the century in accident mortality rates in terms of age, sex and cause of accident. Next, recent changes in accident morbidity based on hospital admission and GP consultation data are examined, and finally, recent changes in road traffic accidents (RTAs), home accidents, work accidents, and sports and leisure accidents are considered.

24.2 Methods

24.2.1 Definitions

In the International Classification of Diseases (ICD) mortality and morbidity arising from accidents (that is, externally

caused unintentional events) are classified both by the nature of the injuries (e.g. fractures, poisonings) and by their external cause (e.g. falls or motor vehicle crashes). In the 9th revision of ICD, Chapter 17 (E800–E999) is used to classify deaths from other violence (that is homicides, suicides, other intentional causes such as 'operations of war', and causes not determined as intentional or unintentional) as well as accidents and accidental poisonings. These deaths are collectively referred to as deaths from injury and poisoning (IP). Where possible we have considered accidents separately from other external causes.

The nature of the injury is coded using N-codes and the external cause using E-codes. There are two separate dimensions to the E-codes, the cause of the accident (e.g. fall) and the place of occurrence or type of accident (e.g. home or work). Since the first edition of the ICD in 1900, successive revisions have more or less managed to encompass the first of these two dimensions using different devices, though in early versions some distinctions were not well made. However, historically the place of the accident was rarely identified. We have therefore examined historical trends in accident mortality using ICD E-codes only with respect to the cause of accident. Discussion of trends in the type or place of occurrence of accidents is based on data collected separately for road traffic accidents (RTAs), home accidents, work accidents, and sports and other leisure accidents. It may be inappropriate to compare rates of occurrence of these different types of accident anyway since the appropriate measures of exposure which could be used to calculate comparative rates may be different. For RTAs, for example, vehicle kilometres or passenger kilometres might be appropriate; for work accidents to employees, the numbers employed; and for home accidents, the whole population.

24.2.2 Data sources

ONS mortality data

The ONS mortality data files for deaths from external causes (IP) for 1901–90 have been examined. This historical data file includes an external cause coded using ICD1 to ICD9, but no nature of injury code, although these are in fact recorded for externally caused accidents. The cause of injury has been classified as accidental (transport, falls, fire and flames, poisoning, drowning/submersion or other), non-accidental, or not known whether accidental or intentional. The ICD E-codes which have been categorised in this way are shown in Table 24.1. This categorisation is not straightforward.

In ICD1–ICD3 (1901–30) accidental falls were distinguished from accidental injury by other forms of crushing, but crushing in transport accidents was not distinguished from crushing in other accidents. Consequently, in ICD1 to ICD3 deaths from falls are identified, but deaths from transport accidents have had to be included in a 'not specified' category. However, in ICD4 (1931–39) deaths from falls and other forms of crushing (including crushing in transport accidents) were not distinguished, the category being

Table 24.1

International classification of diseases codes for injuries and poisoning 1901–91

	ICD 1 1901–10	ICD 2 1911–20	ICD 3 1921–30	ICD 4 1931–39	ICD 5 1940–49	ICD 6 1950–57	ICD 7 1958–67	ICD 8 1968–78	ICD 9 1979–94
Accidents									
Transport					1690-1730	800-866, 960	800-866, 960	800-849	800-849
Poisoning	600, 610, 620, 1820	571, 580, 572, 1650, 1680, 1640	671, 680, 672, 1770, 1810	771, 772, 1780, 1790	781, 791, 782, 794, 795, 1780, 1790	870-895, 691	870-895, 691	860-877	850-869
Falls	1850	1720	1850	1860	1860	900-904	900-904	880-888	880-888
Fire and flames	1810	1660, 1670, 1810	1780, 1790, 1960	1800, 1810, 1930	1800, 1810, 1930	916, 917, 914	196, 917, 914	890-899	890-899
Drownings/ submersions	1830, 1840	1690	1820	1830	1830	929	929	910-915	910-915
Other or not specified elswhere	1750, 1780, 1790, 1860, 1870, 1800, 560, 1760, 1770	1730, 1740, 1530, 1700, 1710, 1750, 1760, 1850, 1770, 1780, 1790, 1800	1800, 1860, 1870, 1760, 1830, 1840, 1920, 1930, 1940, 1950, 2010, 1890, 1880, 1630	1820, 1760, 1840, 1850, 1880, 1890, 1900, 1910, 1920, 1870, 1941, 1942	1740, 1751, 1754, 1760, 1820, 1752, 1753, 1840, 1850, 1880, 1890, 1920, 1900, 1910, 1952, 1953, 1954, 1870, 1955, 1956	910-913, 915, 918-925, 927-928, 930-935, 936, 1940, 1951, 962	910-913, 915, 918-925, 927-928, 930-936, 940-946, 950-959, 962	850-859, 900-909, 930-936, 940-949, 916-928	870-879, 900-909, 930-949, 916-928, 929
Non-accidents									
Suicide	1900	1550, 1560, 1570, 1580, 1590, 1600, 1610, 1620, 1630	4650, 1670, 1680, 1690, 1700, 1710, 1720, 1730, 1740	1630, 1640, 1650, 1660, 1670, 1680, 1690, 1700, 1710	1631-1637 1641-1648	970-979, 963	970-979, 963	950-959	950-959
Homicide	1890	1820, 1630	1620, 1970, 1980, 1990	1720, 1730, 1740, 1750	1680, 1650, 1660, 1670	980-983, 964	980-985, 964	960-969	960-969
Other (e.g. war execution)	1910, 1880		1910, 1900, 2020			926, 984-5, 990-996, 965	926, 990-999	990-999, 970-978	970-978, 990-999
NK accident or non-accident	1870	1860	2030	1950				980-989	980-989

Note: The codes for ICD1 to 5 refer to computer codes used in the ONS historic deaths database.

described as death from 'accidental injury by fall, crushing, etc.' (ICD4 code 186). Consequently the numbers of deaths in the ICD4 period from falls, transport accidents and other not specified crushing causes cannot be identified. From ICD5 (1940–49) onwards, transport accidents were classified properly for the first time, and hence the number of deaths from transport accidents and falls are both recorded and distinguished from deaths from other and unspecified causes.

Some deaths from injuries and poisoning cannot be classi-

fied as accidents because the circumstances were not determined. In ICD9 for example codes E980–E989 are for injuries undetermined whether accidentally or purposefully inflicted. In revisions of the ICD other than the 5th to 7th codes exist for these categories (see Table 24.1). For example, in ICD3 code 203 is for violent deaths of unstated nature. These are important because the numbers assigned to this undetermined category influence the numbers of recorded accidents.

Crude per capita death rates from IP derived from the

mortality data in the ONS historical data file have been computed for 10-year intervals from 1901 to 1990. The rates have also been directly standardised for age, or age and sex, using the 1991 population of England and Wales as the standard. Age-groups in 5- or 10-year bands to age 74, and 75 and over were used for the standardisation. The use of 75 and over, a large age-group for the elderly, does mean that some changes in the numbers of very elderly persons may not be adequately accounted for in the standardisation. Unfortunately population data for early years do not subdivide this elderly group.

Morbidity data

Data on episodes of NHS hospital care for IP have been obtained from the Hospital Inpatients Enquiry (HIPE) (DH and OPCS, 1973, 1982, 1983), and from the Hospital Episode System (HES) (Department of Health 1993b). HIPE was a 10 per cent sample of discharges and deaths from NHS hospitals in England and Wales until 1981 and then, from 1982 to 1985, for England only. HES, available since 1989/90, collects data on finished consultant episodes for in-patients and day cases for England only. Both sets of data contain an ICD code for the nature of injury on admission. We have examined trends in episodes of care for patients with ICD codes for IP (e.g. ICD9 N800–N999), by age and sex.

We have also examined published data from the second (1971/72) (Royal College of General Practitioners, 1974), third (1981/82) (Royal College of General Practitioners, 1984) and fourth (1991/92) (McCormick et al., 1995) General Practice morbidity surveys. These surveys report data relating to patients, consultations and episodes of care classified by ICD coded diagnosis. Again we have examined trends in episodes of care for patients with diagnoses of IP by age and sex.

Place of accident

The General Household Survey (GHS) is a rotating survey of approximately 12,000 households in England and Wales providing continuous data on a range of key socio-economic variables. The GHS reported in 1989 (Breeze et al., 1991) that approximately one fifth of all accidental injuries which resulted in seeing a doctor or going to hospital were RTAs. Accidents in the elderly and very young (0–4 years) tended to occur in the home, and accidents to older children aged 5–15 years occurred mostly in the home or while participating in physical exercise. A relatively high proportion of accidents to men, particularly those aged 16–44 years in manual socio-economic groups, happened during working hours.

Road accident casualty information compiled by the Department of Transport (DoT) is based on accident records referred to as STATS19 forms, which are completed by the police for all road accidents resulting in casualties which are attended by police or notified to them (DoT, 1975–94). STATS19 data have been compiled more or less in their present form since 1949, but we have only examined trends in published data for the last 20 years (1974–93). Casualties are classified by type of road user and by a measure of injury severity (slightly injured, seriously injured, killed). A serious injury is defined as an injury for which a person is detained in hospital as an 'in-patient', or any of the following injuries whether or not they are detained in hospital: fractures, concussion, internal injuries, crushings, severe cuts and lacerations, severe general shock requiring medical treatment, injuries causing death 30 or more days after the accident. An injured casualty is recorded as seriously or slightly injured by the police on the basis of information available within a short time of the accident. This generally will not include the results of a medical examination, but may include the fact of being detained in hospital, the reasons for which may vary somewhat from area to area.

It is interesting to note that death is used as a measure of injury severity in road accident research but more usually as a measure of outcome in health services research. This duality allows us to examine trends in outcome (death) for casualties of given injury severity (killed or seriously injured) in order to make some assessment of the role of tertiary prevention in changing patterns of RTA mortality.

The Consumer Safety Unit located within the Department of Trade and Industry (DTI) has monitored home accidents presenting to Accident and Emergency (A and E) departments in the United Kingdom since 1976 (DTI, 1987, 1993). This Home Accident Surveillance System (HASS) data are compiled from records of first attendances at a sample of A and E departments with more than 10,000 total attendances per annum operating a 24-hour service and taking ambulance cases. The survey has recently been extended to include leisure accidents and road accidents, and also to include data on home accident fatalities. However, we have only examined recent trends in published HASS data for attendances at A and E departments in the United Kingdom for the 8-year period from 1986 to 1993, when reliable national estimates became available. We have also examined ONS mortality data trends over the same period for accidents classified as occurring at home or in residential institutions (ICD9 codes E850–E869, E880–E928).

Health and Safety legislation developed in the United Kingdom in the form of the Factories and various other Acts with different agencies having responsibility for different industries. In 1974 these Acts were consolidated in the Health and Safety at Work et cetera, Act. Since this time responsibility for enforcement of Health and Safety legislation has been divided between the Health and Safety Executive (HSE) and Local Authorities (LA) according to the main activity carried out on the premises (Dewis, 1995). The Health and Safety Commission (HSC) co-ordinates health and safety at work issues overall. The HSE compile annual statistics on fatal and non-fatal accidents occurring as a result of work activities from several different sources. The numbers reported by the HSE are not identical to those reported by ONS in the annual publications on mortality from injuries and violence. For example, persons other than the self-employed or employees who are fatally injured 'as a result of work accidents' are reportable as work fatalities to the HSE but are not usually included as such in ONS statistics. Thus, for example, deaths of spectators at professional football games are counted as work-related fatalities by HSE but as leisure fatalities by ONS. We have therefore examined recent trends in numbers and rates of fatal and non-fatal injuries in the period 1981–92/3 using the HSE statistics (HSE, 1988; HSC, 1993, 1995). As the responsibilities for shipping, factory and other industrial processes before 1974 were covered by different legislation, the fatal accident data are not comparable with recent figures. The longer-term perspective is therefore presented using statistics from the Department of Employment (DoE) (DoE and Productivity, 1971).

Comparisons of accidents occurring as a result of work activities are difficult. The under-reporting of non-fatal accidents to employees has been estimated to be 57 per cent and is reported to be higher in some sectors, for example, in construction and in agriculture, and considerably lower in energy (Stevens, 1992; DoE and HSE, 1992) . The reporting of fatal injuries, however, is believed by HSE to be virtually complete. Definitions used within data collection systems over many years are influenced by factors such as changes in responsibilities and new regulations. The Notification of Accidents and Dangerous Occurrences Regulations 1980 (NADOR), for example, were superseded by the Reporting of Injuries, Diseases and Dangerous Occurrences Regulations (RIDDOR) in 1986 (DoE and HSE, 1989). The definition of a major injury was extended under RIDDOR and the period of data collection also changed from a calendar to a financial year but the continuity of the fatal accident data series would not have been disturbed by the changes.

Statistics on fatal accidents occurring during sports and leisure activities have been compiled by ONS since 1982 (OPCS, 1985–93) from information contained in death certificates or in coroners' reports. The circumstances surrounding death by drowning are often difficult to determine, and as

these have only been classified in the same form since 1984, we have examined trends in these numbers over the period 1984–93. Measures of exposure relating to participation in sports and exercise are not available for the whole of this time period (although some data are periodically available from the GHS), and consequently we have only examined the trends in numbers of fatalities. Reliable information on trends in non-fatal injuries or accidents in sports and leisure activities are not available, although Leisure Accident Surveillance System (LASS) data, compiled along with HASS data by the Consumer Safety Unit of the DTI, will be useful in future studies.

24.3 Deaths from injury and poisoning

The average number of deaths from injury and poisonings has declined from a peak in the 1930s of an average of 25,108 per year to 18,621 per year during the 1980s (see Table 24.2). By 1990 the number of IP deaths in England and Wales had fallen to 17,943, and the most recent data for 1992 show a further fall to 16,681.

The age/sex standardised rate has fallen by approximately half from an average of 761.6 deaths per million persons in the first decade of the century to just 387.0 in the 1980s. The major part of this decline occurred in deaths from accidents, which appear to have fallen from a peak of approximately 18,000 per year during the 1960s to just over 12,000 in the 1980s.

However, this change is made up of two clearly identifiable artificial effects as well as some real improvements. In the first place, the number of all deaths from injuries and

Table 24.2

Deaths from injury and poisoning, 1901–90

Years	All deaths			Accidents			Non-accidents			Undetermined whether accidental		
	Number*	Crude rate**	Standardised rate***	Number*	Crude rate**	Standardised rate***	Number*	Crude rate**	Standardised rate***	Number*	Crude rate**	Standardised rate***
1901–10	19,641	574.2	761.6	15,852	463.5	609.5	3,789	110.7	152.1	0	0.0	0.0
1911–20	21,307	597.1	793.6	15,559	436.1	590.5	3,507	98.3	128.4	2,240	62.8	74.7
1921–30	19,239	493.8	663.5	14,270	366.3	509.2	4,952	127.1	153.7	17	0.4	0.6
1931–40	25,108	618.6	804.1	16,382	403.6	564.4	7,733	190.5	212.1	993	24.5	27.5
1941–50	23,211	576.6	685.2	15,025	373.2	471.5	8,123	201.8	212.4	63	1.6	1.3
1951–60	21,286	476.8	573.1	15,913	356.5	446.0	5,346	119.7	126.5	27	0.6	0.6
1961–70	23,745	497.5	567.5	18,007	377.3	441.5	5,341	111.9	117.6	397	8.3	8.8
1971–80	21,285	430.6	468.4	15,504	313.6	345.8	4,429	89.6	94.0	1,352	27.4	28.6
1981–90	18,621	372.0	387.0	12,297	245.7	249.8	4,482	89.5	100.0	1,842	36.8	37.2

Note: * = Average number per decade.
  ** = Rate per million persons.
  *** = Age/sex directly standardised rate per million persons (1991 population as standard).

Source: ONS historical mortality database

poisonings which were undetermined whether accidental has increased from an average of 397 in the 1960s to 1842 in the 1980s. Thus, the true numbers of accidental deaths in the 1980s could be over 1,500 per year greater than shown in Table 24.2. However, even assuming that the majority of the deaths undetermined whether accidental were in fact due to accidents, the standardised mortality rate from accidents has still fallen from an average of over 600 per million persons in the decade 1901–10 to under 300 in the 1980s.

In the second place, the number of deaths recorded as due to falls showed a steep rise between the 1940s and the 1960s, but recorded numbers have since fallen by 31 per cent from an average of 5,477 per year to 3,769 per year during the 1980s. An examination of the nature of injury resulting in death from falls shows that this decline is almost entirely due to a decline in the number of deaths resulting from limb fractures, while the number of deaths from falls resulting from head injuries and other causes has remained unchanged (see Table 24.3). It is clear that the decline in limb fracture deaths, and hence in falls, is artificial for two reasons. Firstly, the majority of the limb fracture deaths occur in the elderly following fractured femurs and it is known that the incidence of fractured femur was increasing at least until 1980 (Spector *et al.*, 1990; Boyce and Vessey 1985). Secondly, death following fractured neck of femur in the elderly commonly results from complications, such as bronchopneumonia, and there is no consistency in ascribing cause of death in these circumstances. For example, the number of deaths following admission to hospital for fracture of the lower limb recorded in HIPE statistics for 1985 was 6,230; but the number of deaths from lower limb fractures recorded in ONS mortality data was just 2,408. The difference is made up by deaths ascribed to the complications rather than the falls. Some coroners request that all such incidents should be referred to them as accidental deaths; others that these deaths should not be re-

ferred. It seems likely, therefore, that the dramatic decline in limb fracture deaths from falls, which contrasts both with head and other injury deaths from falls and the incidence of fractured neck of femur, is an artefact resulting from an increasing tendency not to ascribe these deaths to the fall but to other complications.

Deaths from falls resulting in head injuries show a surprising consistency during each of the 5 years spanning the four decades we have examined, varying by no more than 6 per cent (see Table 24.3), and there is no evidence that the numbers have shown a declining trend, although the rate per million persons has slowly fallen from 24.5 in 1950 to 20.7 in 1990. If these numbers are reliably recorded, and there is no evidence that they are not, then these data provide little evidence of improvements in either the prevention of these types of accident or of improvement in the management of head injuries.

Table 24.3

Deaths from accidental falls, 1950–90

Year	Pop-ulation (million)	Head injuries Number	Head injuries Rate*	Limb frac-tures	Other injuries	Total
1950	43.8	1,072	24.5	2,494	562	4,128
1960	45.8	1,072	23.4	3,375	818	5,465
1970	48.9	1,063	21.7	3,910	660	5,633
1980	49.6	1,017	20.5	2,578	642	4,237
1990	50.7	1,052	20.7	1,723	622	3,397

Note * = Rate per million persons.

Source: ONS mortality statistics

Table 24.4

Deaths from accidental* causes by sex per million persons, 1901–90

Year	Men Average number per year	Men Crude rate	Men Age standardised rate	Women Average number per year	Women Crude rate	Women Age stadardised rate
1901–10	10,983	664.1	794.3	4,870	275.7	432.9
1911–20	10,955	666.3	782.1	4,604	239.3	407.4
1921–30	9,868	529.5	629.4	4,401	216.6	394.3
1931–40	10,786	556.7	656.3	5,596	263.8	476.9
1941–50	9,522	520.0	561.9	5,503	250.8	385.1
1951–60	9,559	444.8	503.9	6,355	274.5	390.7
1961–70	10,249	442.6	488.7	7,757	315.9	395.7
1971–80	8,630	358.3	384.3	6,883	271.3	309.0
1981–90	7,136	292.5	294.9	5,161	201.1	206.8

Note: * = Excluding not stated whether accidental or not.
Source: ONS historical mortality database

The decline in age-standardised death rates between 1901–10 and 1981–90 has been slightly larger in men than in women, falling by 63 per cent in men and 52 per cent in women (see Table 24.4). Trends in accidental deaths at different ages are particularly interesting. There have been dramatic falls in accidental death rates in both sexes for children (see Table 24.5, Figure 24.1). However, there has been little change in young persons (aged 15–24) of either sex, and the highest rates were seen in the 1960s in men and in the 1970s in women. However, in both sexes these rates have since declined so that the rate during the 1980s was lower than in the first decade in men, though this level has not yet been reached

in women. It is very likely that the peak for men in the 1960s reflects the rapid growth of motor vehicle travel and accidents during the 1960s and 1970s, with the slightly later increase for women reflecting increases in the number of licence-holders The substantial reductions in road traffic accident deaths which have occurred during the 1980s (see below) are probably responsible for the recent downward turn in these rates.

In contrast to both children and young persons, trends in accidental death rates in older age-groups differed between men and women with a comparatively steady decline in men

Figure 24.1

Accidental death rates, by age and sex

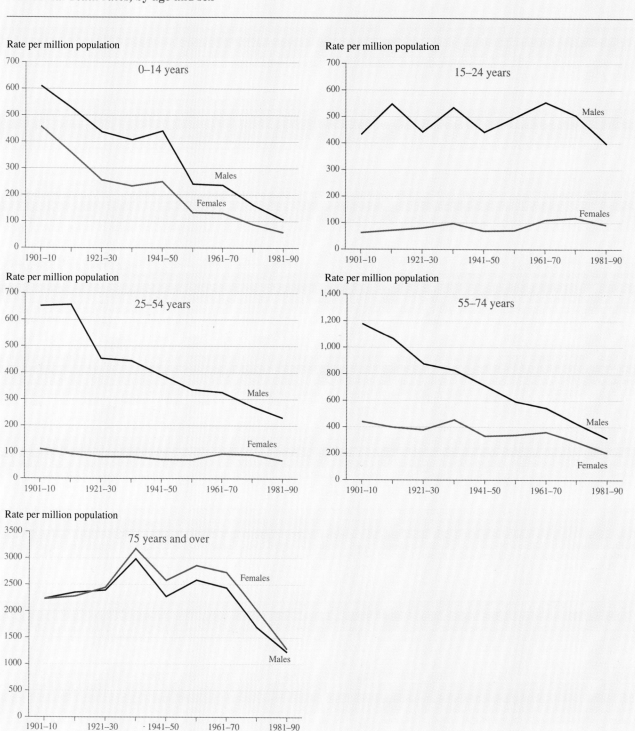

Table 24.5

Accidental death rates per million, by age and sex, 1901–90

Year	0–14		15–24		25–54		55–74		75+	
	M	F	M	F	M	F	M	F	M	F
1901–10	610.5	458.3	432.1	62.3	651.8	112.0	1,178.4	440.3	2,230.9	2,229.6
1911–20	528.5	358.6	547.9	71.3	656.7	94.3	1,065.7	398.1	2,348.7	2,279.8
1921–30	437.3	255.9	442.5	80.2	452.8	82.1	875.2	378.6	2,390.0	2,443.4
1931–40	406.7	233.1	534.8	97.2	444.1	82.2	827.0	453.3	2,979.1	3,176.8
1941–50	440.1	249.5	441.8	69.1	389.6	72.5	710.7	331.6	2,271.3	2,578.2
1951–60	240.7	132.5	497.4	71.4	335.7	71.7	591.3	339.0	2,583.2	2,858.6
1961–70	236.4	130.3	554.9	110.2	325.7	93.9	541.6	361.9	2,436.0	2,730.8
1971–80	161.5	88.1	504.5	118.1	271.8	91.1	424.8	288.9	1,694.3	2,026.1
1981–90	106.0	58.4	396.7	91.7	229.0	68.8	314.1	204.0	1,223.4	1,283.9

Source: ONS historical mortality database

Table 24.6

Deaths from accidental causes, by type of accident, rates per million persons, 1901–90

Year	Transport			Poisoning			Falls		
	Average number per year	Crude	Age/sex standardised	Average number per year	Crude	Age/sex standardised	Average number per year	Crude	Age/sex standardised
1901–10		*(see text)*		611	17.9	22.0	2,585	75.6	188.3
1911–20				1,390	39.0	34.2	3,237	90.7	203.3
1921–30				373	9.6	13.0	3,058	78.5	179.7
1931–40				346	8.5	11.1		*(see text)*	
1941–50	5,278	131.1	148.9	544	13.5	17.0	4,415	109.7	179.5
1951–60	5,956	133.4	148.7	1,130	25.3	31.3	5,130	114.9	176.8
1961–70	7,400	155.1	166.1	1,357	28.4	33.3	5,477	114.8	159.6
1971–80	6,716	135.9	140.5	370	7.5	7.9	4,985	100.8	123.7
1981–90	5,150	102.9	101.8	636	12.7	12.9	3,769	75.3	79.2

Year	Fire and Flames			Drowning			Other and not specified		
	Average number per year	Crude	Age/sex standardised	Average number per year	Crude	Age/sex standardised	Average number per year	Crude	Age/sex standardised
1901–10	2,524	73.8	73.1	4,260	124.6	113.4	5,873	171.7	212.6
1911–20	2,347	65.8	68.5	2,380	66.7	73.1	6,206	173.9	211.4
1921–30	1,625	41.7	50.5	1,594	40.9	43.8	7.637	196.0	222.8
1931–40	1,469	36.2	47.2	830	20.4	20.4	13,736	338.5	485.9
1941–50	1,100	27.3	33.2	1,151	28.6	28.6	2,538	63.0	63.0
1951–60	903	20.2	24.8	907	20.3	20.3	1,888	42.3	43.5
1961–70	931	19.5	22.5	950	19.9	19.9	1,891	39.6	40.2
1971–80	713	14.4	16.1	1,124	22.7	22.7	1,597	32.3	34.4
1981–90	623	12.5	12.9	867	17.3	17.3	1,252	25.0	25.16

Source: ONS historical mortality database

Figure 24.2

Deaths from accidental causes, by type, age-sex standardised rate

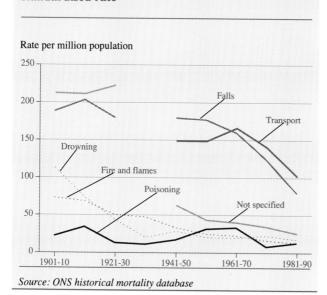

Rate per million population

Source: ONS historical mortality database

aged 25–54 and 55–74, but little change in women until the last 20 years. The decrease in fatal accidents in male employees resulting from work activities in the later part of the century will have had an impact on this pattern. For the elderly aged 75 and over, recorded rates in both men and women increased slightly during the first decades of the century but in both sexes have again fallen sharply in the last 20 years.

Patterns of change during the century in the causes of accidental deaths also show some notable differences (see Table 24.6, Figure 24.2). Standardised death rates from fires have fallen steadily and now stand at just one sixth of the rate at the beginning of the century. Deaths from drowning fell rapidly in the first part of the century but since then have remained nearly constant. Transport accident deaths peaked during the 1960s, as would be expected, but have since fallen by approximately one third. Death rates from both falls and poisonings changed little during the first 70 years, but have fallen by more than half in the last 20 years. The reason for the decline in accidental deaths from poisoning during the 1970s and 1980s may relate to the introduction of better packaging and labelling of medicines and household poisons. As discussed earlier the reason for the similar decline in falls is probably artificial.

24.4 Trends in non-fatal accidents

Casualties from non-fatal accidents are not recorded centrally and trends are therefore difficult to identify. For some types of accident, such as RTAs, home accidents and work-related accidents, records of non-fatal accidents do, however, exist; and trends in morbidity from these types of accidents are described individually in Section 24.5.

Part of the problem with identifying the number of non-fatal accident casualties, i.e. persons injured in accidents, relates

to the difficulty of defining injuries – which can vary from cuts and grazes to major life-threatening trauma. Without a measure of injury severity, therefore, it is not possible to define a casualty, and no adequate scale for measuring the severity of minor injuries exists. It is therefore necessary to take an operational or 'process' approach and define casualties by the consequences of the injury – for example, by whether the injured person sought medical attention, attended an A and E department, consulted a GP, or was admitted to hospital.

The problem with such operational definitions, of course, is that the nature and severity of the injury are not the only determinants of the process of care for, and the outcome of, the injury. The GHS combined data for 1987 and 1989 (Breeze et al., 1991) indicate that medical treatment is sought for a very small proportion of all accidents. Such issues as access to A and E departments, GPs, or other services for the treatment of minor injuries, as well as patient behaviour and expectations, will also play a part in determining the action taken. Among those who reported an accident resulting in seeing a doctor or a hospital visit in the 3 months preceding the interview survey, over 55 per cent presented only to the hospital, compared with 22 per cent who only consulted their GP. Changes in the availability of beds, as well as the technologies available to treat patients, can also result in changes in the numbers admitted as in-patients. Furthermore, casualties (i.e. patients), episodes of care, or consultations could all be counted and may need potentially arbitrary definitions to distinguish them.

Despite all these difficulties, however, we have examined trends during the last 20 years in two recorded aspects of non-fatal accident morbidity: the numbers of episodes of care provided by GPs for conditions classified as IP (N800–N999 in ICD9); and the number of discharges and deaths (and later finished consultant episodes) from NHS hospitals for IP.

24.4.1 Episodes of GP care

The decennial national morbidity surveys (RCGP, 1974, 1984; McCormick et al., 1995) have been examined for estimates of the risk of an episode of GP care per 10^5 persons for conditions classified as IP by age and sex. Data were obtained from the 2nd (1971/72), 3rd (81/82) and 4th (91/92) surveys.

The rate of episodes of GP care per 10^5 persons for IP has risen by over 46 per cent during this 20-year period and the changes have been particularly large in women (over 74 per cent), so that in the most recent morbidity survey the recorded rate of episodes was larger for women than for men (see Table 24.7). The episode rates show the characteristic pattern by age, rising to age 15–24 and then falling before rising again in the elderly aged 75 and over (see Figure 24.3). The increasing episode rate between 1971/72 and 1991/92 was particularly marked for the elderly, and this presumably reflects the change in the age-distribution within this age-group (i.e. more very elderly people) as much as any change

Table 24.7

Episodes of GP care for injury and poisoning;
rates per 10,000 persons at risk by sex

Sex	1971/72	1981/82	1991/92
Men	1,204	1,385	1,505
Women	912	1,279	1,588
Persons	1,052	1,330	1,531

Source: Morbidity statistics from general practice; 2nd, 3rd and 4th national studies

Figure 24.3

Rates of GP episodes for injury and poisonings, by age
1971/72 to 1991/92

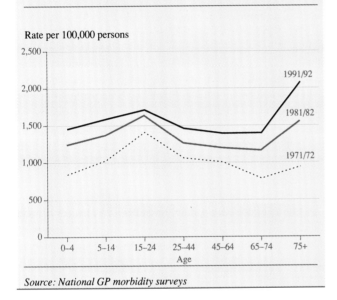

Source: National GP morbidity surveys

in accident risk or tendency for GPs to be involved in the care of elderly accident victims.

24.4.2 Episodes of hospital care

Hospital In-patient Enquiry (HIPE) data for residents of England and Wales for the years 1962–81 show a 51 per cent rise in the numbers of discharges and deaths from NHS hospitals for patients admitted with a diagnosis classified as IP. However, the bulk of this increase had occurred by 1971, and between 1971 and 1981 the numbers increased only marginally from 522,510 to 559,850. HIPE data for English residents show similarly small increases between 1982 and 1985 when HIPE ceased (see Figure 24.4).

Recent changes are more difficult to determine. Hospital Episode System (HES) data for English residents recorded 657,000 finished consultant episodes (FCEs) for IP diagnoses in 1989/90, rising to 677,000 in 1992/93. The ratio of FCEs to discharges and deaths for patients admitted with an IP diagnosis are not known nationally. However, data from Sheffield District Health Authority (Sheffield Health

Figure 24.4

Episodes of hospital care for accidents, poisoning and violence

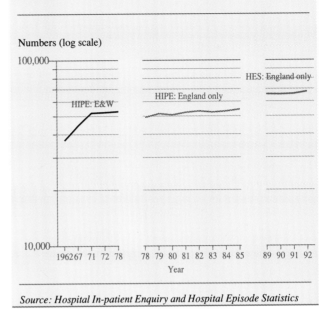

Source: Hospital In-patient Enquiry and Hospital Episode Statistics

Authority, 1995) indicate that this ratio is no more than 5 per cent; and this suggests that the increases in activity of the order of 1 per cent per year seen between 1972 and 1985 continued until 1993.

The rates (per 10,000 persons) of discharges and deaths for men showed little change between 1972 and 1981, although there was a small increase for women (see Table 24.8). The HES data suggest that some increases in both men and women may have occurred between 1981 and 1991/92.

It seems likely that these small increases were principally due to increases in the numbers of very elderly people in the population, as well as increases in the rates in elderly people. For persons aged 75 and over the rates for FCEs recorded in HES for 1991/92 were 60 per cent higher than the rates for discharges and deaths recorded in HIPE in 1972. However, at younger ages these differences ranged from only minus 3 per cent (at ages 0–4) to over 38 per cent (for ages 65–74) (see Figure 24.5).

Table 24.8

NHS hospital episodes for injury and poisoning,
rates per 10,000 population, by sex

Year	Source		Males	Females
1972	HIPE	E&W	1,241	914
1981	HIPE	E&W	1,265	1,005
1982	HIPE	E	1,285	1,003
1991/92	HES	E	1,495	1,253

Source: Hospital In-patient Enquiry Reports for 1972, 1981, 1982, and Hospital Episode Statistics for 1991/92

Figure 24.5

Rates of hospital episodes of injury and poisoning, by age

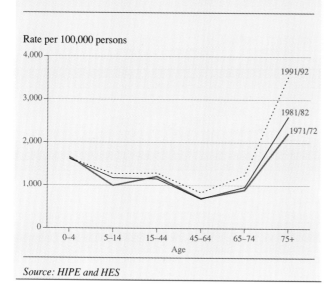

Rate per 100,000 persons

Source: HIPE and HES

24.5 Recent trends in types of accident

24.5.1 Road traffic accidents

In the 20 years between 1974 and 1993 the numbers of fatally injured and seriously injured RTA casualties in accidents reported to the police and recorded in STATS19 data for Great Britain have both fallen by 45 per cent, from 6,876 to 3,814 deaths and from 82,096 to 45,009 seriously injured casualties (see Figure 24.6). In contrast, the numbers of slightly injured casualties have risen marginally from 236,000 to 257,000 (approximately 9 per cent).

During this period the population of Great Britain increased by 2 million (3.7 per cent); the number of motor vehicles

Figure 24.6

Recent trends in road traffic accident casualties

Numbers (thousands)

Seriously injured casualties
Fatalities

Source: Road accidents in Great Britain 1984, 1993

increased by 7.8 million (45 per cent); and an index of all traffic increased by 78 per cent (DoT, 1975–94). Thus with respect to any measure of exposure, the fatal and seriously injured casualty rate has fallen by at least a half within a 20-year period.

Perhaps surprisingly, despite a variety of primary and secondary prevention initiatives aimed at different road user groups, all types of road users have benefited to a similar, though not identical, extent from the 20-year fall in the numbers of road accident casualties. The greatest reduction was seen for car drivers (numbers: 33 per cent; rate: 68 per cent) and the least for pedal cyclists (numbers: 15 per cent; rate: 39 per cent) (see Table 24.9). The discrepancy has been noted before and has raised questions of equity and interpretation of the benefits of legislation and regulations aimed at making car users safer – possibly at the expense of other vulnerable road user groups.

Equally interesting is the proportion of all RTA casualties with severe injuries (i.e. those recorded in STATS19 as killed

Table 24.9

RTA casualties killed or seriously injured by road user type, numbers and rates per 100 million vehicle kilometres, 1974, 1993

Road user type	1974 Numbers	1974 Rate	1993 Numbers	1993 Rate
Pedestrians	23,681		12,658	
Pedal cyclists	4,448	137	3,796	84
TWMV*:				
riders	13,445	418	6,351	152
passengers	1,265		528	
Car:				
drivers	21,468	13	14,278	4.2
passengers	17,774		8,553	
Bus or coach:				
drivers	131	2	59	1.3
passengers	1,488		666	
Light goods vehicle:				
drivers	2,070	4	753	2.1
passengers	1,396		329	
Heavy goods vehicle:				
drivers	1,005	3	535	1.9
passengers	288		100	
All road users	88,979		48,823	

Note: * = Two-wheeled motor vehicle.
Source: Road Accidents Great Britain 1984 and 1993

Figure 24.7

Proportions of seriously injured RTA casualities who died, by user type

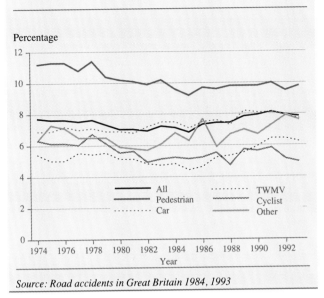

Source: Road accidents in Great Britain 1984, 1993

Table 24.10

Fatal and non-fatal home-accidents, 1974–93

Year	Fatal home accidents, E&W*	Non-fatal home accidents, UK**	
		Estimated attendances at A and E, ('000s)	Estimated inpatient admissions ('000s)
1974	5,747		
1980	5,270		
1986	4,626	1,999	94
1987	4,210	2,102	109
1988	4,274	2,509	113
1989	4,080	2,750	142
1990	4,055	2,596	132
1991	4,078	2,634	140
1992	3,986	2,547	129
1993		2,882	146

Note: * = Source: ONS mortality statistics
** = Source: Home Accident Surveillance System

or seriously injured) who died, which has remained nearly constant during the last 20 years, falling slightly during the 1980s but rising again to its highest level in 1991 (see Figure 24.7). To the extent that the definition and recording of serious injury in STATS19 has remained unchanged during this time, this constant proportion suggests that there has been little improvement in tertiary prevention – that is, in emergency services, medical care and rehabilitative services – during this period.

24.5.2 Home accidents

During the last 20 years the numbers of fatally injured home accident casualties recorded by ONS have fallen by 11 per cent for men and 42 per cent for women, and there are now approximately 4,000 fatal home accidents in England and Wales each year.

This is very similar to the number of fatal road traffic accidents. Part of this recorded decline could be artefactual as a result of declining numbers of deaths following falls at home being ascribed to the fall, rather than other complications, and this could explain the greater reduction for women than for men. However, the reduction in non-fall home accidents (under 25 per cent) has been nearly as substantial as for falls (under 34 per cent), and it seems, therefore, that there has been a real and substantial decline in home accident deaths.

However, in contrast to RTAs, in which the numbers of seriously injured casualties have fallen as dramatically as the number of fatalities, there is no evidence that the numbers of non-fatally injured home accident casualties who attend A and E departments have fallen. Indeed, HASS data suggest that these numbers have been increasing from approximately 2 million per annum in the mid-1980s to 2.9 million in 1993 (see Table 24.10). Because of the changing composition of the HASS survey and changing data collection methods, it is

likely that some of this change is artefactual. Even if only casualties recorded by HASS as admitted to hospital are counted, similar to those classified as seriously injured in STATS19 RTA data, the estimated numbers have increased by 55 per cent from 94,000 in 1986 to 146,000 in 1993.

In addition to the contrast between road and home accidents in the trend in numbers of seriously injured casualties, there is a contrast in the ratio of fatal to serious injuries, which is 7–8 per cent for RTAs compared to 2.5–5.0 per cent for home accidents. This presumably reflects a substantially different injury severity distribution.

By far the largest component of home accident causes are falls and these have remained constant as a proportion of HASS numbers between 1986 (38 per cent) and 1993 (37 per cent).

24.5.3 Work accidents

The data series on fatal accidents was not affected by the introduction of RIDDOR. In the 12-year period between 1981 and 1992/93 (HSE, 1988; HSC, 1995) an average of 593 persons each year were reported by HSE as fatally injured as a result of work activities, which represents approximately 5 per cent of all fatal accidents. There appears to have been a general fall in the number of employees fatally injured at work; an overall increase in the number of work-related deaths in the self-employed; and an erratic but increasing number of fatal injuries to members of the public injured as a result of work activities.

The sharp rises in fatal accidents to members of the public in 1985 and 1989/90 are accounted for by the Bradford Football Club stadium fire and the Sheffield Hillsborough football disaster, respectively (see Figure 24.8).

Figure 24.8

Fatal accidents at work

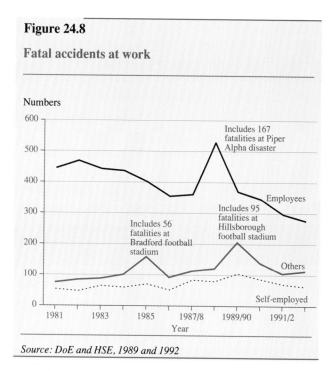

Source: DoE and HSE, 1989 and 1992

Figure 24.9

Fatal and major injury rates per 100,000 employees

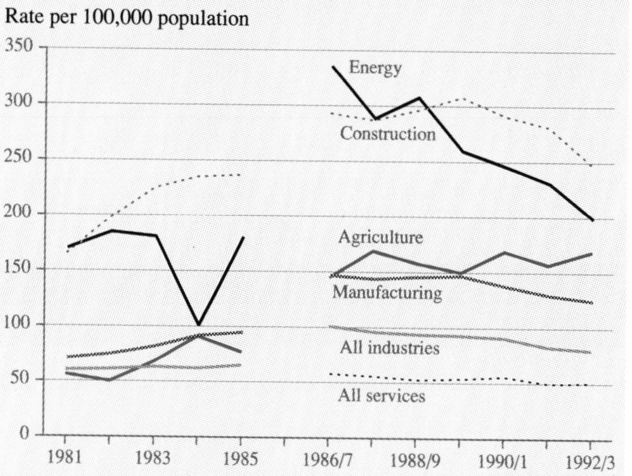

'Energy' includes 167 fatalities in Piper Alpha disater in 1988/89
'Energy' rates for 1984 were affected by industrial dispute in coal mining industry.
Data for 'All services' not included for 1981-85.
Source: DoE and HSE, 1989 and 1992

The overall trend in employee accident rates for fatal and major injuries across all industries increased slightly between 1981 and 1985 (HSE 1988), but between 1986/87 and 1992/93 (HSC, 1993) it has been declining generally. The trends in fatal and major injury rates in energy and construction dropped sharply in 1988 and 1989, respectively (see Figure 24.9). The broad industrial classifications mask variations between industries *within* each classification, but between 1986/87 and 1992/93 the combined fatal and major injury rates among employees in all industrial sectors except agriculture, remained more or less constant or decreased. These rates will be influenced by differences in reporting levels but the patterns can be explained partly by contemporary changes in employment patterns away from hazardous activities like coal mining, and by an expanding service sector where the risks of injury are much lower. In the energy sector, the dip in fatal and major injuries during 1984 resulted, in part, by less exposure to risk caused by an industrial dispute in the coal mining industry, and the rise in 1988/89 is attributable to the Piper Alpha oil-rig disaster.

The overall patterns of work-related injury since 1986/87 have remained constant. Virtually all employees (98 per cent) and all the self-employed who were fatally injured in 1990/91 were men. This reflects the occupational structure and exposure of men to high-risk occupations. In 1990/91, the sector with the highest non-fatal major injury risk for men was construction, with an overall rate of 321/100,000 employees. This was more than four times the rate of the highest risk occupation for women, which was agriculture, where the rate reported for the same period was 77/100,000 employees. These rates which are based on fatal and non-fatal injuries, are likely to be affected by under-reporting which is relatively high in both construction and agriculture. Major injuries in male employees occur predominantly in those aged 25–34, whereas most major injuries in female employees, and fatal injuries in employed and non-employed groups, occur in the age-group 45–54 years (DoE and HSE, 1992).

The most common cause of a fatal injury to an employee was a fall from a height. Slips or falls on the same level were the most common cause of a non-fatal major accident. The most common cause of all accidents to employees as reported are those which occur while handling, lifting or carrying. In 1990/91, approximately three-quarters of all major non-fatal accidents to employees were fractures. Over half of all non-fatal major injuries to employees were to the upper limbs (arms, hands, wrists, fingers). In 1990/91, amputations, mainly of the fingers, accounted for a further 7.3 per cent of all major non-fatal injuries to employees (DoE and HSE, 1992).

Historically, accidents at work accounted for a much higher number of deaths, rising sharply from the mid-nineteenth century and peaking at an average of 4,556 each year between 1910 and 1919 (around the period of the First World War) and rising again temporarily around the Second World War (DoE and Productivity, 1971), presumably reflecting the nature of the workforce and changes in exposure due to the diversification towards industries for military support services and armaments (see Figure 24.10).

Extreme caution has to be exercised in interpreting statistics in the dynamic context of a historical period affected by significant changes in legislation and enforcement practices, contraction and expansion of industries, and considerable variation in reporting of non-fatal injuries. Figures available before 1974 for persons killed in work-related accidents are not directly comparable with recent data, but have been included as background to illustrate that, through regulation and changes in exposure to risk in employees, dramatic reductions in fatal accidents to employees resulting from work activities in Britain have occurred during the twentieth century.

Figure 24.10

Annual average number of fatal accidents at work

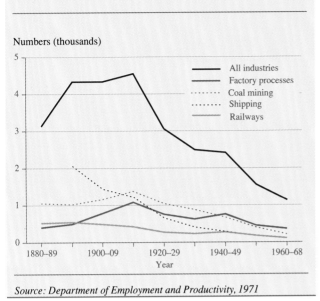

Numbers (thousands)

Legend:
— All industries
— Factory processes
···· Coal mining
···· Shipping
---- Railways

Source: Department of Employment and Productivity, 1971

24.5.4 Sports and leisure

An average of 180 fatal accidents (including deaths by drowning) occurred each year in the period 1986–92 in England and Wales while taking part in sporting and leisure activities (OPCS, 1985–93) (see Figure 24.11). It is estimated that 10 million injuries in sports and exercise occur each year in the United Kingdom population aged 16–45 years which result in some restriction of daily activities (including work) or in treatment being sought from a third party (Nicholl *et al.*, 1993). In fatal and non-fatal sports injuries, young men aged 15–24 predominate. The activities with the highest risk of a fatal accident are air sports and climbing. Most water sports also have a relatively high risk. In popular participation sports, most injuries occur in soccer, but rugby has a substantially higher risk of a fatal or serious injury occurring. Horse-riding has a fairly low risk, but if an injury does occur it is more

Figure 24.11

Fatal accidents (including drowning) occurring in sports and leisure

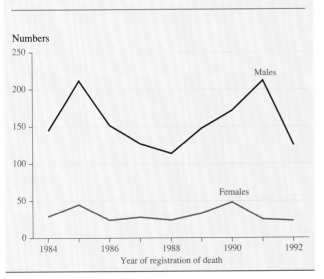

Numbers

Males

Females

Year of registration of death

likely to be serious than in other activities. Only 7 per cent of all sports injuries attend an A and E department and the GP is the medical practitioner consulted most frequently (Nicholl *et al.*, 1993).

The risk of drowning is small but more than three quarters of incidents involve young men aged 15–24 years. Unprotected open water and streams are where more than one third of all incidents occur. The numbers of drowning incidents for the three years 1991 to 1993 were the three lowest ever recorded, but the incidence can be affected by periods of good weather (RoSPA, 1993).

24.6 Discussion

Despite numerous difficulties in interpreting trends in data which have been compiled on accidents there are some clear and striking features.

First, over a long period of time there have been considerable improvements in accident fatality rates, although these have mostly been confined to children 0–14 and men aged 25–74 years. The causes which have seen the most benefits in the long term are deaths from fires, drowning in the early part of the century, and death recorded from falls in the later part, though this may be a largely artificial effect.

In recent years there have also been considerable reductions in accident fatality rates, despite the growth of motor vehicle travel. This has happened largely because substantial reductions in RTA fatality rates per kilometre travelled have outweighed the growth in traffic, and because there have been considerable reductions in both home and work accident fatalities. The reduction in fatalities resulting from work activities in employees, which will have contributed to the trend in men aged 25–74 years, will be associated with the shift away from relatively dangerous heavy industrial occupations, such as coal mining, towards lighter service-types of work where the risk of major injury is much lower, as well as to improvements in safety.

With regard to morbidity, while it is clear that the number of seriously injured RTA casualties has fallen at the same rate as fatalities, this is not so for home accidents. The numbers recorded by HASS as admitted to hospital following attendance at an A and E department as a result of a home accident appear to have been rising slowly in recent years while fatalities were falling. This represents the general picture, which appears to show that in contrast to the mortality data, such morbidity data as there are show that the numbers of patients being treated by GPs and hospitals following injuries and poisonings are not declining at all. In fact, these data on episodes of GP and hospital care appear to suggest that during the last 20 years there has been a steady increase in morbidity from IP. This is in complete contrast to mortality data, which show a reduction from 22,624 deaths in 1971 to 17,943 in 1990. Most of this reduction occurred in accidents with little changes in the numbers of non-accidental causes. There are three possible explanations for the apparent conflict in the morbidity and mortality data. Firstly, decreasing fatality rates, despite increasing numbers of casualties, could be the result of better tertiary prevention – particularly improvements in trauma care services. However, the lack of evidence of any improvement in the RTA case-fatality rate, and only small improvements in the last 40 years in the death rate from head injuries in falls, suggests that improvements in trauma care services are not the main cause.

Secondly, there is a possibility that the casualty severity distribution has changed as a result of the effect of secondary prevention initiatives. Secondary prevention could decrease the numbers of fatalities but leave the number of casualties seeking medical care comparatively unaffected. However, in this case we might have expected improvements in case fatality ratios in RTAs, where there have been numerous secondary prevention initiatives, such as seat belts (Christian and Bullimore, 1989; Harvey and Durbin, 1986) pedal (Wood and Milne, 1988) and motor cycle helmets (Watson *et al.*, 1981), and vehicle engineering (Chinn, 1991; Zadar and Ciccone, 1993) but not in home accidents, where initiatives have been almost exclusively in primary prevention, which would not be expected to alter the case fatality ratio. Since the empirical evidence suggests the opposite effect, with no change in the case-fatality ratio in RTAs and a reduction in home accidents, it is unlikely that this is the explanation of the changing accident mortality and morbidity patterns.

Thirdly, episodes of care could be occurring at a lower threshold of severity of injury, with patients seeking medical attention from both GPs and hospitals with comparatively minor conditions. It is well known, for example, that despite relatively unchanging general mortality levels there is an increasing demand for health services, which may reflect both changing patient expectations and changes in access to services. There is no reason to expect that demand for medical care following accidents should show a different pattern of change.

Finally, there are undoubtedly some problems with the morbidity data themselves. The trend in hospital episode rates are unclear because of changes to HIPE, and then the later introduction of HES. HASS data on A and E attendances have also not been collected in a stable and consistent way for long enough to ensure that the trends are reliably identified. The GP morbidity data have been collected consistently but unfortunately consultations have not been classified by severity of condition consistently over the three surveys.

Plainly the lack of reliable, consistent and accurate data on morbidity following accidents is one of the chief difficulties facing the identification and implementation of successful prevention initiatives. However, it is equally clear from well-documented successes in the primary and secondary prevention of Road Traffic Accidents (Broughton and Stark, 1987; Broughton, 1987; Sabey, 1980, 1995) that a great deal can be achieved in this direction.

Chapter 25

Are we healthier?

By
Karen Dunnell

Summary

- Mortality has been improving throughout the century. The decline continues each decade. Most recently the decline has been greatest for those aged 45–64 and least for those aged 20–44.

- Between 1970 and 1972, and 1990 and 1992, both men and women gained an extra 3 years of life expectancy at age 15 and an extra year at age 65.

- There has been no comparable increase in the number of years of healthy life.

- There has been no improvement in the last decade in the proportion of adults reporting a long-standing illness or short-term illness.

- Over the 4 years of the new national health survey there has been no evidence of any reduction in the proportion of adults with one or more risk factors for heart disease.

- In 1968 almost two fifths of adults had no teeth. This had reduced to one fifth in 1988.

- It is important to monitor health-related behaviour as well as health itself. Cigarette smoking has reduced considerably since the 1970s but there has been little change among men and women aged 16–24 during the last 10 years.

- Alcohol consumption has been reasonably stable among men, but is rising among women.

- There is no evidence that rates of physical activity are currently increasing.

25.1 Introduction

This chapter aims to look at more general measures of health among adults. It tries to answer the question 'Are we healthier?' for different age- and sex-groups within the adult population. A similar approach was taken in the recent review of children's health (Botting, 1995).

Ideally there should be a way of bringing together different measures of health to form a composite index, but this has not, as yet, been achieved. Instead we look at three aspects of health – mortality, morbidity and health status – and some behaviours known to have an impact on health. In general this chapter covers only those statistics which directly measure health, rather than those derived from the use of health services (see Chapter 5). It focuses on the last 10–20 years and uses data from registration systems, sample surveys and the 1991 Census.

Signs of improved health

- all cause mortality for all women and men under 30 and 40 and over
- certain cancers (see Chapter 4 and 17)
- life expectancy at all ages
- dental health
- smoking in older adults

Signs of worsening health

- all cause mortality for men aged 30-34
- certain cancers (see Chapters 4 and 17)
- proportion overweight and obese

Little sign of change in health

- all cause mortality for men aged 35-39
- self-reported acute and chronic morbidity
- healthy life expectancy
- risk factors for heart diseases
- physical activity
- smoking in young adults

25.2 Mortality

All cause mortality has been discussed at length in Chapter 3. This is the measure most commonly used to demonstrate the continuing improvement in population health since death registration began in the nineteenth century. Figure 25.1 and Table 25.1 demonstrate how mortality has improved in just the most recent 10 years. However, as can be seen, not all age- and sex-groups have improved to the same extent. The general pattern for men and women is the same. Those adults aged 15–19 and 45–64 have experienced the greatest improvement in mortality and those aged 20–44 the least.

Apart from the latter group, men's rates have generally declined more than women's. For example, among the youngest men, aged 15–19, the death rate fell by 30 per cent between 1984 and 1994. The comparable figure for young women was 22 per cent. For men and women aged 70–74 the decreases were 17 per cent and 10 per cent respectively. In absolute terms, of course, men, at every age, have higher death rates than women. This can be seen in Table 25.1 and is one clear indication that, in terms of mortality, men have poorer health than women.

The lack of change in mortality among young adults has been the subject of detailed investigation (Dunnell, 1991; Chief Medical Officer, 1993). Among men, deaths related to HIV/AIDs and suicides have largely counterbalanced reductions in deaths from cardiovascular causes and accidents. The picture for women is less clear. However, in the most recent years, mortality for young men and women has generally begun to decline as it had been doing prior to the mid-1980s.

Another way of using death rates to produce a general measure is to calculate life expectancies. These can be calculated from any age after birth. For example, between 1970 and 1972, and 1990 and 1992, life expectancy at birth for males rose from 69 to 73 years and from 75 to 79 for females (OPCS, 1994). Having survived infancy and childhood, life

Figure 25.1

Age-specific death rates for males and females as a percentage of rates in 1984, 1984–94, England and Wales

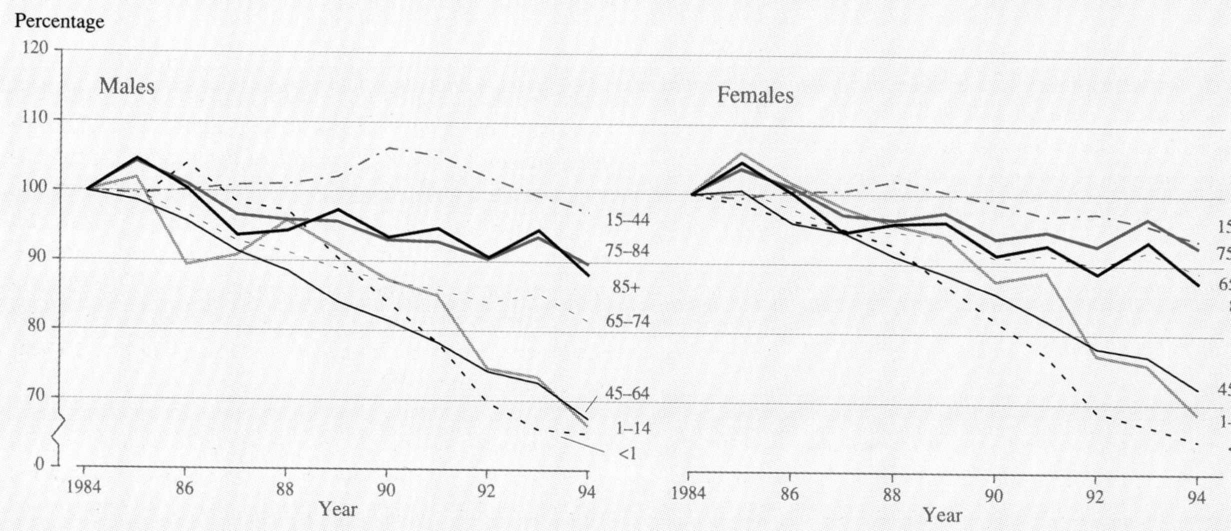

Table 25.1

Deaths rates per 1,000 population by age and sex, 1984–1994, England and Wales [1]

Age group	1984		1994		% change 84/94	
	Males	Females	Males	Females	Males	Females
All ages	11.6	11.1	10.5	10.8	-9.5	-2.8
Under 1 [2]	10.6	8.3	6.9	5.4	-34.7	-35.2
1–4	0.5	0.4	0.3	0.3	-35.9	-29.6
5–9	0.2	0.2	0.2	0.1	-33.9	-38.8
1–14	0.3	0.2	0.2	0.1	-30.8	-30.0
15–19	0.7	0.3	0.5	0.2	-30.2	-22.2
20–24	0.8	0.3	0.8	0.3	-8.3	-8.0
25–29	0.8	0.4	0.8	0.3	-3.0	-18.8
30–34	0.9	0.6	1.0	0.5	7.2	-11.7
35–39	1.3	0.9	1.3	0.8	0.1	-8.9
40–44	2.1	1.4	2.0	1.3	-7.7	-7.8
45–49	4.0	2.5	2.9	2.1	-26.7	-17.0
50–54	7.0	4.3	5.3	3.4	-25.5	-21.4
55–59	12.7	7.3	9.1	5.3	-28.4	-26.6
60–64	21.6	11.5	16.0	9.4	-26.0	-18.4
65–69	34.9	18.4	27.7	16.0	-20.6	-12.7
70–74	54.4	29.1	45.4	26.3	-16.5	-9.6
75–79	84.7	48.1	73.1	43.3	-13.6	-10.0
80–84	129.7	81.4	113.0	72.5	-12.9	-10.9
85+	213.6	167.3	188.5	146.6	-11.8	-12.4

Notes: 1. 1984 rates are based on death registrations;
       1994 rates on death occurrences
       2. Deaths per 1,000 live births

expectancy in males at age 15 in 1990–92 was another 59 years, whilst for females it was 65 years. These compared with 56 and 62 respectively in 1970–72, giving increases of 3 years.

Even at age 65, life expectancy has increased by 1 year for both men and women over the past 20 years. Thus, men aged 65 can expect an average increase in their life expectancy of a further 14 years, from 13 years in 1970–72, contrasting with women's increased expectancy of 18 years, from 17 years in 1970–72. These improvements result from the declining mortality rates in the elderly noted earlier.

25.3 But will we be healthy in old age?

One of the questions raised by continuously decreasing mortality, is whether this merely leads to an increase in the number of years spent with disabling chronic degenerative diseases. For example, if the incidence of stroke remains the same over time, but survival improves, there will be an increase in total life expectancy but no increase in life free of stroke. In recent years, considerable work has been carried out on methods of calculating 'healthy life expectancy' so that trends and comparisons can be drawn. This work has now been drawn together (Bone et al., 1995).

One method of calculation uses information from the ONS General Household Survey (GHS, annual) to determine the prevalence of limiting long-standing illness. The GHS provides statistics for a large sample of the population for each year since the early 1970s. Figure 25.2 shows the trends in life expectancy and healthy life expectancy for men and women at age 65. For men, in contrast to the steady increases in life expectancy, health expectancy remained almost constant between 1976 and 1992, at about 7 years. There may have been an increase from around 9 years to almost 10 years for women in 1991–92.

Thus, the extra years of life gained by the elderly may be extra years with a disability, not extra years of healthy life. This has major implications for the planning of health and social care by services and families of the elderly.

Figure 25.2

Life expectancy and healthy life expectancy at age 65, England and Wales, 1976–92

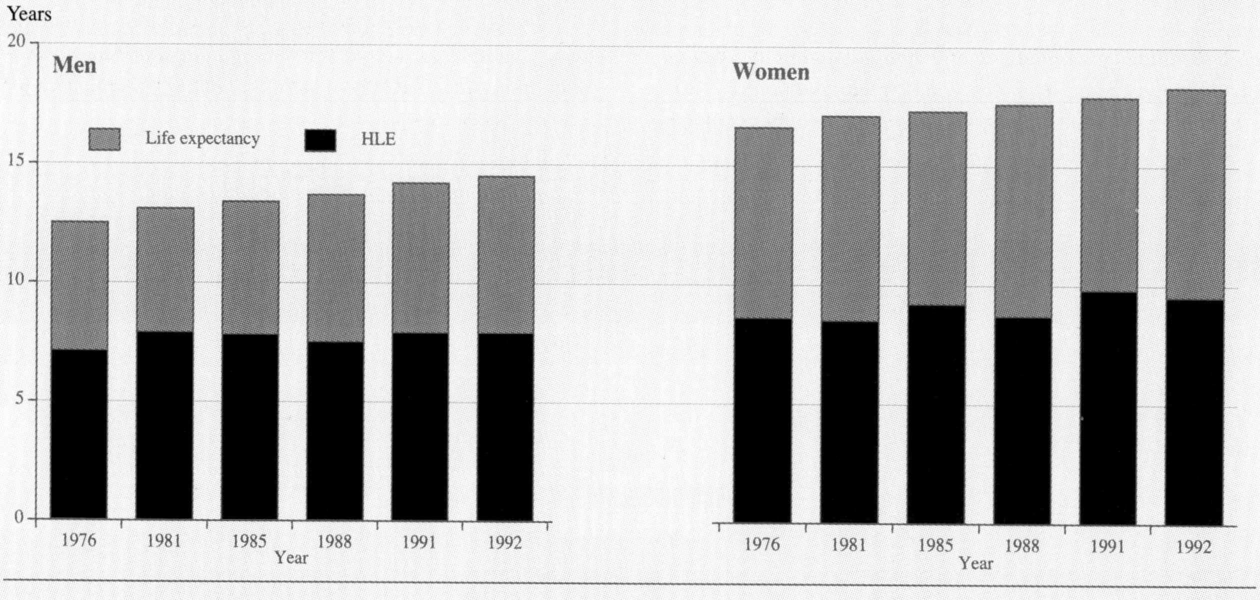

Years

Men — Life expectancy / HLE

Women

Source: Bone et al.

25.4 Morbidity

The previous section has illustrated the importance of measures of ill health and disability in conjunction with our knowledge about mortality trends. Most information about trends in health status comes from large national surveys, most importantly the GHS.

The GHS collects each year information about three types of morbidity:

  (a) the existence of long-standing illness;
  (b) whether this limits peoples' activities at all – limiting long-standing illness;
  (c) acute illness – the restriction of activity in the previous 2 weeks.

Figure 25.3 shows moving 3-year averages for adults from 1979 to 1992. As can be seen, and in contrast to mortality, there has been no overall improvement in health as measured by the GHS questions. Figure 25.3 includes adults under 75 years old; there is no difference between men and women in the proportion reporting a long-standing illness. Also the difference for limiting long-standing illness is small. These findings hold for each age-group and have been remarkably stable over the time period of the survey. Acute illness – measured by 'restricted activity in the last 2 weeks' – is, however, significantly more common among women. This is also true for all age-groups.

Figure 25.4 shows how these three measures of morbidity varied between age-groups in the period 1991–94.

Figure 25.3

Percentage of people with limiting long-standing illness, long-standing illness, and cutting down on usual activities in last 2 weeks (3–year moving average)

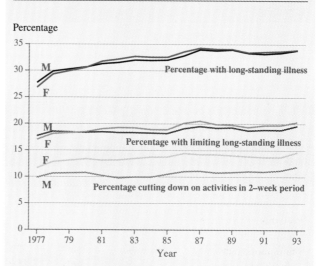

Percentage

Percentage with long-standing illness

Percentage with limiting long-standing illness

Percentage cutting down on activities in 2–week period

Percentage of British population age 15–74, age standardised to standard European population.

Source: General Household Survey, 1975–1994

25.5 Long-standing illness

Figure 25.4 shows the proportions of men and women of different ages who reported a long-standing illness. As can be seen, the prevalence rises in each subsequent age-group from less than a tenth of those aged 16–24 to about six tenths of those aged 85 or more. However, there are no differences between men and women of similar ages except among those aged 75 years and over. This again is in contrast to mortality rate patterns.

In 1988 for the first time for many years, answers to the question 'What is the matter with you?' were coded. Table 25.2 first gives the proportion of men and women in different age-groups who reported a long-standing illness. It then gives the proportions with a long-standing illness affecting four systems of the body: musculoskeletal, circulatory, respiratory and digestive. These were the most commonly reported. Finally it shows the average number of conditions mentioned by those with a long-standing illness. Among women the average number of conditions was 1.2 for those aged 16–44 years, rising to 1.7 for those aged 75 years or more. The pattern for men was similar.

Figure 25.4

Percentage with long-standing illness, 1990–94, by age and sex

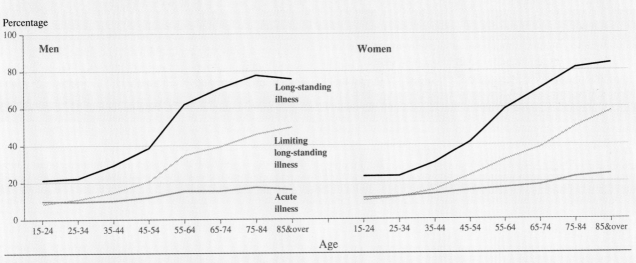

Source: General Household Survey, 1990–1994.

Table 25.2

Long-standing illness among men and women of different ages, Great Britain 1988

	Men				Women			
	Age-group				Age-group			
	16–44	45–64	65–74	75+	16–44	45–64	65–74	75+
Proportion with any long-standing illness, disability or infirmity	25%	44%	59%	61%	24%	43%	60%	71%
Proportion with different types of conditions:								
musculoskeletal	9%	18%	22%	22%	7%	20%	31%	40%
circulatory	2%	14%	25%	22%	2%	11%	23%	26%
respiratory	7%	7%	10%	13%	5%	6%	9%	8%
digestive	2%	5%	8%	9%	2%	5%	7%	10%
Average number of conditions mentioned by those with a long-standing illness	1.2	1.4	1.5	1.6	1.2	1.4	1.6	1.7
Number of people = 100%	4,963	2,700	1,037	582	5,218	2,787	1,283	1,084

Source: Office for National Statistics.

In the GHS, as in the ONS disability survey (Martin *et al.*, 1988), conditions of the musculoskeletal system were the most commonly reported. In the disability survey, where all disabilities were asked about specifically, ear complaints and eye complaints were the next most common, but they were not reported frequently in response to the more general GHS question. The second most common type of chronic illness reported in the GHS was conditions of the circulatory system. These were reported by 2 per cent of adults aged 16–44 years and about one quarter of those aged 65 years or more. Conditions of the respiratory system came next. For men, the proportion with these conditions rose from 7 per cent of those aged 16–44 years to 13 per cent of those aged 75 years or more; the corresponding figures for women being 5 per cent and 8 per cent.

Looking at the proportions of men and women reporting the different types of long-standing conditions, the striking finding is the similarity between them. Two differences stand out. First, 40 per cent of women aged 75 years or more reported a long-standing disease of the musculoskeletal system. This applied to only 22 per cent of men aged 75 years or more. Part of this difference is likely to be related to the relative proportion of very elderly among women aged 75 years or more. Second, these elderly men reported a higher prevalence of respiratory disorder than women aged 75 years or more, 13 per cent compared with 8 per cent. This is likely to reflect differences in lifetime smoking behaviour between men and women.

In 1991 the Department of Health began a new annual health survey in England, which has been repeated every year. Four reports have been published to date. That for 1993 (Bennett *et al.*, 1995) provides preliminary evidence about trends in, for example, blood pressure and obesity. Previous studies have provided comparable measures of overweight adults in the population enabling a longer-term comparison to be made. One of the Health of the Nation targets is to reduce the proportion of adults in the population who are obese.

The recent report (Department of Health, 1995) has drawn together the results of all the surveys. As discussed in Chapter 7 (see Figure 7.15), rather than becoming slimmer, the adult population is becoming more overweight. For example, in 1980, 68 per cent of women were underweight or of acceptable weight. By 1993 this had fallen to 54 per cent. A similar picture exists for men.

The survey measures four major risk factors for cardiovascular disease – current regular smoking, high blood pressure, physical inactivity and raised total cholesterol. One in five men and women had three or four of these risk factors, while only one in 10 had none (Colhoun and Prescott-Clark, 1996). Over the four years that the survey has been carried out, 1991–94, there is no evidence of any reduction in the proportion of the population with one or more risk factors for heart disease. Further annual surveys will provide valuable longer-term trend data about certain specific indicators of morbidity and health status.

25.6 Mental illness

Mental illness is a major cause of morbidity and disability. However, neither the GHS nor the health survey are designed to cover this difficult-to-measure aspect of health. However, in 1993/94 the Department of Health, the Scottish Home and Health Department and the Welsh Office sponsored ONS to carry out a benchmark survey of psychiatric morbidity in adults. The first report (Meltzer *et al.*, 1995) identified considerable morbidity among the population in private households. For example, 18 per cent of women and 12 per cent of men aged 16–64 reported significant neurotic symptoms such as fatigue, sleep problems and irritability. Eight per cent of men and 2 per cent of women were dependent on alcohol.

Figure 25.5 summarises the findings of this prevalence study. It is based partly on an unpublished analysis (Meltzer, personal communication) of the proportion of different age- and sex-groups who were found to have any of the psychiatric disorders measured in the survey. Those included were neurotic and psychotic disorders, and drug and alcohol dependence. Disorders of all levels of severity are included. But some conditions, such as anorexia and bulimia nervosa, presenile dementia, organic psychoses and personality disorders, were excluded. The shaded parts of the histogram represent the prevalence of neurotic disorders.

Among all ages up to 54 the proportion of women reporting neurotic disorders is greater than the proportion of men, around 20 per cent compared with around 13 per cent. For those aged 55–64 the proportions are very similar, around 13 per cent for both men and women. However, this major difference between the sexes is greatly reduced when all psychiatric disorders are considered. This is because

Figure 25.5

Prevalence of any psychiatric disorders, and, within that, any neurotic disorder, by age and sex, Great Britain

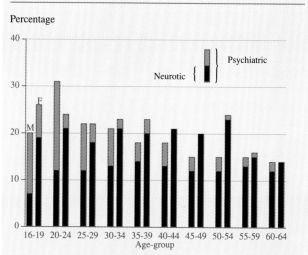

'Psychiatric disorder' includes neurotic disorder in past week, functional psychoses, alcohol dependence in past 12 months.
'Neurotic disorders' include anxiety and depressive disorders, depressive episodes, phobias, obsessive-compulsive disorders and panic disorders

Source: Meltzer et al., 1996 and personal communication

dependence on alcohol and/or drugs is much more common among men than women at all ages. For example, among 20–24-year-olds, men have a higher prevalence of any disorder than do women – but less than half of it is accounted for by neurotic disorders. These account for most of the psychiatric morbidity in all age-groups of women.

25.7 Dental health

Dental health is another aspect of adult health that has been monitored regularly by surveys, including a standardised dental examination as well as questions relating to dental health. The most recent in the series was carried out in 1988 (Todd and Lader, 1991) (see Figure 25.6). The figure takes one indicator of dental health, the proportion with no natural teeth,

and compares it with the situation 10 and 20 years previously.

The proportion of edentulous adults in England and Wales fell from 37 per cent in 1968 to 29 per cent in 1978 and 20 per cent in 1988. This improvement occurred in all age- and sex-groups. In general, women are more likely to lose all their teeth than men. In 1988, 25 per cent of women were edentulous compared with 16 per cent of men.

25.8 Health-related behaviour

People's eating, drinking, smoking and exercise behaviours are known to be related to a wide variety of illnesses and health states. Therefore, it is essential to monitor key aspects of health-related behaviour. Many behaviours affecting health may be influenced by various policy initiatives; for example, smoking may be influenced by health promotion/education, taxation or policy regarding advertising.

The GHS has been the traditional vehicle for some of this monitoring. Smoking has been included since 1972 and consumption of alcohol since 1978. Overall, smoking among both men and women has been decreasing steadily for the last 20 years (see Figure 25.7). But the overall improvement obscures differences in trends between age- and sex-groups. There has been little change among men and women aged 16–24 during the last 10 years.

Smoking rates are now very similar for both men and women in all age-groups. However, men are somewhat more likely than women to smoke 20 or more cigarettes a day – 12 per cent compared with 8 per cent in 1994 (GHS, 1996).

Alcohol consumption is also measured every other year in the GHS. Figure 25.8 summarises the changes in the proportions of men and women drinking more than the recommended sensible levels (these were the levels that applied in 1994). Since 1984, alcohol consumption levels (units per week) have

Figure 25.6

The proportion of edentulous adults in England and Wales, 1968–88 by age

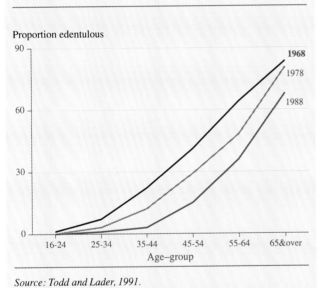

Source: Todd and Lader, 1991.

Figure 25.7

Prevalence of cigarette smoking by sex and age, Great Britain, 1974–94

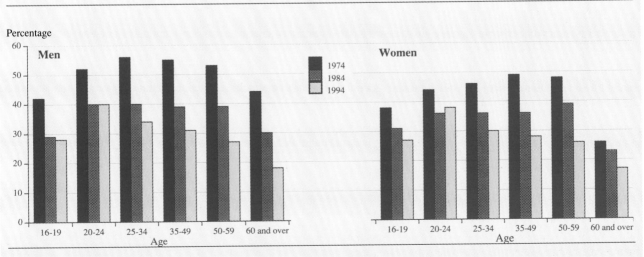

Source: General Household Survey

179

Figure 25.8

Alcohol consumption: percentage of men and women drinking more than the recommended sensible levels, Great Britain, 1984–94

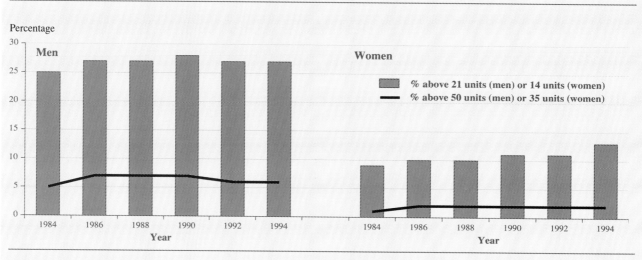

Source: *General Household Survey*

remained fairly constant for men, while for women there has been a gradual shift towards increased levels of consumption. Nevertheless, the latest figures, for 1994, show that women were still twice as likely as men to be non-drinkers (14 per cent compared with 7 per cent) and half as likely to drink more than moderate amounts (13 per cent and 27 per cent respectively). In 1994, just over one in four men drank more than the recommended current sensible level of 21 units per week and one in 20 men drank more than 50 units per week. This masks differences between age-groups; for example, 35 per cent of men aged 18–24 drank more than 21 units per week in 1994 compared with 17 per cent of men aged 65 and over. The comparable figures for women were 20 per cent and 7 per cent.

The 1993 GHS (GHS, 1995) reviews trends in participation in sports games and physical activities (in the last 2 weeks). Among women, walking, keep-fit/yoga and swimming are the three most common activities for all age-groups. For men aged 16–19 the top three are cue sports (snooker/pool/billiards), walking and soccer; among ages 45–59 walking, cue sports and swimming are preferred. Vigorous activities and sports were generally played by small proportions of people. For example, in 1993, 7 per cent of men had done running, 9 per cent soccer and 3 per cent squash. The figures for women were 2 per cent running and 1 per cent squash. In contrast, 45 per cent of men and 37 per cent of women had done any walking. (Walks were recorded if they were 2 or more miles and walking for the sake of walking.) Figure 25.9 shows trends over time for different age-groups; Table 25.3 gives more details for men and women.

Following a significant increase between 1987 and 1990, overall rates of participation in sport in 1993 were similar to those reported in 1990. The proportion of adults who said that they had participated in at least one activity in the 4-week reference period rose from 61 per cent in 1987 to 64 per cent in 1990 and remained at a similar level in 1993.

Figure 25.9

Trends in 4–week participation rates by age, Great Britain, 1987, 1990 and 1993

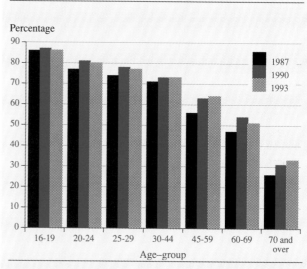

Source: *General Household Survey,*

25.9 Summary

This chapter has not sought to put forward a particular health definition nor attempted to provide a single measure of health. Rather, it has taken examples from the wide range of indicators available at national level to try to answer the question 'Are we healthier?' At a simple level, the answer could be that almost universal improvements in mortality rates and increasing life expectancy suggest that we are indeed healthier. However, surveys of reported and measured health status suggest there is no comparable general improvement in health. In addition, several behaviours related to poor health show little sign of change. The answer to the question can only be that some things are better, some worse and some have stayed the same.

Table 25.3

Trends in participation in sports, games and physical activities in the 4 weeks before interview by sex: Great Britain ,1987, 1990 and 1993

persons aged 16 and over

Active sports, games and physical activities*	Men			Women		
	1987	1990	1993	1987	1990	1993
	Percentage parcipating in the 4 weeks before interview					
Walking	41	44	45	35	38	37
Any swimming	..	14	15	..	15	16
Swimming: indoor	*10*	*11*	*12*	*11*	*13*	*14*
Swimming: outdoor	*4*	*4*	*4*	*3*	*4*	*3*
Snooker/pool/billiards	27	24	21	5	5	5
Keep fit/yoga	5	6	6	12	16	17
Cycling	10	12	14	7	7	7
Darts	14	11	9	4	4	3
Weight lifting/training	7	8	9	2	2	3
Golf	7	9	9	1	2	2
Running (jogging etc.)	8	8	7	3	2	2
Any soccer	10	10	9	0	0	0
Tenpin bowls/skittles	2	5	5	1	3	3
Badminton	4	4	3	3	3	2
Tennis	2	2	3	1	2	2
Fishing	4	4	4	0	0	0
Lawn/carpet bowls	2	3	3	1	1	2
Squash	4	4	*3*	1	1	*1*
Table tennis	4	3	2	1	1	1
Horse riding	0	1	0	1	1	1
Cricket	2	2	2	0	0	0
At least one activity (exc. walking)†	57	58	57	34	39	39
At least one activity†	70	73	72	52	57	57
Base = 100%	*9,086*	*8,119*	*8,062*	*10,443*	*9,455*	*9,490*

* Includes only activities in which more than 1.0% of all adults participated in 4 weeks before interview in 1993.
† Total includes those activities not separately listed

Source: General Household Survey

Chapter 26

The health and health care of older adults in England and Wales, 1841–1994

By
Emily Grundy

Summary

- In 1841 the over-55s accounted for 10 per cent and the over-75s for 1 per cent of the population. In 1991 these proportions were 26 per cent and 7 per cent.

- Much of this change has been due to long-term falls in fertility, but falls in death rates are now an increasingly important cause of further population ageing.

- Over the period as a whole, survival to and beyond 55 and 75 has increased dramatically. Over half the girls born in 1911 survived to age 75, compared with fewer than a fifth of those born in 1841.

- Mortality rates began to fall in the early twentieth century. For men improvement was slower and more intermittent – until recently – than for women.

- Recent improvements in mortality have been substantial. Between 1971 and 1991, two and a half years was added to men's further life expectancy at age 55 – the same as the gain between 1851 and 1961.

- Health care for the elderly has changed dramatically over the period, with hospitals replacing workhouses, pensions replacing Poor Law relief and with the establishment of the NHS and development of geriatric medicine.

- The rate of institutionalisation among elderly people, whether due to poverty or ill health, rose from 1841 up to the first quarter of the twentieth century, since when it has generally fallen – except in the past decade.

- Although their mortality is lower, women report more ill health than men and rates increase with age.

- Reported rates of long-term illness since the early 1970s show no improvement, but this may be due to changes in health expectations. There is some suggestion that rates of serious disability may have fallen.

- There is a need for more data on the health of the elderly, with consideration taken of individuals' history and environment.

26.1 Introduction

Many of the health problems of older adults may have more to do with a poor environment and cumulative exposure to various hazards than with the effects of ageing (senescence) alone. In this chapter our primary concern is with documenting and interpreting trends and differentials in the health of adults aged 55 and over, rather than distinguishing these separate contributions, but they cannot be ignored altogether. Changes in the absolute and relative size of the older population, and in its demographic composition, are also discussed, particularly given current concerns about the implications of population ageing for family support of older people and health care expenditures.

26.2 Ageing and senescence

26.2.1 Background

The conventional meaning of senescence relates to changes which are particularly associated with the post-reproductive period of life, and which threaten the viability of the organism. Senescence is associated with reduced physiological adaptability and the eventual outcome of this process is death. Its start remains debatable, but many authorities suggest adolescence or early adulthood, largely because the risk of death increases exponentially with age throughout adult life (Evans, 1985; Kirkwood, 1988; Olshansky and Carnes, 1996). However, this pattern is less evident in cohort than in period mortality data, and weakens in extreme old age (Grundy, 1992a; Barrett, 1985, 1986; Thatcher, 1981). The pace of deterioration of different body systems varies considerably, and ageing is a process involving social and behavioural, as well as biological change, hence defining its onset is problematic (Shock, 1983). Selective survival further complicates the study of age-related change.

Indeed it may not be possible, or appropriate, to distinguish 'normal', 'healthy' and 'pathological' ageing. Progressive degenerative processes, such as loss of muscle strength with ageing, may be slowed or reversed through physical training (Aniannsson and Gustafsson, 1981). Longitudinal studies have shown that there are groups of elderly people whose function improves over time (Strawbridge, *et al.*, 1992). Our ability to distinguish between 'intrinsic' and 'extrinsic' factors, and their interaction in disease processes, is also limited by the extent of current scientific knowledge.

However, although chronological age itself is not a very reliable predictor of performance or health in individual adults, age may be a quite sensitive indicator at the population level (Siegel, 1992).

26.2.2 Defining later life

In this chapter we consider the health of adults aged 55 and over. Where possible, and appropriate, those aged 55–74 are distinguished from those aged 75 and over. This differs from the usual choice of 60 or 65 to distinguish elderly and other adults, coinciding with retirement age, currently 60 for women and 65 for men in England and Wales. Townsend and others have argued that old age, or at least dependency in old age, is primarily a social construction peculiar to advanced industrial societies, which is largely imposed through compulsory retirement at fixed ages (Townsend, 1981; Walker, 1980; Phillipson, 1982). This has been challenged by Johnson (1989), but most agree that social mores influence perceptions of the age at which others, if not oneself, become elderly. However, the 60–65 boundary has blurred with the spread of early retirement and unemployment. Over 70 per cent of 64-year-old men were working or seeking work in 1977 (Parker, 1980). In 1988 there was a much greater spread of retirement ages and only a third of men aged 64 were economically active (Bone *et al.*, 1992). The usefulness of retirement age as a boundary is also limited here, because our investigation spans a century and a half, and there have been major changes in working patterns and pension schemes.

The age of 60 or 65 is no watershed from a health or health services perspective, at least in contemporary England and Wales. Reported long-standing illness shows gradual increases throughout adulthood, with a more rapid escalation after the ages of 70 or 80. Other indicators, such as hospital admission rates, start to increase from about the age of 50 (Evans *et al.*, 1992). Most departments of geriatric medicine which operate an age-related referrals policy define their target population as those over 75 or even 80 (Horrocks, 1982).

Clearly on any criteria (for example, income and marital status) there is a huge difference between contemporary people at ages 55 and 75. The concept of a 'Third Age' has recently gained prominence, intermediate between a 'Second Age' dominated by the concerns of paid work and child-rearing, and a 'Fourth Age' of increasing dependence and frailty (Laslett, 1989). While the 'Third Age' is functionally, rather than chronologically, defined, the age-group 50–74 or 55–74 is often used as an age-bounded equivalent, as in the recent Carnegie Inquiry into the Third Age (Carnegie Inquiry, 1993). The concept of a Third Age has been challenged, however, because it is unclear how distinctive within adult life it is, and because many of the negative stereotypes about ageing and old age are merely transferred to an older age-group (Bury, 1992).

Such a stage of life is a contemporary phenomenon and historically would have been enjoyed by at most a small privileged elite. F B Smith has argued that in the nineteenth century 'middle age settled into old age around 45' (Smith, 1979, p. 316). Bourdelais has also argued that age cannot be regarded as an ahistorical variable and that 'as the nature of old age has changed, so the calculation of the proportion of "elderly" persons must depend on a changing threshold of entry to old age' (Bourdelais, 1993, p. 178). Similarly, some commentators on ageing in contemporary less developed societies have suggested adopting a lower threshold for 'old age' (Tout, 1989).

Figure 26.1

Age at which 15 years of life remain, by period and sex

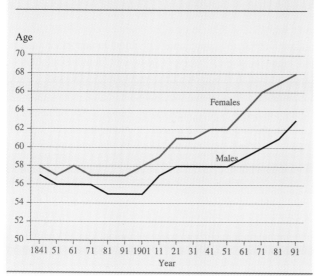

Other commentators, however, caution against assuming that people in the past were 'old' when still young, and studies of health in later life in contemporary less developed countries show a picture of age-related change fairly similar to that in England and Wales and other developed countries (Smith, 1991; Heikkenen *et al.*, 1996). Undoubtedly, however, attitudes to ageing, as well as the experience of later life, have changed considerably, even recently. As one 70-year-old respondent in a 1965 survey commented:

> *I remember my mother as a little old lady in black with a white cap – yet at the time she could only have been forty. Nowadays they are still young at sixty.*
> (Harris, 1987, p. 479).

Siegel has suggested a measure of 'old age' based on average years of life remaining (Siegel, 1992). If the age at which, on average, 15 years of life remain is chosen, then 'old age' for men in the mid-nineteenth century began at 55 or 56, compared with 58 for most of the first half of the twentieth century and 60 in 1971 (see Figure 26.1). Among women in the nineteenth century this 'threshold' was about 2 years higher at 57 or 58; in 1921 it had reached 61 and by 1971 it was 66.

26.2.3 Population ageing and demographic transition

Chapter 3 shows that in 1841 those over 55 accounted for 10 per cent, and those over 75 only 1 per cent of the population of England and Wales, compared with 26 per cent and 7 per cent respectively in 1991. Increases in the absolute number of older people are more striking still. Chapter 27 discusses the even greater growth in the numbers of centenarians. This change in the distribution by age is more important than changes in absolute numbers, since it has a close association with the overall pattern of health and health care need and the capacity of a population to meet the needs of its oldest members (Preston, 1976). Nevertheless, changes in absolute numbers also merit attention, and indeed, in terms of short-

term planning, may have the greatest impact (Gonnot, 1992).

Essentially, the number of people aged 75 and over depends on the number of births 75 and more years earlier, and their subsequent survival. Past fluctuations in the numbers of births in England and Wales have been considerable, as shown in Chapter 6, and are reflected in the numbers in older age-groups many decades later. Early in the next century there will be renewed growth in the numbers over 65 as survivors of the 'baby boom' cohorts attain this age, a phenomenon currently of concern in most Western countries. Changes in the other main determinant of the numbers of older people, survival to and beyond later life, have been very substantial, as discussed in Chapter 3. Declines in the mortality of older age-groups, particularly for men, although evident since the turn of the last century, were, until relatively recently, less substantial and more prone to fluctuation. As Table 26.1 shows, there have been major increases in the proportions of birth cohorts surviving to and beyond the age of 55. While only 19 per cent of girls born in 1841 survived to age 75, projections suggest survival to this age for two thirds of the girls born a century later. Fewer than 10 per cent of the boys born in the 1970s are expected to die before the age of 55, compared with half of those born in the 1870s.

It has been demonstrated, both empirically and theoretically, that it is long-term decline in fertility which is the cause for what may be termed 'primary' population ageing – the initial shift to an older age-structure, because of larger generations being succeeded by smaller ones (Notestein, 1954; Carrier, 1962). In England and Wales the total period fertility rate (TPFR) fell from 4.8 in 1871 to 3.5 in 1901–05 (OPCS, 1987). There have been substantial fluctuations since then, but no return to nineteenth-century or pre-industrial levels. In the 1930s the TPFR fell to 1.8, at the height of the postwar baby boom in 1964 it reached 2.9, but since 1973 it has remained below replacement level and relatively stable at 1.7 to 1.9.

Declines in mortality among those with reproductive potential influence not just the size of the age-group affected at the time, but also the size of succeeding generations. Werner, for example, estimated that, had the 1841 female birth cohort suffered only negligible mortality before the age of 45, children born to the cohort would have averaged nearly 5 per woman, as compared with the 3 per woman actually achieved (Werner, 1987). While historically, falls in fertility led to population ageing, changes in mortality at older ages may influence the structure and the size of the older population (Benjamin and Overton, 1981). In populations with low mortality, and with fertility at or below replacement level (TPFR = 2.1), mortality changes may cause further population ageing from the apex rather than the base of the population pyramid, as in England and Wales today (Bourgeois-Pichat, 1979). Mortality rates at young ages are now so low that any further improvement will have negligible demographic impact, and the bulk of deaths occur in older age-groups (see Chapter 3). Benjamin has estimated that some 38 per cent of the increase in the proportion of elderly people in the United Kingdom between 1951 and 1981 was due to mortality change, compared with 21 per cent during the period 1911–51 (Benjamin, 1987).

Table 26.1

Survivorship out of 100,000 births to, and further expectation of life from, age 55 and age 75, by year of birth, England and Wales, 1841–1981

| Year of birth | Survivorship | | | | Expectation of life | | | |
| | to age 55 | | to age 75 | | at age 55 | | at age 75 | |
	Males	Females	Males	Females	Males	Females	Males	Females
1841	40,295	44,898	13,992	18,975	16.08	17.80	6.30	7.22
1861	44,899	49,770	18,420	25,456	17.35	19.80	6.28	7.72
1881	53,982	59,923	24,207	35,944	18.45	22.10	7.08	8.98
1901	60,593	66,415	27,517	45,107	18.92	24.60	7.67	10.43
1911	67,730	72,838	34,216	51,475	20.18	25.70	8.56	11.30
1921	73,282	79,215	41,023	57,484	21.54	26.40	9.37	11.93
1931	79,447	84,390	48,620	63,347	22.89	27.20	9.79	12.21
1941	84,263	88,757	53,716	67,855	23.56	27.60	9.98	12.34
1951	88,584	92,609	57,390	71,288	23.80	27.80	10.06	12.39
1961	89,592	93,465	58,703	72,334	23.96	27.80	10.06	12.39
1971	91,171	94,309	60,020	73,216	24.05	27.90	10.06	12.39
1981	92,518	95,230	60,916	73,938	24.05	27.90	10.06	12.39

Note: figures below the dotted lines are projections.
Source: ONS

26.2.4 Mortality, morbidity and the health transition

The enormous redistribution of deaths from younger to older age-groups, discussed in Chapters 3 and 4, is important demographically as a prerequisite of the 'population ageing from the apex' phenomenon. It has also been associated with a transformation in major causes of death and pre-death morbidity. It is also important from a sociological perspective, as death has become increasingly associated with later life, and the young and middle-aged can confidently expect to survive to and beyond their sixth decade. Not only has the distribution of deaths by age changed, so too has the ratio of male to female deaths. Although in the nineteenth century women had higher mortality than men in some age-groups, today women are advantaged at all ages, particularly among young adults and those aged 50–74.

Mortality has conventionally been used as an indicator of population health, but now that chronic degenerative diseases predominate this is becoming less appropriate (Ruzicka and Kane, 1990). New approaches partition life expectancy into 'healthy' or 'disability free', and 'unhealthy' or 'disabled', components (Robine et al., 1992; Bone et al., 1996; Boshuizen and van de Water, 1994). These require data on health status which are often lacking in contemporary, let alone historical, populations. The new developments arise largely from uncertainties about the possible changing relationship between health (at the population level) and death, particularly in the older population.

At the individual level, the best predictors of mortality in elderly people are markers of disease or disability (Campbell et al., 1985; Ruigomez et al., 1993). However, selective survival may result in the deterioration in the health of the older population, as larger proportions with unfavourable health characteristics survive to older ages (Vaupel et al., 1979; Verbrugge, 1984). Some have argued that the declines in mortality at older ages in the 1970s may have been achieved through the prolongation of pre-death morbidity in those with health impairments, rather than through the extension of 'healthy' life (Gruenberg, 1977; Kramer, 1984; Verbrugge, 1984). The survival of old people with dementia, for example, seems to have increased (Blessed and Wilson, 1982; Christie, 1983; Gruenberg and Hagnell, 1987). However, this may reflect elderly people with dementia sharing the improvements in life expectancy experienced by the general population, rather than any 'excess' increase in survival (Wood et al., 1991). Increases in the incidence of fractured neck of femur have also been associated with decreases in mortality, possibly suggesting that an increased survival of frailer groups may be partly responsible (Finsen, 1988). Population surveys in Britain, France, Canada and the United States do show increases in the reported prevalence of chronic conditions (Colvez and Blanchet 1981; Robine et al., 1992). As a result, calculations of disability-free life expectancy generally show an unfavourable balance between years of 'disabled' life gained and years of 'active' life, at least if *all* degrees of disability are considered. However, this apparently unfavourable trend may reflect changes in health expectations, rather than in health status itself.

Riley has suggested a more general negative relationship between population morbidity and mortality, due to increased survival of frailer members and greater accumulation of health insults in longer-surviving groups (Riley, 1990). A more optimistic argument is that the lifespan is biologically fixed, and that future improvements in health will result in a 'compression of morbidity' as the onset of morbidity, but not death, is delayed (Fries, 1980). However, even if there is a fixed limit to the lifespan, which many dispute, it has been argued that recent mortality data show a wider dispersion by age, rather than signs of increasing concentration as hypothesized by Fries (Gavrilov and Gavrilova, 1991; Rothenberg *et al.*, 1991). Wilmoth *et al.*'s (1995) analysis of mortality data from Sweden, Japan and the United States indicates that mortality *has* been compressed and survival curves become more rectangular, but that this process has recently slowed down or been reversed. Moreover, a compression of mortality does not necessarily imply a compression of morbidity, or a change in the association between morbidity and mortality.

Manton pointed out that, although the arguments of Fries on the one hand and Gruenberg on the other seemed irreconcilable, both interpretations shared an assumption that the relationship between morbidity and mortality was changing (Manton, 1982). He concluded that the prevalence of chronic diseases was increasing, not as a result of the postponement of lethal sequelae, but rather because the rate of progression of certain degenerative diseases had slowed down, partly as a result of medical interventions. This had resulted in a 'dynamic equilibrium' between mortality and morbidity. In fact, later work suggests a recent improvement in the ratio of active to total life expectancy in very old age-groups (Manton and Stallard, 1994).

Strong relationships have been suggested between health in early and later life, particularly nutritional influences, and the possible adverse consequences of early nutritional deprivation followed by relative affluence (Barker, 1992; Forsdahl, 1977, 1978). A link between health in early and later life seems highly plausible, although some ecological analyses of this issue have been criticised (Elo and Preston, 1992). Since living conditions and nutrition have improved, some predict that more recent cohorts with a better health legacy will enjoy better health in old age.

26.2.5 Data sources

Many sources of data on the older population are restricted to those over 65 or over retirement age. There is a lack of quality data on morbidity, particularly in the earlier part of the period covered. Age-, sex- and cause-specific mortality data are available for the whole of the past 150 years and constitute a major source.

General issues about data quality are considered in Chapter 2, but misreporting of age is a particular problem when the health of the older population is under investigation. Even in recent censuses, age inflation in the oldest age-groups has been found to be extensive and the problem was worse in nineteenth-century and early twentieth-century censuses (Thatcher, 1981). Lee and Lam investigated the age-distribu-

tions recorded in English censuses from 1821 to 1931 (Lee and Lam, 1983). Women aged 55–59 were under-enumerated by over 10 per cent in the 1851–71 censuses, with over-enumeration of women aged 70 and over, increasing with age from 3–4 per cent at ages 70–74 to some 45 per cent for those aged 80 or more. These problems were worst early on, causing miscalculation of population sizes. Their results suggest over-enumeration of those aged 80 and over by 12 per cent in 1911–21 and by between 7 and 9 per cent in 1921–31. The effect of these errors will be to under-estimate mortality rates in over-enumerated groups (those over 70 and particularly those over 80) and vice versa. The mortality data for those aged 85 and over, for the period 1841–1960, have been adjusted in the Government Actuary's Department life tables used in Chapter 3. No adjustment has been made to the data for people aged 70–84, and these unadjusted data are used here.

Cause of death data present further problems because of changes in the quality of diagnosis and coding practices. Again these are particularly serious in older age-groups, because of difficulties in identifying the major underlying cause of death in those with multiple pathologies, the often atypical presentation of such pathologies in old people, and a tendency not to bother very much with establishing the cause of their death. ONS, for example, concluded that the reported increase in mortality from respiratory diseases among elderly people in 1951–75 was largely due to the increased proportion of deaths occurring in hospital (OPCS, 1981). Cause of death was recorded by (often junior) hospital doctors who were more likely than general practitioners to ascribe deaths among elderly people to bronchopneumonia. A change in coding practices also resulted in a substantial drop in deaths assigned to respiratory diseases in 1983 (OPCS, 1985, 1986) – see Chapter 2.

Morbidity data available are even more restricted. For the nineteenth century the only national sources available are data on sickness spells collected by Friendly Societies, census data on specific infirmities, and evidence from the surveys conducted by Charles Booth and other social reformers (Booth, 1894). Some of these are collated in the reports of various Royal Commissions. Data for the early and mid-twentieth century are also limited; they include results from the survey of sickness conducted 1944–51 and results from the first enquiry into morbidity statistics from general practice 1955–56 (GRO, 1958).

A wider range exists for the past three decades, including Hunt's study of the elderly at home and Townsend's and Wedderburn's national survey of elderly people (Hunt, 1978; Townsend and Wedderburn, 1965). Since 1971 additional sources of data are available. These are the General Household Survey (GHS) (OPCS, 1973 to 1993), the recent ONS surveys of disability (Martin *et al.*, 1988), and the Second, Third and Fourth GP morbidity studies (RCGP *et al.*, 1974, 1979, 1982, 1986, 1990; McCormick *et al.*, 1995; Logan and Cushion, 1958).

In the following sections we look separately at the period from 1841 to the 1920s, and at the more recent past.

26.3 The health of older adults in the late nineteenth and early twentieth centuries

26.3.1 Mortality

Table 26.2 shows further expectation of life at age 55 for men and women for decennial years between 1841–43 and 1921–23, based on period mortality. There was no improvement in expectation of life until the end of the period, and even some deterioration for men.

Chapter 3 shows trends in mortality for ages 55–64, 65–74 and 75–84. Declines evident at the end of the nineteenth century accelerated in the early twentieth century, particularly for women. Mortality at ages 75–84 rose in 1915, and was higher during 1915–17 than during the post-First World War influenza pandemic. Possible reasons for this increase, which also affected infants, are wartime privations, a reduction of support from younger relatives and the disruption of medical services, with a third of all hospital and infirmary beds taken over for the armed forces (Abel-Smith, 1964). However, mortality rates fell for other age-groups (Winter, 1985).

These data suggest no improvement, and indeed some deterioration in the health of older adults, until late in the nineteenth century, followed by a period of quite rapid progress in the early twentieth. Data limitations severely restrict investigations of specific causes, largely because of the high proportion of deaths at older ages which are assigned to ill-defined causes, and uncertainty about the effects of changes in classification, coding and diagnostic accuracy (see Chapter 4, Figures 4.3 e and f). Gage partitioned male mortality 1861–1964 into biologically interpretable components (Gage, 1993). He concluded that later nineteenth century increases in senescent (age-related) mortality were partly due to the emergence of Asian influenza viruses, to senescent forms of tuberculosis, and to one or more of the degenerative causes of death. The decline in senescent mortality during the 1901–21 period, he suggested, was associated with changes in the age-distribution of deaths from influenza, pneumonia and bronchitis.

26.3.2 Morbidity: evidence from data on sickness spells

Of the limited data available for the end of the nineteenth and early twentieth centuries, returns of sickness benefits paid by Friendly Societies constitute one of the best known sources. A number of investigations into the sickness and mortality rates of Friendly Society members were carried out by contemporaries (see, for example, Ratcliffe, 1850, and Humphreys, 1885). Information derived from returns from the largest society, the Manchester-based Independent Order of Odd Fellows (IOOF), was used to calculate contribution rates when the first compulsory national insurance scheme (for workers earning less than £160 per annum) was established in 1911. More recently, Alter and Riley have used IOOF data, relating to periods between 1846–50 and 1893–97, to examine the relationship between male mortality and morbidity in all adult age-groups (Alter and Riley, 1989). They concluded that between the 1860s and 1890s morbidity rates increased while mortality fell, and used a model which incorporated both selective survival and insult accumulation to account for this.

Friendly Society and other insurance-based data have a number of strengths but also some weaknesses. Until 1911 membership of Friendly Societies was voluntary, and applicants were self-selected. Members were predominantly better-off manual workers in their twenties and thirties (Smith, 1979). Further selection occurred at admission, when the chronically ill were excluded, and some societies also excluded those in hazardous occupations. Long-term members (likely to include many of the older members) represent an even more selected group, as membership turnover was high and those who remained in membership were likely to differ from those who dropped out, although the effects of these selective processes undoubtedly changed over time as membership grew (Humphreys, 1885; Smith, 1979). A further problem arises from possible age-related and other influences on actual claims by members. Some societies appear to have made payments to older members as a form of pension, rather than as sick pay (Helowicz, 1987).

These problems complicate the interpretation of differentials by age in sickness, as recorded by Friendly Societies over time. Figure 26.2 shows weeks of sickness per thousand, by age, for the periods 1834–40 to 1921–23. The data may not be entirely comparable over time, being drawn from Alter's and Riley's (1989) presentation of IOOF data compiled by Watson in 1903, from Neison's compilation of returns from all England Friendly Societies, and from Friendly Societies' administration of benefits payable under the compulsory national insurance scheme. However, the returns for all the periods considered show very strong relationships between age and weeks of sickness.

Table 26.2

Expectation of life at age 55, by period of death and sex, England and Wales, 1841–1921

Year	Males	Females	Difference
1841	16.3	17.3	1.0
1851	15.6	16.6	1.0
1861	15.9	16.9	1.0
1871	15.5	16.8	1.3
1881	15.4	16.8	1.4
1891	15.3	16.8	1.5
1901	15.5	17.1	1.6
1911	16.3	18.2	1.9
1921	17.5	19.6	2.1

Source: ONS

Figure 26.2

Weeks of sickness per 1,000 weeks at risk, Friendly Society members, male

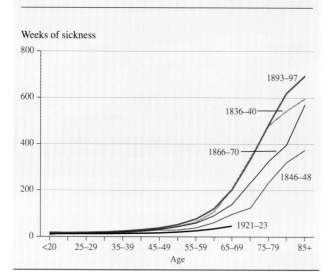

Alter and Riley have drawn attention to the increase in sickness rates between 1866–70 and 1893–97 and they note that this was particularly marked among those aged 70 and over. They suggest that this was due to increased survival of the frail, together with a greater accumulation of insults resulting from previous illnesses among these survivors. It seems equally probable that either changes in the procedures of the IOOF, or in the membership, account for the apparent rise in morbidity. Membership of Friendly Societies and other benefits societies grew rapidly during the second half of the nineteenth century; the IOOF had some 60,000 members in 1836, nearly a quarter of a million in 1844, and by the 1890s nearly a quarter of adult males were members of some society (Humphreys, 1885; Smith, 1979).

At face value, these data imply a decrease in the morbidity of older men between the 1840s and 1860s, an increase between

then and the 1890s, and a substantial improvement in the health of men aged 55–64 during the first two decades of the twentieth century (when mortality rates in this age-group were falling). However, it is likely that these apparent trends are strongly influenced by data biases; perhaps what is of greater interest is the consistent relationship between age and health.

26.3.3 Morbidity in the late nineteenth and early twentieth centuries: evidence from census data on impairments

Blindness and deafness and muteness

From 1851 to 1911 the decennial censuses included questions on blind and 'deaf and dumb' people. Table 26.3 shows the proportions identified as having these impairments in the age groups 45–64 and 65 and over during the period 1851–1911 Alternative age-groupings are not available in the published reports, but Farr's more detailed breakdown of results on blindness from the 1861 Census is shown in Table 26.4 (Humphreys, 1885).

Blindness is still strongly age-related, reflecting the importance of cataracts. As in most contemporary less-developed countries, the prevalence of blindness in the 45–64-year-old group, and, early in the period, among those aged 65 or more, was higher among men than women; from 1871, however, rates for women in the 65 and over age-group slightly exceeded those for men. The 1861 rates are comparable with rates recorded for contemporary Mali, which itself has particularly high rates of blindness (US Bureau of the Census, 1992).

Blindness is still an important cause of disability worldwide: in Bangladesh blindness is the predominant reported cause of disability for 40 per cent of the elderly disabled population (United States Bureau of the Census, 1992). Historical English data show a fall in the prevalence of blindness in the later nineteenth century, and a further drop between 1901 and

Table 26.3

Blind and 'deaf and dumb' persons per thousand population aged 45–64 and 65 and over, England and Wales, 1851–1911

Year	Blind persons per 1,000				'Deaf and dumb'* persons per 1,000			
	45–64		65+		45–64		65+	
	M	F	M	F	M	F	M	F
1851	2.2	1.6	8.9	8.4	0.6	0.5	0.5	0.4
1861	2.0	1.5	7.8	7.7	0.7	0.6	0.6	0.5
1871	2.0	1.5	7.2	7.5	0.6	0.5	0.5	0.4
1881	2.0	1.3	6.9	6.9	0.6	0.5	0.6	0.5
1891	1.9	1.3	6.0	6.1	0.6	0.5	0.5	0.4
1901	1.7	1.2	5.6	5.7	0.6	0.5	0.5	0.6
1911	1.5	1.1	5.1	5.2	0.6	0.5	0.5	0.4

* *Including those returned as dumb only, 1871–1911.*
Sources: Census data

Table 26.4

Prevalence (per thousand population) of blindness among adults by age and sex, England and Wales, 1861

Age–group	Males	Females
15–24	0.5	0.4
25–34	0.8	0.4
35–44	1.0	0.6
45–54	1.5	1.0
55–64	2.6	2.2
65–74	5.6	5.0
75–84	12.2	12.3
85+	24.7	23.2
All ages (including children)	1.1	0.9

Source: 1861 Census data reported by Farr (Humphreys, 1885, p. 59)

Figure 26.3

'Deaf and dumb' persons by age-group, England and Wales, 1851–1911

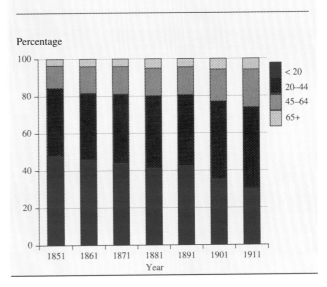

1911. This latter drop may partly reflect a change in the census question from 'blind' to 'totally blind'. Improvements in hygiene, declines in infectious diseases and possibly advances in treatment reduced prevalence rates. Smith reports that successful cataract operations were carried out in the 1840s, and a number of eye hospitals were opened in the mid-nineteenth century (Smith, 1979). By 1866 there were six eye hospitals and seven ophthalmic clinics in London alone (Abel-Smith, 1964).

The prevalence of deaf-muteness above age 45, by contrast, showed little variation by age in the nineteenth century and only very small changes in prevalence. However, as attributed in the 1911 Census, 'modern educative methods' of helping deaf children to learn to speak resulted in a change in the age-distribution of the 'deaf and dumb' population (see Figure 26.3), and the prevalence of muteness would be expected to be lower in cohorts reaching older age-groups later in the twentieth century.

Mental impairments

The censuses of 1871–1911 also asked for the identification of 'idiots, imbeciles and lunatics' in both private and non-private households. Under-reporting was a problem. Logan and Brooke noted that matching mental hospital admissions records with census returns showed that many of those admitted had not been identified as 'defectives' in the census (Logan and Brooke, 1957). From 1901 the term 'feeble-minded' was substituted for 'idiot' to encourage reporting, and from 1921 the question was dropped altogether.

The prevalence of mental health problems shown in Table 26.5 is broadly comparable with results from some of the early studies of mental health, based on surveys of whole populations (Lin, 1953). However, these surveys (and presumably the census) identified only the most serious cases. More detailed studies in the mid-twentieth century in Britain

estimated the prevalence of mental disorders among elderly people to be at least ten times higher. Kay *et al.*, for example, reported that over 5 per cent of elderly people in Newcastle upon Tyne had moderate or severe dementia and nearly 3 per cent had a functional psychosis (Kay *et al.*, 1964). Most subsequent surveys, in a range of locations, have estimated the prevalence of severe or moderately severe dementia, in populations aged 65 and over, to be in the range of 3–7 per cent (Cooper, 1991). Recent estimates of the prevalence of severe clinical depression range between 1–5 per cent, with a further 10–15 per cent affected by substantial depressive symptoms which today would merit intervention from psychiatric services (Bowling *et al.*, 1992).

The census data show the relationship between age and mental infirmities noted in more recent enquiries, and they also show the higher prevalence of mental health problems among women. The data also show an increase in reported prevalence between the late nineteenth and early twentieth centuries. As illustrated for men in Figure 26.4, this was due to the enormous increase in the proportions in lunatic asylums; the prevalence of identified mental health problems in the private household population remained unchanged. As a result, while in 1871 53 per cent of the male 'idiot, imbecile and lunatic' population was enumerated in asylums and other specialist institutions, by 1911 this proportion had increased to 73 per cent. It seems probable that the increase in reported prevalence of mental health problems reflects the overall growth in institutionalisation during this period, coupled with increased awareness of mental illness and the growing trend towards segregation of the mentally ill (Arie and Isaacs, 1978).

Table 26.5

'Idiots, imbeciles and lunatics' per thousand population aged 45–64 and 65 and over, England and Wales, 1871–1911

| | Age-group and sex | | | | | |
| | 45–64 | | | 65 and over | | |
Year	Males	Females	Persons	Males	Females	Persons
1871	5.7	6.6	6.2	6.2	7.6	7.0
1891	7.1	8.5	7.8	7.4	9.5	8.6
1901	8.3	9.7	9.0	10.5	12.9	11.9
1911	8.9	10.1	9.5	10.3	13.0	11.8

Source: Census reports

Figure 26.4

'Idiots, imbeciles and lunatics' per 1,000 population, 1871–1911

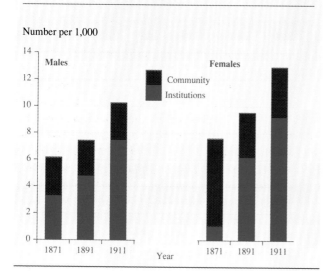

Number per 1,000

26.3.4 Use of health and related services

Even now the inferences about health status that may be drawn from service-use data are severely limited. This is because the availability of services, as well as the lay and professional expectations of health and health services, exert strong influences on patterns of use. For the late nineteenth and early twentieth centuries drawing such inferences is even more of a problem, as the main 'services' with which elderly people had contact were those administered by Poor Law Boards of Guardians. The provision of care to elderly people with health problems was closely bound up with policy on pauperism.

The New Poor Law was introduced with the 1834 Poor Law Amendment Act. This had as its guiding principle the deterrence of pauperism among the able-bodied, i.e. reliance on payments from the poor rate, and this was realised largely through application of the 'workhouse test'. The destitute, or near destitute, were to be offered relief 'in the house', and out-relief payments were to be curtailed. Between 1852 and 1892 the numbers receiving outdoor relief (in all age-groups)

fell from 45 per thousand to 19 per thousand, while the number of indoor paupers per thousand remained largely unchanged (fluctuating between 6 and 7 per thousand) – see Chapter 6. The Royal Commission on the Aged Deserving Poor noted this fall with satisfaction and attributed it to both rising living standards and to the effectiveness of the new administrative arrangements (RCADP, 1895, vol.1, p. ix).

The Poor Law Guardians also had responsibility for the 'impotent' poor – those unable to support themselves as a result of age or infirmity. Many Poor Law unions seem to have counted all paupers over 60 or 65 as 'not able-bodied', although practice varied and sometimes involved an assessment by a medical officer (RCADP, 1895, vol.1).

Widespread payment of out-relief to the aged seems to have continued after the 1834 Act, at least until the last decades of the century, when there was a renewed campaign against out-relief (Quadagno, 1982; Thomson, 1984). Between 1872 and 1892 the number of 'not able-bodied' outdoor poor (in all age-groups) fell from 16.2 to 8.8 per thousand population (RCADP, 1895, vol.1, p. x). Census data show that the proportion of older people in workhouses (including sick beds) increased dramatically in the last decades of the nineteenth century (see Table 26.6). In the 1901 Census, for example, 9 per cent of men aged 75 and over were enumerated in workhouses, compared with fewer than 5 per cent in 1851.

This increase in institutionalisation was principally due to the harsher implementation of the Poor Law (Quadagno, 1982), and so reflects a change in the economic status of the elderly population, rather than its health. The Royal Commission on the Aged Deserving Poor concluded, however, that most elderly pauper inmates would have been unable to care for themselves outside 'the house'.

The latter nineteenth century saw the rise of voluntary hospitals, which by 1921 accounted for a quarter of all beds in hospitals and related institutions for the physically sick (Pinker, 1966). These hospitals, however, excluded those with chronic illnesses and those with infectious diseases. Some provision for the latter group was made in specialist municipal hospitals out of public health necessity (Abel-Smith, 1964).

Table 26.6

Inmates of workhouses per thousand population among those aged 55 and over, England and Wales, 1851–1921

| | Age-group and sex | | | | | |
| | 55–74 | | | 75 and over | | |
Year	Males	Females	Persons	Males	Females	Persons
1851	20.8	12.9	16.6	48.7	31.6	39.1
1861	20.5	12.9	16.5	55.6	33.0	42.9
1871	25.3	13.5	19.0	64.0	35.4	47.9
1891	30.8	16.8	23.2	78.3	48.1	60.9
1901	34.9	17.1	25.3	92.2	56.0	71.0
1911	40.5	15.3	26.9	74.1	43.1	55.3
1921	18.7	9.0	13.5	47.4	33.2	38.7

Source: Census data

Some information on the gradually changing balance of provision in institutions for elderly people, and the extent of overall institutionalisation, is available from the decennial censuses. The census reports from 1851 to 1921 (excepting 1881) published tabulations on workhouse inmates by age (or inmates of poor law institutions in 1921); not all provide age-specific data on inmates of other institutions, including hospitals and lunatic asylums. Estimates of the age-distributions of hospital inmates in 1911 have been made on the basis of the published age-distributions available for 1871 and 1921. The total proportions of persons aged 55 and over enumerated in the census years in all institutions, including hospitals and 'homes', are shown in Table 26.7 (including the approximated data for 1911). This illustrates the marked rise in overall institutionalisation rates between the mid-nineteenth and early twentieth centuries. Not all of these inmates were permanent residents, since workhouses often seem to have been used as a temporary last resort (Thomson, 1984). Comparison with Table 26.6 shows the dominant, although declining, role of the workhouse. In 1851, 96 per cent of all institution inmates aged 75 and over were in workhouses. By

1921 this had declined to under 80 per cent and this would have included a much larger proportion in specialist infirmaries.

The late nineteenth and early twentieth centuries were thus marked by greater institutionalisation of elderly people, accompanied by a growth in specialist types of institution (including hospitals), and by notions of acute and chronic illness. In 1929 the Poor Law Unions were replaced by Public Assistance Committees and local authorities were empowered to take over poor law institutions. Many that did so converted the old workhouse into a hospital for the chronic sick, while the infirmary became the general hospital (Pinker, 1966). Even these general hospitals remained the poor relations of the voluntary hospitals.

Outside of institutions, health care in this period was rudimentary. Voluntary hospitals provided out-patient clinics, and in some areas Poor Law dispensaries existed. Members of Friendly Societies were entitled to medical consultations with 'club' doctors. With the implementation of the 1911 National Insurance Act, insured workers were entitled to free consul-

Table 26.7

Inmates of all institutions per thousand population among those aged 55 and over, England and Wales, 1851–1921

| | Age-group and sex | | | | | |
| | 55–74 | | | 75 and over | | |
Year	Males	Females	Persons	Males	Females	Persons
1851	24.3	15.7	19.8	50.2	33.1	40.5
1861	24.8	16.6	20.5	57.9	35.1	45.1
1871	31.1	16.5	23.4	67.3	36.9	50.2
1911*	50.5	26.1	36.1	82.3	54.0	63.4
1921	27.6	19.3	23.1	55.3	44.4	48.6

* Age-distribution of hospital inmates estimated by applying weighted average of 1871 and 1921 age distributions to 1911 total.
Source: Census data

tations with 'panel' doctors and free medicines. This entitlement extended beyond the age of eligibility for a pension, but applied only to insured workers so that women were largely excluded. Contact with Poor Law medical officers was probably more usual prior to 1913, and for women and other uninsured elderly people thereafter (Honigsbaum, 1979). These officers could prescribe 'medical out-relief', which might include food and drink as well as medicine. The cost of medicines prescribed had to be paid for by the medical officers themselves. A return made in 1892 showed that, on one day in that year, 268,397 people aged 65 and over were in receipt of medical relief – some 15 per cent of the elderly population (RCADP, 1895, p. xii).

26.4 The health of older adults since 1921

26.4.1 Mortality

Table 26.8 shows further expectation of life at ages 55 and 75, for decennial years 1921 to 1991, based on mortality rates for that period. For men there was no improvement until after 1951 and the same was true for women aged 75. The expectation of life for women aged 55, however, increased steadily from 1931. The maximum difference between female and male expectation at age 55 was reached around 1971, since when it has diminished. Of note is the extent of recent change in the further life expectation of older adults. Life expectancy for men aged 55, for example, increased by 1.6 years during the 1980s, compared with an increase of only 1.3 years between 1921 and 1971 (see also Chapter 3).

The trends in Table 26.8, particularly the apparent deteriorating survival prospects of older men between 1941 and 1951, partly reflect the choice of years shown. 1951 was a year of particularly high mortality (there were over 100,000 more deaths in that year than in 1952), as were 1929 and 1940. Figure 3.6 of Chapter 3 shows there was a drop in mortality among adults aged 75 and above during most of the Second

World War period, which has been attributed to enhanced social cohesion and to the effective, and relatively equitable, distribution of resources (Winter, 1985).

As shown in Figure 26.5, the probability of surviving from age 75 to 80 or 85 (based on period mortality rates) increased for men from 1951 and for women from 1961. Projections suggest that women aged 75 in 1991 have a 75 per cent chance of living to the age of 80 and nearly a 25 per cent chance of reaching the age of 90.

26.4.2 Morbidity 1921–94 – sources of data

During the 1920s and 1930s survey techniques developed. However, the main focus was still poverty, and national data on the health of elderly people during this period are lacking (Abrams, 1951). The first official survey of hospital beds,

Figure 26.5

Probability of survival from age 75 by period, males and females

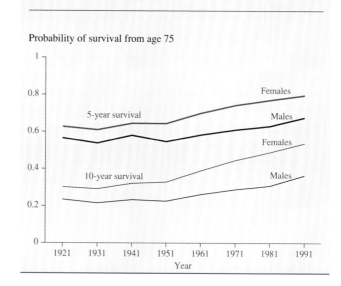

Probability of survival from age 75

Table 26.8

Expectation of life at age 55 and age 75 by period of death and sex, England and Wales, 1921–91

| | Expectation of life | | | | | |
| | at age 55 | | | at age 75 | | |
Year	Males	Females	Difference	Males	Females	Difference
1921	17.5	19.6	2.1	6.3	7.2	0.9
1931	17.3	19.4	2.1	5.9	6.8	0.9
1941	17.4	20.3	2.9	6.1	7.3	1.2
1951	17.3	21.0	3.7	5.9	7.2	1.3
1961	18.1	22.7	4.6	6.5	8.3	1.8
1971	18.8	23.9	5.1	7.0	9.3	2.3
1981	19.7	24.6	4.9	7.2	9.7	2.5
1991	21.3	25.7	4.4	8.0	10.6	2.6

Source: ONS

undertaken in 1938, revealed the inadequacies of much hospital accommodation. In January 1944 the Survey of Sickness was initiated, and those over 65 were included from December 1944 (Stocks, 1949; Logan and Brooke, 1957). This survey continued until 1951 and so straddles the immediate pre- and post-NHS period. A resurgence of interest in elderly people was reflected in the Nuffield Foundation's survey committee on the Problems of Ageing and Care of Old People, which oversaw social surveys conducted in seven areas between 1945 and 1947. One of these, in Wolverhampton, was followed up with a linked medical survey, which provides some local benchmark data for the mid-century (Sheldon, 1948).

Townsend and Wedderburn compiled a selected list of 33 social surveys of elderly people conducted between 1945 and 1965 (Townsend and Wedderburn, 1965). Most of these were fairly small, restricted to one locality and often to one particular group of older adults (for example, those in receipt of services); few used standardised measurements. Townsend and Wedderburn's own 1962 survey, however, was a national one and is particularly useful because of their pioneering efforts in classifying functional disabilities. Tinker updated Townsend and Wedderburn's list to 1992 (Tinker, 1992). Notable inclusions were the first survey of disability (Harris, 1971), Hunt's 1976 study of the elderly at home, and the mid-1980s ONS surveys of disability (Martin *et al.*, 1988). Since 1971, General Household Survey (GHS) data are available and, despite the exclusion of the institutional population, they are invaluable in providing trend data for the past 20 years based on a large national sample. The decennial censuses also include data on residents of institutions, as they did in the nineteenth century.

26.4.3 Reported sickness: the Survey of Sickness and General Household Survey

Respondents to the Survey of Sickness were asked about periods of sickness, days of incapacity and medical consultations in the previous 2 (initially 3) months. Table 26.9 shows the percentage reporting one or more episodes of sickness in a month, by sex and age-group. Reported sickness was higher among women than men and increased with age. Although the rates of sickness reported appear very high, respondents included minor complaints. In 1947, 87 per cent of those over 65 who reported some sickness had not actually experienced any days of incapacity as a result, and only 6 per cent had been incapacitated for longer than a week (Stocks, 1949). In all age-groups shown, the level of reported sickness for both men and women was higher in 1949–51 than in 1947–48.

The proportion of older adults, including those aged 75 or more, reporting any illness, was generally higher in 1951 than in 1947 (Table 26.9), yet among women aged 75 or more the number of days of, incapacity reported fell, from 29.7 in 1947–48 to 21.4 in 1950–51 (not shown in table). This implies a reduction in the incidence, progression to, or duration of, incapacitating illness, perhaps due to treatment in the new NHS or the new therapies, such as antibiotics, which became available.

In Table 26.10, days of incapacity reported in the Survey of Sickness 1947–51 are compared with days of restricted activity reported in the General Household Survey 1975–94. The Survey of Sickness data are not fully comparable with those from the GHS, and there was clearly some under-reporting (Stocks, 1949). In particular, the longer reference period used in the survey of sickness (2 to 3 months) as against that used in the GHS (2 weeks), means that respondents' recall of days of illness is likely to be lower.

The GHS data show higher levels of this type of reported morbidity, and also an upward trend in reported restricted activity, although this seems to have recently levelled off among those aged 75 and over. In all periods, people over 75 experienced more acute illness than did those aged 65–74, and, among women, those aged 65–74 had more days of incapacity than those aged 55–64 (see also section 26.5 for discussion of this gender difference).

Table 26.9

Reported monthly sickness (% reporting one or more episodes of sickness) England and Wales, 1947–51, males and females aged 55 and over

	Males			Females		
Year	55–64	65–74	75 and over	55–64	65–74	75 and over
1947	67	75	81	78	84	89
1948	68	74	82	79	84	88
1949	70	76	83	81	86	89
1950	71	76	85	80	86	92
1951	72	79	85	80	86	91

Source: Logan and Brooke (1957), Table 4

Table 26.10

Days of incapacity per person per year, 1947–51, and days of restricted activity per person per year, 1975–94 among males and females aged 55 and over.

Years	Age-group and sex					
	Males			Females		
	55–64	65–74	75 and over	55–64	65–74	75 and over
1947–51	19.2	18.6	20.7	14.7	19.2	25.7
1975–79	27.3	26.3	34.5	25.1	32.1	42.2
1980–84	31.4	33.8	45.6	33.7	43.9	55.7
1985–89	34.4	36.5	52.3	35.4	48.0	66.2
1990–94	37.6	39.2	49.3	39.7	45.9	65.4

Sources: 1947–51 (England and Wales), Logan and Brooke (1957) Table 4; questions relate to previous 2 months
1975–1994 General Household Survey (OPCS, 1973–96); questions relate to previous 2 weeks. (1991 unpublished table ELDACSCK)

26.4.4 Other survey evidence

Serious restrictions on mobility

Sheldon *et al.* and Hunt all collected data on mobility which allowed comparison of the numbers of people confined to bed and those who were housebound (Sheldon, 1948; Townsend and Wedderburn, 1965; Hunt, 1978). However, Sheldon's study was small and geographically restricted, Townsend and Wedderburn asked about ability to go outside the building rather than the dwelling, and the categorisation of the temporarily bedfast or housebound in these earlier surveys is unclear. The classification of those with less serious mobility problems varies so substantially that comparisons are difficult. However, Table 26.11 shows the results from

these three studies on the extent of confinement to bed or to dwelling (or building in 1962). The table suggests a decline in the prevalence of very severe mobility restrictions between the mid-1940s and the mid-1970s. This is supported by Harris's 1965 study, which found that between 8 and 11 per cent of those surveyed in nine areas were bedfast or housebound (Harris, 1968). An earlier study conducted in 1966 also found that 8 per cent of housewives aged 65 and over were bedfast or housebound (Harris, 1970). Changes in the management of illness in elderly people may partly account for this trend, with the acceptance that, for elderly people, bed-rest was generally dangerous rather than beneficial (Warren, 1946).

It was reported from a study conducted in and around Aber-

Table 26.11

Percentage of elderly people bedfast and housebound, 1945–47, 1962 and 1976

		Bedfast			Housebound		
		1945-7[1]	1962[2]	1976[3]	1945–7[1]	1962[2]	1976[3]
Males	65–74	1.0		0.0	3.4		1.5
	75+	5.5		0.2	12.7		8.2
	65+	2.8		0.1	7.0		3.4
Females	65–74	1.7		0.0	4.7		2.0
	75+	2.1		1.2	22.3		9.4
	65+	1.9		0.4	10.9		4.7
Persons	65–74	1.5		0.0	4.2		1.9
	75+	3.4		0.8	18.8		9.0
	65+	2.2	2.1	0.3	9.5	10.6 [4]	4.2

(1) Wolverhampton.
(2) Britain.
(3) England.
(4) Confined to building rather than house.

Sources: Derived from Sheldon (1948), Townsend and Wedderburn (1965), Hunt (1978)

deen that mobility and other indicators of health status were associated with social class, social class of origin and circumstances of upbringing, specifically whether raised by natural parents or others (Richardson, 1964). Comparable data for earlier and later periods are lacking, but these results point again to the influence of early environmental factors on health in later life.

Dental health
The Aberdeen study, referred to above, also reported that 90 per cent of the respondents had no natural teeth (edentulous) (Richardson, 1964). Results from national dental surveys and the General Household Survey show an enormous improvement since then. Between 1968 and 1988 the proportion who were edentulous, in England and Wales, fell from 64 per cent to 36 per cent for people aged 55–64, from 79 per cent to 56 per cent for those aged 65–74, and from 88 per cent to 80 per cent for people aged 75 or more (OPCS, 1990). Changes in dental practice are undoubtedly a major influence on this pattern, but it also suggests an improvement in health status (not least because dentition itself is an important influence on nutrition). Marked regional and social class differentials in the prevalence of edentulousness persist.

Use of health services
The mid-twentieth century saw several major developments of medical and other services for elderly people, with the introduction of the National Health Service, and with the National Assistance Act in 1948 requiring local authorities to provide residential services to those in need, including disabled elderly people.

In 1947 the British Geriatrics Society was established and the British Medical Association issued a report on The Care and Treatment of the Elderly and Infirm. This report emphasised the need for co-coordinated care of elderly people, involving inter-disciplinary and inter-agency collaboration (Barker, 1987).

Warren demonstrated that, with multi-disciplinary assessment and active rehabilitation, many aged patients of the infirmary could become independent enough to be discharged (Warren, 1946, 1948). The enthusiasm of others for a specialist geriatric service was rooted in self-interest. As one commentator noted in 1985:

> Geriatric medicine came into the world because of the hardness of men's hearts ... the British medical establishment of the 1950s saw the speciality as no more than a device for coping with the old workhouse hospitals and their unfortunate residents. (Anon, 1985)

The principles of the new geriatric medicine speciality undoubtedly took some time to diffuse. An influential survey conducted in the early 1960s demonstrated that many elderly people had health problems unknown to their general practitioners (Williamson et al., 1964).

Table 26.12 shows data on medical consultations per person per annum drawn from the Survey of Sickness, the GHS, and the morbidity surveys in general practice. These data are not strictly comparable, but suggest a slightly rising trend in GP

consultations among men during the late 1940s, and a fluctuating, but lower, level of consultations since 1971, with possibly a further rise in the 1990s. Under-reporting of consultations was presumably greater in the Survey of Sickness than in the GHS, because of the longer reference period used. This suggests that the true difference between consultation rates may be even greater.

Previous work based on the first and second National Surveys of Morbidity in General Practice showed a drop in consultation rates between 1955–56 and 1970–71. The Birmingham Research Unit of the Royal College of General Practitioners reported that the main change was a drop in the number of consultations per episode, rather than in episodes of illness or proportion of patients ever consulting. This was attributed to better management of episodes of illness, greater use of ancillary staff (for example, practice nurses) and a relative increase in consultations for minor conditions (BRU, 1976).

26.4.5 Consultations by diagnosed cause – comparisons between the National Surveys of Morbidity in General Practice

These surveys are known as the Morbidity Statistics from General Practice (RCGP et al., 1974, 1979, 1982, 1986, 1990; McCormick et al., 1995). They define consultations by the number of diagnoses recorded during a contact between a patient and a general practitioner. This leads to a measure of the prevalence of a condition, or group of conditions (patient consulting rates), based on the number of patients consulting for that condition at least once during the year.

Patient consulting rates (prevalence) for patients aged 65 and over, divided by diagnostic group (ICD chapter) as based on the GP's diagnosis, are shown in Table 26.13 . These data are taken from the first, second, third and fourth National Morbidity Surveys. The figures illustrate the limitations of using mortality data alone to make inferences about health. Circulatory and respiratory diseases feature prominently in both these morbidity and in mortality data, but musculoskeletal disorders (ICD Chapter XIII) and mental illness (Chapter V) are far more important reasons for consultation than they are as causes of death. Conversely, patient consulting rates for neoplasms (Chapter II), which are a major cause of death, are relatively low, but much of the medical care for these patients is provided by hospitals rather than GPs.

Changes in diagnostic practice and awareness of particular conditions obviously influence the apparent differences between time points. The enormous increase between 1955–56 and 1970–71 in patients consulting for mental illness (largely due to increases in consultations for depressive illness), and the drop in diagnoses of diseases of the nervous system (ICD Chapter VI) is a good example of this. It is perhaps surprising that patient consulting rates for mental illness have changed very little since. The lower rate of patients consulting for respiratory diseases (Chapter IX) in the second survey, as compared with the first, may reflect changes in air quality. The prevalence of respiratory diseases has subsequently increased again. The prevalence of circulatory dis-

Table 26.12

Average number of GP consultations per persons per year, males and females aged 65 and over, 1947–94

		Age and sex					
		Males			Females		
Year	Source	65–74	75 and over	65 and over	65–74	75 and over	65 and over
1947	SoS	6	7	7	7	9	8
1948	SoS	7	9	7	7	10	8
1949	SoS	8	9	8	7	9	8
1950	SoS	9	10	9	8	10	8
1951	SoS	8	11	8	8	10	8
1955/56	MSGP1	-	-	6	-	-	6
1970/71	MSGP2	3	5	6	4	4	4
1971	GHS	5	7	4	5	7	6
1976	GHS	4	5	6	4	5	5
1981	GHS	4	6	4	5	6	5
1981/82	MSGP3	4	5	5	5	6	5
1986	GHS	5	8	4	6	7	6
1991	GHS	5	7	6	6	6	6
1991–2	MSGP4	4	6	5	5	6	5
1994	GHS	5	5	5	6	6	6

GHS data: Britain; other data: England and Wales.

Sources and notes:
1947–51 Survey of Sickness (Logan and Brooke, 1957), based on patient-reported consultations in prior two months
1955–56 MSGP1 (Logan and Cushion, 1958) based on GPs' reports of patient consultations
1970/71, 1981/82, 1991/92 MSGP2, MSGP3, and MSGP4; OPCS data, definition as for MSGP1
1971, 1976, 1981, 1986, 1991 and 1994 GHS data from published and unpublished (1991) tables. Based on reported patient consultations in prior 2 weeks

eases has risen since 1955–56, particularly among men. In 1991–92 nearly a third of the population aged 65 and over consulted a doctor in connection with circulatory diseases. Among women the biggest increase, nearly all occurring since 1970–71, has been in consultations for musculoskeletal disorders. Between 1981–82 and 1991–92 there were also marked increases in consultations for circulatory and respiratory diseases (ICD Chapters VII and VIII) and diseases of the nervous system and sense organs. Patient consulting rates for both infectious diseases and ill-defined conditions have also increased. In fact, the prevalence of some serious infectious diseases, notably respiratory tuberculosis, has fallen steeply. However, between 1955–56 and 1970–71 the prevalence of intestinal infections increased, and, in the third survey, the prevalences of fungal infections, and of particular diseases which have a cyclical pattern, such as mumps, were higher than in the second. Increases in the prevalence of ill-defined conditions may partly reflect an increase in consultations for relatively trivial complaints.

The use of these broad groupings obscures changes in the prevalence of particular conditions. Among men aged 65 and over the prevalence of malignant neoplasms of the lung, bron-chus and trachea, for example, doubled between 1955–56 and 1970–71, rising from 3.7 to 7.4 per 1,000 (BRU, 1976). However, this trend was partly offset by a decline in the prevalence of other cancers (for example, those of the stomach).

As a source of information on health these data are, of course, imperfect, because access to medical services, expectations, and attitudes, as well as health status, are known to influence consultation patterns. In 1980–81, for example, men aged over 65 from Social Classes IV and V had a standardised patient consulting ratio for neoplasms of only 75 (McCormick and Rosenbaum, 1990). Analyses of data from the ONS Longitudinal Study, however, show that men classified as Social Class IV and V in 1971 had above average mortality from malignant neoplasms during the subsequent 10 years. Indeed, differences in the point at which patients consult doctors are likely to account for some of the differences between social classes in survival with cancer (Kogevinas, 1990).

26.4.6 Use of hospitals and other institutions

The number of beds in hospitals and related institutions continued to grow in the inter-war period; by 1938 there were

Table 26.13

Patient consulting rates per 1,000 in 1955–56, 1970-71, 1981–82, 1991–92, ages 65 and over

	Rate per 1,000 person-years							
	Males				Females			
ICD Chapter	1955–56	1970–71	1981–82	1991–92	1955–56	1970–71	1981–82	1991–92
All diseases and conditions	684	666	740	846	727	670	772	866
I Infectious and parasitic diseases	20	28	49	70	18	27	59	86
II Neoplasms	30	39	39	56	25	24	30	45
III Endocrine, nutritional, metabolic, immunity	32	33	50	81	53	42	58	86
IV Blood and blood forming organs	14	13	13	19	33	31	22	30
V Mental disorders	28	70	77	73	63	142	146	127
VI Nervous system and sense organs	151	117	162	223	153	110	160	227
VII Circulatory system	186	216	281	330	227	238	283	325
VIII Respiratory system	260	232	248	294	226	175	210	289
IX Digestive system	134	96	116	154	119	79	111	152
X Genitourinary system	43	41	59	75	46	51	66	118
XII Skin and subcutaneous tissue	68	76	100	137	69	78	110	148
XIII Musculoskeletal system and connective tissue	119	123	186	239	165	177	257	307
XVI Symptoms, signs and ill defined conditions	110	157	184	192	137	167	228	228
XVII Injury and poisoning	66	53	85	120	85	78	131	169

Source: MSGP surveys 1955–56, 1971–72, 1981–82, 1991–92

6.4 beds per thousand population in public and voluntary hospitals, compared with 6.0 in 1921 (Pinker, 1966). However, elderly people were still treated in the old Poor Law institutions, and pioneering improvements in treatment and care were not yet widespread. During the Second World War attention was drawn to the poor standards in many hospitals (Abel-Smith, 1964). Honigsbaum argues that elderly people's access to specialist hospital services actually deteriorated after 1948, as NHS consultants who worked in upgraded poor law hospitals were no keener than their colleagues elsewhere to treat elderly people with chronic illnesses (Honigsbaum, 1979).

Hospital In-Patient Enquiry (HIPE) data for the period 1949– 74 has been analysed by Adelstein and Ashley (1980). The analysis shows huge increases in discharges per thousand population aged 65 and over, and this trend has continued (Bosanquet and Gray, 1989; McPherson and Coleman, 1988). GHS data show that, in the private household population, the percentage of people aged 75 or more with at least one in-patient stay in the previous 12 months increased from 13 per cent in 1982 to 18 per cent in 1994.

Changes in hospital activity data do not necessarily reflect changes in health status, but they are useful in illustrating changes in the incidence of particular conditions which normally require hospital treatment. The huge increase in cases of fractured neck of femur among elderly people during the postwar period is a good example of this (Adelstein and Ashley, 1980). Reasons for this increase are not wholly clear, although it has been observed in other countries as well (Svanborg, 1988). Probable contributions are the increase in smoking and in alcohol consumption (which are both risk factors for osteoporosis) particularly among women, and also a decline in the level of customary physical activity.

Table 26.14 shows the proportion of men and women aged 55 or more who were enumerated in non-private households in the censuses of 1921 to 1991. This includes residents and visitors in institutions of all kinds, together with groups such as campers, vagrants and those on board ship. (It is not possible to subdivide this group by type of institution in all the years considered.)

Trends in the proportions in these non-private households vary markedly by age and sex. In general, the proportion of inmates of institutions has fallen among men and women aged 55–69, and among men (but not women) in their seventies. Among women aged 75 and over, and men over 80, however, the proportion of inmates of institutions has increased. Before 1922 the proportion of men in non-private households was higher than the proportion of women, whereas today, among those aged 75 and over, women far exceed men.

These trends point to changes in the reasons for admission to institutions. They also reflect policy changes affecting the relative balance between institutional and community care. Developments in chemotherapy (for example, for tuberculosis sufferers in the mid-century and more recently for those with certain mental illnesses) are also involved. As a result, the prevalence of institutionalisation has become much more strongly associated with age and with health status. Townsend pointed out that poverty or inadequate hous-

Table 26.14

Persons enumerated in non-private households per thousand population, by age and sex, England and Wales, 1921–91

Year	Sex	Age-group					
		55–59	60–64	65–69	70–74	75–79	80 and over
1921	M	17.3	25.1	37.2	45.8	51.9	61.1
	F	14.4	17.8	22.4	28.6	37.4	54.5
1931	M	19.5	26.0	34.4	39.3	49.2	63.8
	F	14.6	17.2	21.3	26.9	36.8	61.1
1951	M	18.4	21.4	26.1	34.7	49.1	75.2
	F	16.9	20.4	25.0	34.2	50.1	94.2
1971	M	23.5	24.9	28.2	37.0	52.2	109.7
	F	20.5	22.1	26.4	38.4	61.4	156.3
1981	M	19.1	19.3	21.4	27.7	42.4	98.0
	F	14.5	15.7	19.4	29.4	54.2	156.0
1991	M	14.8	18.2	22.0	31.4	45.7	120.2
	F	10.9	14.7	20.2	31.3	55.1	199.2

Sources: Census Reports; 1991 Census SARs

ing was often the predominant reason for admission after 1948 (Townsend, 1962). More recent studies indicate that the majority of people in institutions are moderately or seriously disabled (Wilkin et al., 1978; Gilleard et al., 1980; Martin et al., 1988).

Rates of residence do not simply reflect chronic disease and disability, however, and some elderly people in private households are more incapacitated than residents of homes or hospitals. In the ONS Disability Surveys, 40 per cent of those in the most severely disabled group identified, and who were aged 70 and over, were living in private households (Martin et al., 1988). Analyses of data from the ONS Longitudinal Study have shown socio-demographic differences in the proportions of elderly people moving from private to non-private households between 1971 and 1981, which could not wholly be explained by differences in health status (Grundy, 1992b). The rise in the prevalence of institutionalisation in the oldest age-group, shown in Table 26.14, is also evident in the USA (Siegel, 1992). This rise cannot be interpreted as an indication of an increased prevalence of serious disability, even though it is consistent with such a trend. There have been very large changes in the residence patterns of elderly people in the postwar period, with considerably fewer elderly people living with younger relatives (Grundy, 1992c, 1993; Murphy and Grundy, 1993). It is highly probable that the increase in institutionalisation at least partly reflects this. Changes in access to institutional care and to support services at home are also important influences. The rise in institutionalisation in the 1980s, for example, reflects the growing availability of means-tested Social Security payments to fund residential care in the private sector. This led to a phenomenal expansion of the provision of profit-earning residential care, with a resultant increase in the level of overall provision (DHSS, 1989; Laing and Buisson, 1991). The escalating cost of this provided a major impetus for the 1990 Community Care Act (DHSS, 1989).

26.5 Recent trends in health: 1971–92

The chief source of data on trends in health status in the past two decades is the General Household Survey. The findings on restricted activity and GP consultations were discussed in section 26.4. In most years, questions about long-standing illness, and long-standing illness which limited activities, have also been asked. These data constitute the major national source of subjective information on trends in chronic illness in private households, though they inevitably exclude many people in the poorest health. They have been used to study differences in the prevalence of long-standing illness in age-groups over 65 by social class, which is assigned on the basis of last job or, in the case of married women, the husband's last job (Grundy, 1987; Victor, 1989). The extent of limiting long-standing illness estimated in the 1991 GHS was higher than that reported in the census. This is because of differences in the way the information was elicited. However, the difference decreased progressively with age, and in the group aged 85 and over the census prevalence is slightly higher than the GHS estimate (OPCS, 1993).

Figure 26.6

Limiting long-term illness by sex, age and residential status, Great Britain, 1991

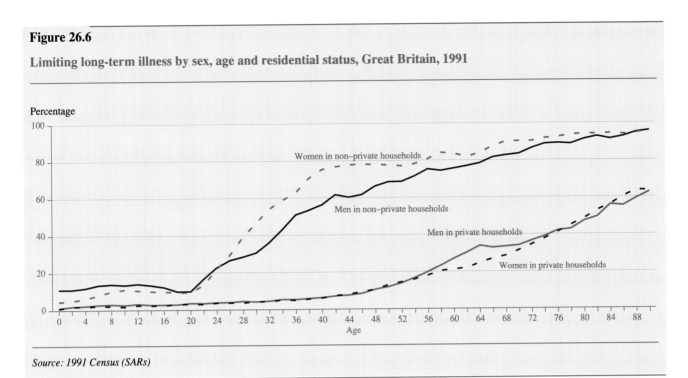

Source: 1991 Census (SARs)

A different pattern was revealed by a comparison between results from the 1985 GHS and the ONS Disability Surveys, which was based on much more detailed questioning about ability to undertake a range of activities (Martin et al., 1988). This showed that the GHS estimates of disability were higher than those from the Disability Survey up to the age of 75, while above this age the GHS estimate was markedly lower. This difference almost certainly reflects under-reporting of long-standing limiting illness by the oldest respondents in the GHS, who attribute their limitations of activity to age rather than to illness.

The relationship between age and health is also weakened in the GHS by the exclusion of the institutional population. Figure 26.6 shows the prevalence of limiting long-term ill-

ness reported in the 1991 Census, by age and sex, for the private and non-private household populations. Reported long-standing illness is very much higher in the non-private household group. Thus, the omission of this group leads to an underestimation of the prevalence of long-term illness. In addition, it can distort the relationships between variables such as marital status and health, since the probability of residence in an institution is associated with these and other factors.

These differences between the GHS and other sources do not in themselves cast doubt on the validity of trend data from the GHS (although for the oldest age-groups they will be influenced by changes in the relative size of the institutional population). But they strongly suggest that apparent trends may be influenced by changes in, for example, health expec-

Figure 26.7

Percentage with long-standing illness, 1975–94

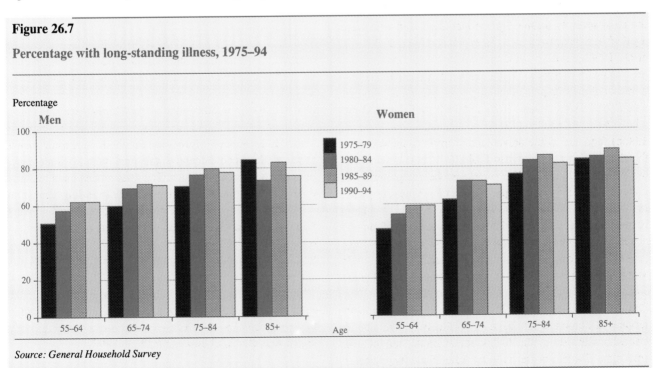

Source: General Household Survey

Figure 26.8

Percentage with limiting long-standing illness, 1975–94

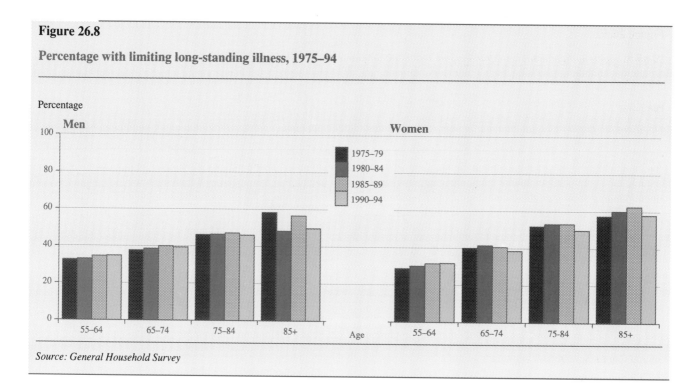

Percentage

Men   Women

1975–79
1980–84
1985–89
1990–94

Source: General Household Survey

tations and awareness, both among the general public and among general practitioners. Changes in health expectations have been suggested as the explanation for generally rising rates of morbidity reported from the GHS and equivalent surveys in other countries.

In Figures 26.7 and 26.8 data are presented for long-standing illness and limiting long-standing illness for 1975–79, 1980–84, 1985–89 and 1990–94. The data for women show a stronger relationship between age and long-standing, particularly limiting long-standing, illness, than do the data for men. There is little change in the prevalence of limiting long-standing illness in the 65–74 and 75–84 year old age-groups over time, and, in all periods, the rates are higher for women

than for men. Among those aged 55–64, long-standing and limiting long-standing illness are more prevalent among men than among women and appear to have risen over time. These differences may be influenced by labour market factors. Rates of reported morbidity are often higher among men than for women in the 'pre-retirement' age-band. This may be because men who have retired early for health reasons are particularly conscious of health limitations and so are more likely to report them (Grundy, 1992a). This can be seen clearly in Figure 26.6, which, as it is based on the Census SARs, permits desegregation by single years of age. The proportion of men leaving the labour market before the age of 65 rose very substantially between the mid-1970s and early 1990s, with invalidity benefits often 'bridging the gap' between the end

Figure 26.9

Percentage with long-standing illness reporting health as 'not good'

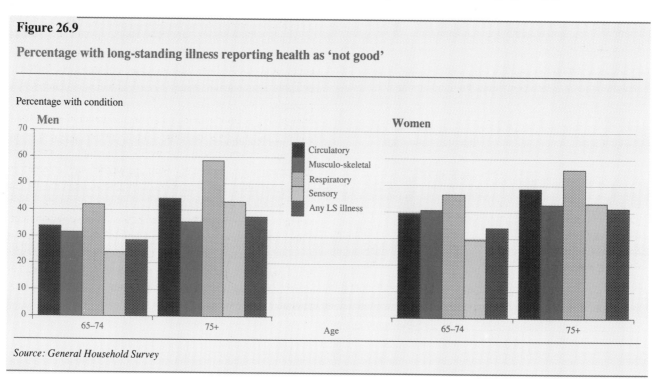

Percentage with condition

Men   Women

Circulatory
Musculo-skeletal
Respiratory
Sensory
Any LS illness

Source: General Household Survey

Figure 26.10

Percentage usually unable to manage going outdoors and down the road on their own

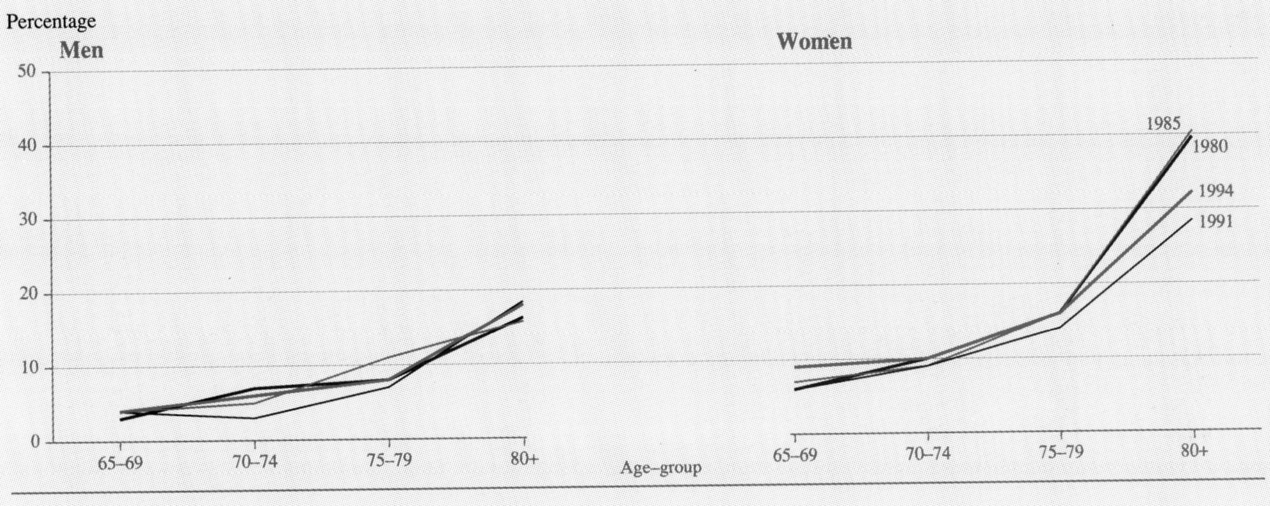

Source: General Household Survey

of work and pensionable age (Henretta, 1994). This may also have led to increases in the proportions reporting long-standing illness.

The major causes of long-standing illness reported by respondents in the 1989 GHS are shown in Table 26.15. Circulatory and musculoskeletal disorders predominate, with the latter being particularly prevalent among women aged 75 and over. Although fewer of the respondents reported that they were suffering from long-standing respiratory diseases, those who did so were particularly likely to assess their health as 'not good', as is shown in Figure 26.9.

In 1980, 1985, 1991 and 1994 the GHS collected more detailed information on ability to undertake various activities of daily living (ADL) and instrumental activities of daily living (IADL), including questions on mobility and on domestic and personal care tasks. Such data are widely used to compute indices of functional disability (Katz et al., 1983). These measures have the advantage of being more sensitive than general questions on overall activity and of being easily interpreted. They are also relevant to considerations of policy for health and social care (Bowling, 1991; Donaldson, 1992). In addition, they correlate reasonably well with other indicators of health status, such as mortality and institutionalisation (Branch and Jette, 1982; Warren and Knight, 1985).

However, ADL scales lack specificity in that, often, respondents have no opportunity to indicate how difficult they find a task, as opposed to whether they find it difficult at all. They also ignore important aspects of health such as psychosocial well-being (Bowling, 1991). Responses are also dependent to some extent on cultural norms about behaviour appropriate to a particular age and gender, and changes in these attitudes may lead to changes in ADL-based measures. For example, until 1994 the GHS showed that the proportion of men unable to cook a main meal, or to wash clothes by hand unaided, was higher than the corresponding proportion of women. This was despite the well known higher prevalence of disability among elderly women, which was reflected in the higher proportions of women unable to perform all the other activities that were queried. Ability to undertake a particular task also depends to some extent on the environment. Thus, ability to get around the house will reflect not just a respondent's health status, but also the design of the dwelling. Large differences between studies in the assessment of functional disability have been reported, probably for these reasons (Weiner et al., 1990).

Table 26.15

Proportion (%) of males and females aged 65 and over reporting long-standing illness, by major cause group, Great Britain, 1989

Cause group	Age-group and sex			
	65–74		75 and over	
	Males	Females	Males	Females
Circulatory	25.0	22.3	21.9	26.2
Musculoskeletal	21.0	29.0	23.8	38.9
Respiratory	10.2	8.2	11.8	8.2
Sensory (eye and ear)	9.1	8.2	11.5	18.4
Any long-standing illness	58.0	58.7	60.4	69.7

Source: OPCS data from 1989 GHS HLI14

201

Table 26.16

Proportion (%) of men and women aged 65 and over unable to perform four activities of daily living (ADLs) independently, 1976–94

Age and sex		Unable to perform ADLs independently				
		1976	1980	1985	1991	1994
65–69	M	4	4	4	2	4
	F	6	4	3	3	6
70–74	M	8	6	3	4	5
	F	15	8	6	3	7
75–79	M	18	8	11	5	6
	F	22	10	9	6	9
80–84	M	25	18	15	9	13
	F	36	13	19	7	15
85+	M	43	13	23	20	18
	F	54	36	33	21	25

Sources: Bebbington's analysis of data from the 1976 Elderly at Home Survey, (Bebbington and Darton, 1996) and the 1980, 1985, 1991 and 1994 rounds of the GHS (Bone et al., 1996).

Bebbington has compared information on the ability to undertake specific activities in the GHS and in the 1976 Survey of the Elderly at Home (Bone et al., 1996; Hunt, 1978). There was a marked drop in the proportions unable to undertake four activities of daily living without assistance (see Table 26.16). This, together with the earlier results on mobility, restrictions (see Table 26.11), suggests a reduction in the extent of serious disability. However, the GHS data on, for example, the proportions unable to go outside and down the road on their own (see Figure 26.10) show no consistent trend. A number of other European countries, and the United States, have reported reductions in the extent of serious disability but an increase in the prevalence of mild health impairments (Boshuizen and van de Water, 1994; Crimmins et al., 1989).

Results from the GHS and other surveys suggest a similar pattern in Britain.

26.6 Discussion and conclusions

During the period 1841–1991 there was a substantial increase in survival to and beyond the age of 55. Cohort changes in survival to the ages of 55 and 75 are shown in Figure 26.11. Fewer than a fifth of the women born at the start of the period reached their 75th birthday; 57 per cent of those born in 1921 will celebrate this birthday in 1996. Corresponding changes among men are less marked and the major difference is be-

Table 26.17

Estimates of the prevalence of disability and serious disability in the private household and total population aged 50 and over, England and Wales, 1984–85

Age-group	Prevalence of disability per 1,000					
	All levels of disability (1–10)			Severe disability (9–10)		
	Private household population	Total population	Difference	Private household population	Total population	Difference
50–9	131	133	2	6	7	1
60–9	236	240	4	13	16	3
70–9	395	408	13	23	32	9
80+	674	714	40	85	133	48

Source: OPCS Disability Surveys (Martin et al., 1988)

tween those born in the nineteenth century and those born in the twentieth. Changes in the probability of survival from age 55 are shown for the whole period in Figure 26.12.

The mortality regime of 1991 implies survival for a further 20 years for 70 per cent of women, compared with only 40 per cent for most of the second half of the nineteenth century. Among men, changes are slighter but still pronounced, and much of this improvement has occurred relatively recently. In comparison with recent changes, the extent of earlier improvement at older ages among men appears very modest, and the restriction or concentration of change to the first two decades of the twentieth century is also puzzling. It is possible that the late nineteenth-century pattern was influenced by the emergence of new viruses, while later in the twentieth century, economic problems, an increase in exposure to cigarette smoking and unfavourable health legacies impeded further progress (Gage, 1993). Among older women, the early twentieth century was also a period of particular improvement in survival, but gains continued throughout the 1920s and 1930s.

How were these changes related to changes in morbidity or in health? Census data suggest a decline in the prevalence of blindness, which, although fairly small, is a positive indicator. It may also indicate an improvement in the nutritional status of the population reaching old age. The incidence of mental illness appears to have increased, but undoubtedly the epidemic here was in institutionalisation rather than madness.

Data from the middle of the twentieth century point to the high prevalence of self-reported illness, much of it minor, and to the large use of doctors by older people. Rates of medical consultation have fallen from the levels recorded in the 1950s, reflecting improvements in therapies and in medical management. However, rates of self-reported long-standing illness have not fallen, and in some cases have increased.

The lack of major improvement in the mortality of older men in the middle decades of the twentieth century was, until relatively recently, interpreted by some as indicating little scope for further improvement in life expectancy, once the virtual eradication of infectious disease mortality had been achieved through improvements in public health and living conditions. Certainly, in the context of the major changes in the health care of older people, this lack of improvement for men appears disappointing. However, from the late nineteenth century onwards, increasingly larger proportions of men have been exposed to cigarette smoking. This has undoubtedly had a major influence on the mortality levels and patterns of health of men as compared to women (Alderson and Ashwood, 1985; Waldron, 1986).

Since 1971 there have been further major changes in the delivery of health and welfare services, important socio-economic changes and the further development of medical interventions, including drugs. This period has seen quite substantial falls in death rates at older ages, but, according to the results from the General Household Survey, no decrease in reported long-term illness. This might suggest an altered relationship between mortality and morbidity at the population level, but other interpretations are also possible. These include an increase in health expectations and changes in the threshold for reporting health limitations. The data are also limited due to the exclusion of the institutional population who, in the oldest age-groups, comprise a large proportion of those with serious health problems (see Table 26.17). More optimistically, patchy evidence from a few mid-century surveys, and from the 1970s onwards, suggest a decline in very serious mobility and other functional restrictions. Similar findings have been reported from other developed countries. These results would seem most consistent with Manton's thesis of delays in the rate of progression of degenerative diseases (Manton, 1982).

The inability to draw firm conclusions about even recent trends in morbidity and its relationship with mortality points to an urgent need for better data. A new national health survey, including both objective as well as subjective measures of health, was instituted in 1991, and this should provide a surer basis on which to review trends in the 1990s. However, even the most comprehensive contemporary datasets are unlikely to reveal all we would wish to know about future trends in the health of the older population, simply because the foundations of this may have been laid many decades in the past.

Figure 26.11

Cohort survivorship to ages 55 and 75, men and women born 1841–1921

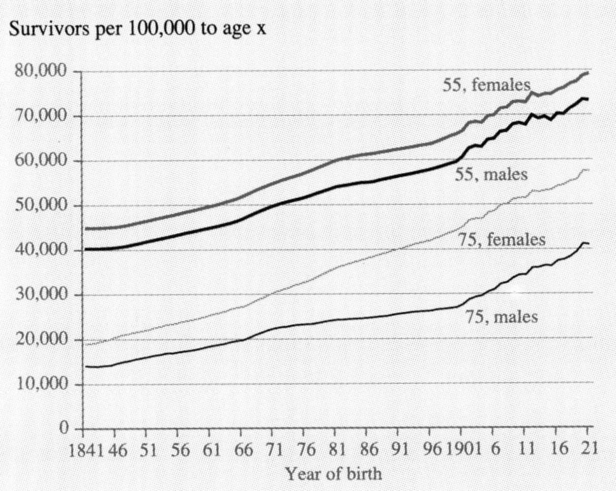

Survivors per 100,000 to age x

Figure 26.12

Probability of survival for age 55 (period life tables)

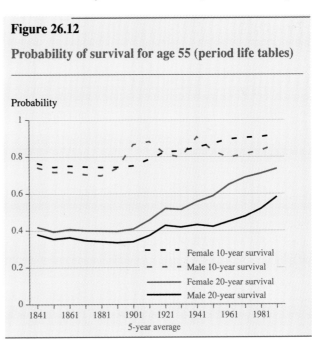

Chapter 27

Trends and prospects at very high ages

By
Roger Thatcher

Summary

- Over the last 50 years falling death rates and rising numbers in the age-groups 80–99 have had a greatly magnified effect on the numbers of centenarians.

- Since the 1950s the number of centenarians has increased at a rate of about 7 per cent per year, faster than most other age-groups.

- Accurate data for numbers and death rates at very high ages can be found by using the so-called 'method of extinct generations'. Rising numbers of centenarians are represented by a shift in the statistical frequency distribution towards the higher ages. The shift is most clearly visible at the upper tail of the distribution.

- Death rates at very high ages, including centenarians, have been falling, particularly since the Second World War. The fastest fall has been between the 1970s and 1980s.

- The increases in expectations of life at very high ages have not been very large. They are measured in months rather than years.

- The highest ages recorded for men and women in Britain are showing a spectacular increase. There has been an increase of 6 years in the highest ages reached by both men and women in the cohort born in 1871–80 compared with that born in 1841–50.

- Population projections prepared by the Government Actuary's Department, which assume continually falling death rates, show a 10-fold increase in the number of centenarians in Britain between 1991 and 2031.

- Centenarians are far more likely to be women than men. The majority of the whole age-group are widowers or widows.

- There have been no systematic surveys of the physical and mental health of centenarians in England and Wales.

27.1 Introduction

A previous chapter by Emily Grundy has considered elderly people. In this chapter we shall be concerned with the very highest age-group, namely the centenarians. This group is growing at a spectacular rate. It is not very large numerically, so in economic or social terms it is not very important in its own right, but it is a very sensitive indicator of what is happening at lower ages. Changes such as falls in death rates and rising numbers in the age-groups 80–99 have a greatly magnified effect on the numbers of centenarians. In contrast, the annual numbers of births occurring more than 100 years previously play a small part in dictating changes in the numbers of centenarians, at least over the next 20 years or so (Thatcher, 1981; Craig, 1983).

The trends for centenarians are also important for another reason. Changes in the nineteenth and twentieth centuries have transformed the death rates at young and middle ages, so that the shape of the survival curve now looks much more like a rectangle. If there are further falls in death rates, but if there is a more or less fixed upper limit to the length of life, then this process of 'rectangularisation' will continue to the point where deaths will eventually be compressed into a narrower range of ages. On the other hand, if the upper limit to life (supposing that it exists) is much higher than the maximum ages currently achieved, there will be less 'rectangularisation' and less compression of the ages at death, but people will live even longer.

The group of centenarians contains people who have attained exceptional longevity. There is a natural human interest in the maximum length of life, the highest ages which have been reached so far and the prospects for longevity in the future.

The aim of this chapter is to bring together the data which are most relevant to the trends at these very high ages, and to discuss current projections for the future. There is also a short postscript on the characteristics and health of centenarians. Here too their experience may be relevant to discussion about the 'compression of morbidity' (Fries, 1980): as people live longer, are their illnesses also postponed to the time around when they die, or are the years of life gained marred by increased ill health (Perls, 1995; Grundy, 1984)?

27.2 Background

In the 1911 Census of population, the number of persons in England and Wales who were recorded as being aged 100 and over was 128, out of a total population of 36 million. These centenarians were a great rarity. They had all been born before the official registration of births began in 1837, so there were often doubts about their exact ages and whether they were true centenarians.

Since then, the picture has changed beyond recognition. Since the 1950s the number of centenarians has increased dramatically, at a rate of about 7 per cent per year.

This is much faster than the rate of most, if not all, other age-groups. By 1991 the number of centenarians had reached 4,400. Most of this increase has been due to falling death rates at lower ages, so that more people have survived to reach age 100; but even at age 100 there are indications that death rates have been falling and that the expectation of life (at least for women) has risen a little. The highest recorded age in England and Wales has increased from 106 to 112 for men, and from 109 to 115 for women.

27.3 Methodology

It is not easy to compile accurate data for numbers and death rates at very high ages. Unfortunately, there are errors in many of the very high ages recorded in the censuses of population. Above the age of 85 it is difficult to produce accurate estimates of death rates at individual years of age by the traditional method of combining data from death registrations with data from censuses. At these very high ages, better results are obtained (at least retrospectively) by using death registrations alone. The principle behind the calculations is that once all the members of a given birth cohort have died, their dates of birth and death (as recorded at the death registration) give enough information to reconstruct the numbers who were alive at earlier dates, provided that we confine ourselves to ages which are high enough for international migration to be negligible. This is the so-called 'method of extinct generations'.

For the most recent cohorts, which are not yet quite extinct, the data on deaths can be supplemented by data on the number still surviving, obtained from the 10 per cent sample of pensioners which is analysed by the Department of Social Security.

A full account of the methods used in this section, including sources, references and a discussion of the reliability of the data, will be found in Thatcher (1992).

27.4 Rising numbers

The trends in numbers at the highest ages can be seen from Table 27.1. In order to set the changes at ages 100 and over in perspective, we show also the corresponding numbers at ages 80–89 and 90–99.

Since 1911, the numbers at ages 80–89 have been growing at a reasonably steady rate of between 2 and 3 per cent per annum. At ages 90–99, the rate has been somewhat faster, particularly in the second half of the period. At ages 100 and over, however, although the numbers are small, the percentage rate of growth has been spectacular. Between 1951 and 1991 the total number of centenarians (men and women) grew from 300 to 4,400. This is a rate of increase of 7 per cent per annum, roughly doubling every 10 years.

It may seem surprising that the fastest percentage rate of growth should occur at the highest ages of all. There is, however, a simple explanation. As death rates have fallen and

Table 27.1

Numbers at high ages in England and Wales, estimated from death registrations in 1911–90 and numbers of pensioners in 1990–91

Period	Aged 80–89	Aged 90–99	Aged 100 and over
Men		*thousands*	
1911	74.8	4.3	0.0
1921	88.2	4.3	0.0
1931	112.4	5.4	0.0
1941	150.0	6.4	0.0
1951	224.9	10.7	0.0
1961	285.9	16.3	0.1
1971	305.2	24.8	0.2
1981	356.4	28.8	0.3
1991	524.7	41.8	0.5
Women			
1911	122.3	9.3	0.1
1921	157.7	10.8	0.1
1931	203.9	14.4	0.1
1941	272.8	18.6	0.1
1951	406.5	31.5	0.3
1961	582.4	50.0	0.5
1971	733.1	86.1	1.1
1981	908.0	119.0	2.0
1991	1,166.5	183.7	3.9

Source: Thatcher (1992)

people have lived for longer, the statistical frequency distribution of ages has shifted towards the higher ages. This shift produces its largest proportionate effect at the upper tail of the distribution, where the absolute numbers are relatively small.

27.5 Falling death rates

The trends in death rates at very high ages can be seen very conveniently from Table 27.2. This shows the probabilities of dying within 12 months (q_x in the actuarial notation), averaged over successive decades. The steady progression from column to column shows very clearly how the death rates have been falling, particularly since the Second World War.

It is worth noting that the falls have extended right up the age scale, even as far as the centenarians. For example, the probability that a female aged exactly 100 will die before reaching age 101 has fallen during the period covered by the table from 0.43 to 0.36.

The annual percentage rates of decrease in the death rates between successive decades are summarised in Table 27.3. Although these figures have margins of error, and those for ages 100–104 are less reliable than the rest, they are the best

indicators of the detailed rates of change which are at present available.

It will be noted that the fastest falls have been in the most recent period, between the 1970s and the 1980s, when they averaged about 1 per cent per annum for men and nearer 1.5 per cent for women. There is no indication here that the trend is slowing down.

27.6 Expectations of life

By using the 'method of extinct generations', it is possible to estimate the cohort expectations of life which were actually achieved by the cohorts born between 1841 and 1880. Earlier cohorts, born before the official registration of births began, have been omitted. The results are shown in Table 27.4 and speak for themselves.

Owing to the way that demographic arithmetic works, falling death rates have a larger numerical effect on the expectation of life at low ages than at high ages, because younger people gain the benefit of increased expectations at all ages greater than their own. The falling death rates have indeed increased the expectations of life as shown in Table 27.4, but at these very high ages the increases have not been very large. They are measured in months rather than years.

27.7 The highest ages recorded

Although the expectation of life at age 100 has increased by only a few months for women, and has hardly changed for men, there has nevertheless been a spectacular increase in the highest ages recorded. Table 27.5 (for men) and Table 27.6 (for women) show the numbers in the relevant birth cohorts who survived to reach higher ages. For example, the first column of Table 27.5 shows that, of the men born in 1841–50, there were 215 who survived to reach age 100, of whom 135 survived to reach age 101, and so on, until the last two survivors died at age 106.

The tables show that for the cohorts born in 1841–50, the highest ages which were reached were 106 for men and 109 for women. For the cohorts born in 1871–80, the highest ages reached were 112 for men and 115 for women. Thus for each sex, the highest age increased by 6 years. We can be confident that this 6-year increase is genuine, because all the entries in the tables at ages 110 and over have been individually verified, by tracing their original birth registration, to check that the age recorded at death was consistent with the birth entry. Only the verified cases are included in the tables.

A very large part of this 6-year increase can be explained simply by the fact that the numbers reaching age 100 have increased by factors of 6.3 for men and 7.6 for women. The statistical theory of extreme values shows how an increase in the numbers is itself sufficient to increase the maximum age which will be reached, even if the death rates and expectations of life at high ages do not change at all.

Table 27.2

Probabilities of dying (q_x) in England and Wales estimated from death registrations in 1930–90 and numbers of pensioners in 1990

Age	1930–40	1940–50	1950–60	1960–70	1970–80	1980–90
Men						
85	0.212	0.196	0.194	0.179	0.172	0.157
86	0.231	0.215	0.214	0.197	0.186	0.172
87	0.246	0.231	0.229	0.211	0.199	0.180
88	0.255	0.238	0.244	0.224	0.213	0.195
89	0.276	0.264	0.261	0.243	0.227	0.207
90	0.290	0.275	0.275	0.252	0.243	0.222
91	0.300	0.286	0.290	0.266	0.259	0.234
92	0.314	0.304	0.313	0.294	0.279	0.255
93	0.344	0.321	0.332	0.306	0.295	0.270
94	0.376	0.352	0.352	0.324	0.314	0.293
95	0.374	0.371	0.382	0.341	0.335	0.307
96	0.410	0.388	0.400	0.374	0.355	0.328
97	0.403	0.405	0.408	0.378	0.374	0.342
98	0.415	0.427	0.436	0.400	0.396	0.369
99	(0.495)	(0.468)	0.479	0.405	0.403	0.371
100			(0.448)	0.451	0.433	0.406
101				(0.500)	0.485	0.416
102					(0.424)	0.407
103						(0.431)
Women						
85	0.174	0.159	0.152	0.137	0.126	0.108
86	0.190	0.174	0.168	0.152	0.139	0.121
87	0.203	0.186	0.179	0.164	0.150	0.131
88	0.215	0.197	0.192	0.175	0.163	0.143
89	0.231	0.217	0.210	0.191	0.179	0.159
90	0.247	0.232	0.223	0.206	0.195	0.172
91	0.252	0.240	0.234	0.218	0.208	0.186
92	0.277	0.260	0.256	0.239	0.228	0.204
93	0.295	0.280	0.273	0.258	0.248	0.222
94	0.317	0.296	0.291	0.273	0.264	0.237
95	0.334	0.317	0.307	0.291	0.282	0.251
96	0.347	0.343	0.332	0.316	0.301	0.273
97	0.365	0.363	0.352	0.323	0.316	0.287
98	0.405	0.401	0.371	0.351	0.337	0.301
99	0.415	0.414	0.393	0.346	0.348	0.327
100	0.433	0.430	0.406	0.386	0.371	0.358
101	0.481	0.401	0.429	0.403	0.403	0.377
102	(0.441)	(0.468)	0.445	0.406	0.397	0.393
103			(0.500)	0.465	0.417	0.401
104				(0.444)	0.475	0.437
105					(0.483)	0.476
106						(0.467)
107						(0.495)

Figures in parentheses are based on fewer than 200 (but more than 100) deaths.
Source: Thatcher (1992)

Table 27.3

Average annual percentage rates of decrease in death rates between successive decades in England and Wales

Period	85–89	90–94	95–99	100–104
		Ages		
Men				
1910s to 1920s	0.1	0.1	0.2	-0.6
1920s to 1930s	-0.2	-0.6	-0.7	0.9
1930s to 1940s	0.9	0.8	0.5	0.1
1940s to 1950s	0.0	-0.2	-0.4	-0.9
1950s to 1960s	0.9	0.9	1.2	-0.2
1960s to 1970s	0.6	0.4	0.3	0.9
1970s to 1980s	1.0	1.1	1.0	1.3
Women				
1910s to 1920s	0.2	0.0	0.0	1.2
1920s to 1930s	0.1	-0.2	-0.3	-1.7
1930s to 1940s	1.1	0.8	0.6	0.8
1940s to 1950s	0.4	0.2	0.4	0.3
1950s to 1960s	1.0	0.8	0.7	0.8
1960s to 1970s	0.9	0.5	0.4	0.3
1970s to 1980s	1.5	1.3	1.2	0.6

Note: The rates of decrease are derived from death rates (m_x), age-standardised within each 5-year age-group, in the decades 1911–20, 1921–30,..., 1981-90.

Source: ONS

Table 27.4

Cohort expectations of life (England and Wales)

Cohorts born in	80	85	90	95	100
		Expectation of life at age			
Men					
1841–50	4.77	3.46	2.63	1.98	1.76
1851–60	4.86	3.60	2.72	1.99	1.65
1861–70	5.11	3.67	2.77	2.12	1.60
1871–80	5.28	3.92	2.99	2.22	1.71
Women					
1841–50	5.56	4.06	3.05	2.28	1.82
1851–60	5.81	4.32	3.24	2.38	1.81
1861–70	6.18	4.48	3.36	2.54	1.97
1871–80	6.53	4.82	3.59	2.63	2.00

Table 27.5

England and Wales
Men survivors reaching given ages

Reaching age	1841–50	1851–60	1861–70	1871–80
		Cohorts born in:		
100	215	339	720	1,364
101	135	184	397	774
102	73	106	204	401
103	32	51	104	231
104	19	25	51	115
105	8	9	20	66
106	2	7	10	30
107	0	2	4	16
108		1	1	10
109		1	1	4
110		1	0	1
111		1		1
112		0		1
113				0

Source: ONS

Table 27.6

England and Wales
Women survivors reaching given ages

Reaching age	1841–50	1851–60	1861–70	1871–80
		Cohorts born in:		
100	1,085	2,122	4,233	8,273
101	615	1,272	2,616	5,186
102	379	720	1,563	3,115
103	213	396	955	1,846
104	107	196	535	1,080
105	63	107	287	610
106	31	49	132	319
107	17	23	70	172
108	5	12	34	84
109	2	6	15	27
110	0	3	7	12
111		1	5	7
112		0	2	4
113			0	4
114				2
115				1

Source: ONS

27.8 Prospects

Nobody can foresee with certainty the course which death rates at high ages will take into the distant future. This is, in fact, a matter of very considerable controversy. On the one hand, there are those who believe that medical advances are imminent which will offer the prospect of new cures for many forms of cancer, the postponement of deaths from heart disease and other major changes. These, particularly if combined with improvements in lifestyle, could transform the position and lead to substantially lower death rates at high ages than those observed at present. On the other hand, there are those who foresee that economic pressures may make it difficult to increase indefinitely the amount of resources which can be allocated to the care of the old, and to pay for increasingly expensive treatments for continuingly increasing numbers of old people.

Even more pessimistically, there are those who think that the environment is starting to deteriorate and that, at some stage during the twenty-first century, pressures generated by the world population explosion will eventually make matters worse, with resulting repercussions on health. These are, however, problems which, if they materialise, will affect mortality at all ages, not just at high ages. Demographic historians will recognise that these conflicting modern views are remarkably similar to those advanced by Condorcet and Malthus a long time ago.

However, these are unresolved arguments about the long-term future. For the present, the position is that there is a strong and well-established downward trend in death rates, apparently extending to ages even above 100, not only in England and Wales but also in many other countries. There are no medical or biological reasons to expect this trend to be halted in the immediate future, though how long it will continue is obviously a matter for debate.

The latest national population projections (OPCS, 1993), prepared by the Government Actuary and covering the period up to 2031, assume that death rates will continue to diminish, though at a declining pace. The projected rates of mortality at ages 85–100 show average rates of decrease, over each of the four decades between 1991 and 2031, which almost all fall between 0.5 and 1.5 per cent per annum. The projected increases in the numbers at high ages are shown in Table 27.7.

These projections show a further 10-fold increase in the number of centenarians (from 4,400 in 1991 to 45,000 in 2031), which is even larger than the six-to-eightfold increases in the particular past period covered in Tables 27.5 and 27.6. Also, the death rates are projected to continue to fall at rates which are not very different from the past. Clearly, these projected changes between the years 1991 and 2031 are likely to produce a further increase in the maximum recorded age at death. If it were not for the presumption that death rates at ages 115–120 will be higher than at ages 110–115, the projected changes in numbers and death rates might be expected to produce another 6-year increase (give or take a year or two) in the maximum recorded age. There are uncertainties here, but on the information available at present it is reasonable to expect that the maximum recorded age for women in England and Wales (at present 115) will reach at least 118 or 119, or possibly even more. In France, where the expectation of life is higher, the age of 121 has already been attained.

27.9 Postscript on the characteristics of centenarians

This chapter has been primarily concerned with the trends in numbers and lengths of life of centenarians, but we may add a little information about their characteristics.

In this age-group, women currently outnumber men in a ratio of more than seven to one. The official statistics give analyses by marital status. For example, of the centenarians who died in England and Wales in 1990, only 3 per cent of the men and 16 per cent of the women had remained single. Eighteen per cent of the men but only 0.5 per cent of the women had surviving spouses. Only 1 per cent of each sex were divorced or 'not stated'. All the rest, the overwhelming majority of the whole age-group, were widowers or widows.

In England and Wales there have, so far, been no systematic surveys of the physical and mental health of centenarians, like those which have been conducted in France and Finland. In those countries, it was found that centenarians were generally less fit than they had been in their nineties, and that almost all had some form of physical disability. As a broad generalisation, about a third were relatively healthy and about a third were definitely ill. (This last does not seem surprising, when it is remembered how many of the centenarians were near the end of their lives.) In Finland, about 20 per cent of the male and 50 per cent of the female centenarians

Table 27.7

Government Actuary's 1991-based projection of future numbers at high ages in England and Wales

	Aged 80–89	Aged 90–99	Aged 100 and over
Men		*thousands*	
1991	543	45	1
2001	637	83	1
2011	760	115	3
2021	918	158	5
2031	1,259	243	8
Women			
1991	1,161	178	4
2001	1,245	292	9
2011	1,297	367	19
2021	1,334	415	30
2031	1,812	494	37

Source: GAD

suffered from dementia. At the other extreme, there were many centenarians who were reported to be alert and to have good memories, particularly about family matters and the events of their youth. Often they were reported to have strong characters. A very curious and unexpected find in the French survey was that the proportion of centenarians with blue, blue-grey or green eyes was much higher than in the population as a whole.

Acknowledgement

This chapter includes material from Thatcher (1992) which was written as part of the Project on Maximal Length of Life of the Cambridge Group for the History of Population and Social Structure. Thanks are due to **Population Studies** for permission to reproduce Tables 27.1, 27.2 and 27.4.

Appendix A

International Classification of Diseases (ICD) codes used to define the diseases examined in chapters 16 to 22

CHAPTER 16

	1901–10 ICD1	1911–20 ICD2	1921–30 ICD3	1931–39 ICD4	1940–49 ICD5	1950–57 ICD6	1958–67 ICD7	1968–78 ICD8	1979– ICD9
Gonorrhoea	030	038.1-3	040.1-2, 039	035.1-2	025	030-035	030-035	098.0-9	098.0-9
Syphilis	029, 085, 091	037, 062, 067	038, 072, 076	034.1-2, 080, 083	030.1-5	020-029	020-029	090-097	090-097
PID	–	–	–	–	–	–	–	098.1, 612-614 615.1, 622	614.0-5, 614.7-9

CHAPTER 17

	1958–67 ICD7	1968–78 ICD8	1979–92 ICD9
All malignant neoplasms	140-207.1, 292.3, 294	140-209	140-208.9, 238.4, 289.8
Cancer of oesophagus		150	150
Cancer of stomach		151	151
Cancer of colon and rectum		153.0-8, 154	153, 154
Cancer of lung		162	162
Malignant melanoma of skin		172.0-4, 172.6-9	172
Cancer of breast (female)		174	174
Cancer of cervix		180	180
Cancer of ovary		183	183
Cancer of prostate		185	185
Cancer of testis		186	186
Cancer of nervous system		191, 192.0-3, 192.9	191, 192
Non-Hodgkin's lymphoma		200, 202	200, 202
Hodgkin's disease		201	201
Multiple myeloma		203	203
Leukaemia		204-207	204-208
Cancer of unspecified site		195, 199	195, 199

CHAPTER 18

Ischaemic heart disease

1921-30	ICD3	
	Fatty heart	90(5)
	Other unspecified myocardial disease	90(7)
	Arteriosclerosis without record of cardiovascular lesion	91(b)(2)
	Angina pectoris	89

1931-39	ICD4	
	Acute myocarditis	93a
	Fatty heart	93b(1)
	Cardio-vascular degeneration	93b(2)
	Other myocardial degeneration	93b(3)
	Myocarditis, not returned as acute or chronic	93c
	Diseases of the coronary arteries, Angina pectoris	94
	Arterio-sclerosis without record of cerebral lesion	97(3)

1940-49   ICD5

Acute myocarditis	93a
Chronic myocarditis specified as rheumatic	93b
Cardio-vascular degeneration	93c(1)
Myocardial degeneration described as fatty	93c(2)
Other myocardial degeneration	93c(3)
Myocarditis not distinguished as acute or chronic	93d
Diseases of the coronary arteries	94a
Angina pectoris without mention of coronary disease	94b

1950-57   ICD6

Arteriosclerotic heart disease, including coronary disease	420
Heart disease specified as involving coronary arteries	420.1
Angina pectoris without mention of coronary disease	420.2
Other myocardial degeneration	422
With arteriosclerosis	422.1
Other	422.2
Arteriosclerosis	450

1958-67   ICD7

Arteriosclerotic heart disease, including coronary disease (as stated)	420
- specified as involving coronary arteries	420.1
- Angina pectoris without mention of coronary disease	420.2
Other myocardial degeneration - Fatty degeneration	422
- With arteriosclerosis	422.1
- Other	422.2
Arterio-sclerosis	450

1968-78   ICD8

Acute myocardial infarction	410
Other acute and subacute forms of ischaemic heart disease	411
Chronic myocardial infarction	412
Angina pectoris	413
Asymptomatic ischaemic heart disease	414

1979-92   ICD9

Acute myocardial infarction	410
Other acute and subacute forms of ischaemic heart disease	411
Chronic Old myocardial infarction	412
Angina pectoris	413
Other forms of chronic ischaemic heart disease	414

Cerebrovascular disease

1901-10   ICD1

Apoplexy, hemiplegia	1070*
Cerebral haemorrhage, cerebral embolism	1060*
Softening of brain	840*

1911-20   ICD2

Apoplexy	64a
Serous apoplexy and oedema of brain	64b
Cerebral congestion	64c
Cerebral atheroma	64d
Cerebral haemorrhage	64e
Softening of brain	65
Hemiplegia	66a

1921-30   ICD3

Cerebral haemorrhage so returned	74a(1)
Apoplexy (lesion unstated)	74a(2)
Cerebral embolism	74b(1)
Cerebral thrombosis	74b(2)
Hemiplegia	75a
Cerebral softening	83
Arteriosclerosis with cerebral vascular lesion	91b(1)

1931-39 ICD4

Cerebral haemorrhage so returned	82a(1)
Apoplexy (lesion unstated)	82a(2)
Cerebral embolism	82b(1)
Cerebral thrombosis	82b(2)
Cerebral softening	82b(3)
Hemiplegia	82c(1)
Other paralysis of unstated origin	82c(2)
Arteriosclerosis, with cerebral haemorrhage	97(1)
Arteriosclerosis with record of other cerebral vascular lesion	97(2)

1940-49 ICD5

Cerebral haemorrhage	83a
Cerebral embolism, thrombosis and softening	83bc
Arteriosclerosis (ex. coronary or renal sclerosis or cerebral haemorrhage)	97

1950-67 ICD6 and ICD7

Subarachnoid haemorrhage	330
Cerebral haemorrhage	331
Cerebral embolism and thrombosis	332
Spasm of cerebral arteries	333
Other and ill-defined vascular lesions affecting central nervous system	334
Other cerebral paralysis	352

1968-78 ICD8

Psychosis associated with other cerebral condition	
– with cerebral arteriosclerosis	293
– with other cerebrovascular disturbances	293.1
Cerebrovascular disease	430-438
Other cerebral paralysis	344

1979- ICD9

Cerebrovascular disease	430-438
Arteriosclerotic dementia	290.4
Hemiplegia	342
Other paralytic syndromes	344

* No numbering was used for ICD1. The codes given are the computer codes used in the ONS historic deaths database

CHAPTER 19

	1901–10 ICD1	1911–20 ICD2	1921–30 ICD3	1931–39 ICD4	1940–49 ICD5	1950–57 ICD6	1958–67 ICD7	1968–78 ICD8	1979– ICD9
Parkinson's disease	–	–	084.4	087.3	087.3	350	350	342	332.0
Post-encephalitis Parkinsonism	–	–	023	017	032.2	083.0	083.0	066	310.8, 332.1
Motor neurone disease	–	–	–	081.1, 081.4	082.1	356	356	348	335.2
Dementia, including Alzheimer's disease	–	068, 154	164	084.2, 162	084.4, 162	304-306, 309, 794	304-306, 309, 794	290, 299, 794	290, 298.9, 331, 797
Senility without mention of psychosis	–	154.2	164.2	162.2	162.1, 162.3	794	794	794	797
Multiple sclerosis	–	–	084.3	087.4	087.4	345	345	340	340
Guillain-Barre syndrome (acute, infective or post infective polyneuritis)	–	073.2	082	087.2	087.2	364	364	354	357.0
Epilepsy	088	069	078	085	085	353	353	345	345
Myasthenia gravis	–	–	–	156.2	156.2	744.0	744.0	733.0	358.0

CHAPTER 20

	1901–10 ICD1	1911–20 ICD2	1921–30 ICD3	1931–39 ICD4	1940–49 ICD5	1950–57 ICD6	1958–67 ICD7	1968–78 ICD8	1979– ICD9
COPD									
Bronchiectasis						526	526	518	494
Bronchiectasis, bronchial catarrh, other bronchitis		89, 90							
Bronchitis, chronic and unqualified								490, 491	490, 491
Chronic bronchitis and bronchitis not distinguished as acute or chronic			99b, c, d	106b, c	106b, c				
Chronic bronchitis, bronchitis with emphysema, bronchitis (unqualified)						501, 502	501, 502		
Emphysema								492	492
Emphysema without mention of bronchitis							527.1		
Other obstructive airways disease								519.8	496
Pulmonary emphysema		97	106	113	113				
Asthma									
Asthma		96	105	112		241	241	493	
Asthma, unspecified									493.9
Asthma with 'flu as contrib. or secondary cause					112.1				
Asthma without any of above complications					112.6				
Emphysema, asthma	119								
Extrinsic asthma									493.0
Intrinsic asthma									493.1
Pneumonia									
Acute interstitial pneumonia								484	
Bronchopneumonia		91	100	107		491	491		
Bronchopneumonia (unspecified)								485	485
Bronchopneumonia with 'flu as a secondary or contributary cause					107.1				
Bronchopneumonia without 'flu					107.2				
Lobar pneumonia		92.1	101.1	108		490	490		
Lobar pneumonia with 'flu					108.1				
Lobar pneumonia without 'flu					108.2				
Other bacterial pneumonia								482.0-2, 482.4-9	482.0-4, 482.8-9
Pneumococcal pneumonia								481	481
Pneumonia - broncho	38								
Pneumonia - epidemic	37								
Pneumonia - lobar	36								
Pneumonia - not defined	39								486
Pneumonia (not otherwise defined)				109					
Pneumonia (other & unspecified)						493	493		
Pneumonia - other specified organism								483	483
Pneumonia (type not specified)		92.2	101.2						
Pneumonia (unspecified)								486	
Pneumonia (unspecified) with 'flu					109.1				
Pneumonia (unspecified) without 'flu					109.2				
Primary atypical pneumonia						492	492		
Staphylococcal pneumonia								482.3	
Viral pneumonia								480	480.0-2, 480.8-9
Lobar and pneumococcal pneumonia	36	92.1	101.1	108	108.1-2	490	490	481	481

CHAPTER 21

ICD revision, years covered:

(1)	1901-10
(2)	1911-20
(3)	1921-30
(4)	1931-39
(5)	1940-49
(6)	1950-57
(7)	1958-67
(8)	1968-78
(9)	1979-

Nephritis nephrosis nephrotic syndrome

ICD1	1430, 1440
2	1190, 1201, 1202, 1222, 1223
3	1280, 1290
4	1300, 1310, 1320
5	1300, 1311, 1312, 1313, 1320
6	590-4
7	590-4
8	580-4
9	580-7,589

Infection

ICD2	1221
3	1331 (cystitis)
4	1331 (pyelitis)
5	1351 (cystitis) 1331 (pyelitis)
6	600 (infection) 605 (cystitis)
7	600 (infection) 605 (cystitis)
8	590 (pyelitis) 595 (cystitis)
9	590 (pyelitis) 595 (cystitis)

Uraemia

ICD6	792 (uraemia nos coma) 788.9 (uraemia extrarenal)
7	792, 788.9
8	792, 788.9
9	792, 788.9

Other

ICD1	1470
2	1224
3	1310
4	1332
5	1332
6	603
7	603
8	593
9	593

ICD1	1560
2	1381, 1382, 1383
3	1480
4	1460.2
5	1401, 1442, 1470, 1480
6	640, 641, 642, 680, 685
7	640, 641, 642, 680, 685
8	635 636, 637, 639.9
9	635, 636, 639.3 642.1, 642.4-7, 646.2, 646.5, 646.6, 669.3

Tuberculosis

ICD1	0520 (TB other)
2	0343 (TB other)
3	0364 (TB Genitourinary)
4	0300 (TB Genitourinary)
5	0200 (ditto)
6	016 (ditto)
7	016
8	016
9	016

Calculus

ICD1	1450 (all)
2	1230 (all)
3	1320 (all)
4	1341 (ureter/kidney) 1342 (bladder) 1343 (unspec)
5	1341 (ureter/kidney) 1342 (bladder) 1343 (unspec)
6	602 (ureter/kidney) 604 (other)
7	602 (ureter/kidney) 604 (other)
8	592 (ureter/kidney) 594 (other)
9	592 (ureter/kidney(594 (other)

Prostate hyperplasia

ICD1	1460	(diseases of bladder prostate)
2	1260	(diseases of bladder prostate)
3	1350	(diseases of prostate)
4	1370.1	(diseases of prostate)
5	1371.2	(hyperplasia of prostate)
6	610	(ditto)
7	610	(ditto)
8	600	(ditto)
9	600	(ditto)

Prostatitis

ICD5	1372
6	611
7	611
8	601
9	601

Diabetes with renal disease

ICD8	250.5
9	250.3

Hypertension and renal

ICD8	403
9	403

Hypertensive heart and renal

ICD8	404
9	404

Congenital renal

ICD5	1583
6	752
7	757
8	753
9	753

Pueperal renal

Hydronephrosis

ICD6	601
7	601
8	591
9	591

CHAPTER 22

	1901–ICD1	1911–ICD2	1921–ICD3	1931–ICd4	1940–ICD5	1950–ICD6	1958–ICD7	1968–ICD8	From 1979 ICD9
Gastric ulcer/peptic ulcer	1250	1020	1111	1171	1171	540	540	531,533	531,533
Duodenal ulcer	–	1048	1112	1172	1172	541	541	532	532
Appendix acute	1310	1080	1170	1210	1211	550	540	540	540
Appendix, other	–	–	–	–	1212	551-553	541-543	541-543	541-543
Diverticular disease of colon	–	–	–	1232	1231	572.1	572.1	562.1	562.1
Irritable bowel disease and other non-infective non-ulcerative disorders	–	–	1131-1132	1191-1192	1191-1192	572.2	572.2	563.1	556
CD	–	–	–	–	–	572.0	572.0	563.0	555
Biliary tract disease Gall stones/Gall bladder disease	1370	1140	1230	1261-1262	1260	584-585	584-585	574-575	574-575
Other biliary disease	–	–	–	1271-1272	1271-1272	586	586	576	576

	ICD7 1958–67	ICD8 1968–78	ICD9 1979–
Abdominal pain	785.5	785.5	780.0
Rectal and anal pain	–	–	546.6
Anal fistula, fissure perianal abcess	574-575	565-566	565-566
Bleeding per rectum	–	–	569.3
Constipation	573.0	564.0	564.0
Irritable colon	573.1, 573.2	564.1	564.1, 564.5
Hiatus hernia	560.4	551.3	553.3
Haemorrhoids	461	455	455
Disorders of function of the stomach	544	536	536

Appendix B

Chronology of major events

Although this report covers health from 1841 to 1994, the likelihood of a person succumbing to disease may depend on previous experiences. For example those dying in 1841 may have been affected by disability and unemployment caused by the Napoleonic Wars, previous periods of hardship, and other factors. Thus this chronology begins some time before 1841. It has been constructed in the main to place major events that may have influenced health or health statistics in time. A few other well known events have been added for interest.

1802	Act introduced to limit the employment of children to under 12 hours per day.
1806	Installation of first steam-operated loom.
1819	Peterloo Massacre. Factory Act forbade the employment of children under the age of 9 in cotton mills. Queen Victoria born.
1825	First public steam railway – Stockton to Darlington.
1830	Publication of William Cobbett's *Rural Rides* describing the plight of the rural poor.
1832	Cholera arrived in GB for first time (from India) and 22,000 died by June. Reform Act (abolition of rotten boroughs, franchisement of new industrial towns).
1833	Factory Act legislation banned any employment of children under 9, restricted working hours of older children, appointed factory inspectors. First government grant to education.
1834	Poor Law Amendment Act passed – benefits for the poor reduced and workhouses established. Tollpuddle Martyrs convicted.
1836	Births and Deaths Registration Act and Marriage Act established Office of Registrar General. Enabled first national statistics on numbers of births, deaths and marriages to be produced. Thomas Lister appointed the first Registrar General.
1837	Victoria's reign began. Registrar General introduced births, deaths and marriages registrations from 1 July.
1839	William Farr introduced the first classification of causes of death, published in the Registrar General's first report.

——————— BEGINNING OF PERIOD COVERED BY THIS VOLUME ———————

1841	First census of population to be conducted by Registrar General
1842	Anaesthesia first used in an operation. Chadwick's *Report on the Condition of the Labouring Population of Great Britain. Coal Commission Report* published. *Children's Employment Commission Report* published.
1843	Royal Commission into state of large towns (reported 1844-45).
1844	Legislation extending protection of workers into mines and other industries.
1846	Corn Laws repealed. The office of Medical Officer of Health instituted in local authorities - responsible for producing an annual report (posts abolished 1974).
1848	Further major cholera outbreak (50-70,000 deaths, 14,000 in London). Public Health Act which created a central Board of Health, and empowered individual towns to set up local Medical Officers of Health. *The Communist Manifesto* was published.
1851	Lodging Houses Act – checked the worst abuses. The Great Exhibition. The 1851 census of population was the first to ask marital status and relationship to head of household.
1853-56	Crimean War.
1853	Smallpox vaccination of children within 4 months of birth made compulsory.
1854	Dickens published *Hard Times*. 10,675 cholera deaths in London.
1855	General Register Office (Scotland) established. London's "great stink".
1856	First synthetic dye produced. Bessemer converter invented for cheap steel production.
1860	Florence Nightingale published her *Notes on nursing,* set up training school for nurses.
1861	Semmelweis published research results linking dirt with infection (discovered 1848).
1862	Pasteur demonstrated link between bacteria and disease, invented pasteurization.
1865	Mid-year population estimates first produced for large towns.
1866	Public Health Act. Local Authorities to improve sanitation and appoint sanitary inspectors. London cholera epidemic – 5,000 died within 3 weeks.

1867	Passing of second Parliamentary Reform Act. Lister introduced antiseptic surgery, using carbolic acid. Marx published *Das Kapital*.
1868	Trades Union Congress founded.
1869	Lister introduced antisepsis into surgery – surgical mortality fell by two thirds.
1870	Foster's Education Act, providing virtually free elementary education for anyone wanting it. Schools financed in part from the rates. Major smallpox outbreak, 40,000 died, 10,000 in London.
1872	Public Health Act.
1874	Factory act introduced a 10 hour day, and raised age of employment of children to 10. Trade Unions acquired legal right to strike. Births and Deaths Registration Act transferred the obligation to register births and deaths from the registrar to the person directly concerned; certification of cause of death by a doctor now required.
1875	Public Health Act – set standards for sanitation in new houses. Compelled notification of all cases of cholera. Artisan's Dwelling Act – gave local authorities the power to clear slums.
1876	Robert Koch identified bacteria that cause tuberculosis, anthrax and cholera. Bell invented the telephone.
1880	Education up to age 10 years of age was made compulsory.
1881	Census of population. Mid-year population estimates produced for **all** registration counties and large towns.
1882	Koch discovered tuberculosis bacillus.
1883	Klebs and Loffler discovered diphtheria bacillus, leading to development of antitoxin.
1881-85	Cell division described by Walther Fleming. Pasteur used attenuated bacteria to confer immunity against rabies and anthrax. Motor cars invented by Karl Benz.
1889	Notification of certain infectious diseases made compulsory in London. Sterilisation of surgical instruments by dry heat introduced.
1892	Diphtheria antitoxin isolated by Paul Ehrlich.
1883	Government established special education for blind and deaf children.
1884	Passing of third Parliamentary Reform Act.
1895-96	Roentgen discovers X-rays. Diesel invented the diesel engine. Becquerel discovered radioactivity.
1897-98	Ronald Ross discovered that malaria was transmitted by the mosquito. Beijerinck discovered viruses. Aspirin first marketed.
1899	Boer War. Notification of infectious diseases made compulsory in **every** urban, rural and port sanitary district in England and Wales. Local authorities given powers to provide special schools for the "educable mentally subnormal".
1900	Seebohm Rowntree investigated poverty in York.
1901	Queen Victoria died. Age of employment for children raised to 12. ABO blood grouping discovered.
1903-06	First sustained flight (Wright brothers). Einstein's special theory of relativity. Vitamins recognised as essential to health. Charles Booth - *Life and Labour of the People in London* (1891-1903).
1908	Old Age Pensions Act
1909	Chromosomes established as carriers of heredity.
1911	National Health Insurance Act. Census of population - first to ask fertility questions. Registrar General's "social classes" introduced as means of analysing population statistics according to the general standing in the community of occupation/employment groups. Second revision of the International list of causes of deaths adopted by the Registrar General.
1914-1918	First World War
1917	Bolshevik Revolution in Russia.
1918	Representation of People Act. Gave the vote to all males over 21, and females over 30 with property qualifications.
1919-38	Great Depression. 2.8 million unemployed in 1932.
1919	Ministry of Health established.
1920	Age of employment of children raised to 14.
1922	Insulin isolated, and used for the first time to treat diabetics.
1926	General Strike. First Adoption of Children Act. Legitimacy Act. Births and Deaths Registration Act – made it unlawful to dispose of a body before the registrar's certificate or coroner's order had been issued. Also required the registration of stillbirths.
1927	Still births first registered.
1928	Universal adult suffrage. Anti-bacterial activity of penicillium mould was discovered by Alexander Fleming (but not made stable enough for medical use until 1939).
1929	Marriage Act – increased the minimum age from 12 for girls and 14 for boys to 16 years for both.
1931	Census of population – "usual address" question introduced.
1932	Sulphonamide antibiotic discovered, shown to be effective against streptococcal septicaemia. Modern drip methods perfected, enabling advanced surgery.
1934	First radioisotopes produced by the Curies.

1939-1945	Second World War. First nuclear reactor. Penicillin used for first time. Kidney machine invented. DDT invented. Synthetic fertilisers produced. First nuclear bombs used in war.
1939	National Registration Act – provided for establishment of a national register of the entire population maintained by GRO. Identity cards were issued. Penicillin manufactured in quantity.
1940s	Mass immunisation against diphtheria in Britain.
1941	Wartime Social Survey formed. National Insurance Act – compensated for "industrial diseases and injuries".
1944	Disabled Persons Act. Streptomycin discovered – active against tuberculosis.
1948	National Health Service Act. World Health Organisation established. Cancer registration scheme introduced. National Assistance Act – gave local authorities responsibility for providing accommodation and welfare services for people in their area who required it on account of age, infirmity and other circumstances.
1950s	BCG vaccination against tuberculosis introduced in Britain. Betablockers developed for treating hypertension. Ultrasound developed.
1951	Census of population – questions about household amenities (e.g. WCs) introduced.
1952-55	Food rationing ended. Polio vaccine developed. Oral contraception introduced. Link between smoking and lung cancer proposed.
1952	National Health Service Central Register set up from National Registration records.
1953	Hospital In-patient Enquiry first carried out.
1956	Clean Air Act, after 4,000 died in 1952 London smog.
1957	Family Expenditure Survey started on behalf of Department of Employment.
1960s	Kidney machine developed. Benzodiazepines developed. First renal transplants undertaken. Cytotoxic chemotherapy became standard for a number of cancers including leukaemia and Wilms' tumour.
1961	Census of Population – some small area statistics published for first time.
1962	Royal College of Physicians report on *Smoking and Health* recommended restrictions on tobacco advertising, increasing taxation on cigarettes, etc. Doll and Hill published their findings linking cigarettes to lung cancer in the mid 1960s.
1964	Congenital malformations reported for first time on national basis.
1966	First heart transplant. Sample census – questions on car availability and means of transport to work introduced.
1967	Penicillin nucleus isolated, leading to new antibiotics.
1968	Legal abortions statistics collected for first time. Regional population projections started.
1969	Family Law Reform Act reduced age of majority from 21 to 18.
1970	General Register Office and Government Social Survey combined to form the Office of Population Censuses and Surveys – OPCS. The General Household Survey began. Chronically Sick and Disabled Persons Act – to help families cope with appreciably or severely handicapped members at home (unemployable and employable treated the same for first time).
1973	Britain joined European Community (EC). OPCS Longitudinal Study set up.
1975	Live birth weight information collected by OPCS.
1977	British scientist discovered complete genetic structure of a virus.
1978	British first test tube baby born.
1979	"Thatcher Revolution" – powers of unions curbed, number of home owners increased, Monetarism, privatisation.
1981	Industrial Diseases (Notification) Act – certification of deaths and recording of information relating to industrial diseases. Brixton and Liverpool riots. Over 3 million unemployed. First reported AIDS cases in UK. First heart-lung transplant. WHO published *Global Strategy for Health for All by the Year 2000*.
1982	Falklands War.
1983	Seat belts made compulsory. Labour Force Survey expanded to become annual and continuous.
1984	Coalminers' strike. Famine in Ethiopia.
1986	Chernobyl nuclear reactor meltdown. Greater London Council abolished.
1987	Regan and Gorbachev agreed to begin nuclear disarmament. Gorbachev began reforms of Soviet Union.
1989	Berlin Wall demolished. Fall of communist governments in Poland, East Germany, Hungary, Czechoslavakia, Bulgaria and Romania.
1991	Germany reunited. Gulf War. Census of population – introduced new questions on ethnicity and limiting longstanding illness. Communism collapsed in the USSR. Treaty of Maastricht signed. Green Paper – *Health of the Nation* – published.

Appendix C

Referees

The Authors would like to thank the following people for being referees:

Dr John Ashley
Dr John Ashton
Roger Black
Nick Bosenquet
Bev Botting
Carol Brayne
Peter Burney
Janet Cade
Mike Catchpole
Susan Cole
Michèl Coleman
Derek Cook
Cyrus Cooper
Mike D'Souza
Tim Devis
Stuart Donnon
Karen Dunnell
Grimley Evans
Douglas Fleming
Spence Galbraith
Adrian Gallop
Eileen Goddard
Jan Gregory
Andy Hall
Walter Holland
Jen Hollowell

Derek Jewell
Heather Joshi
Ken Judge
Sue Kelly
David Kerr
Tim Key
Johan Mackenbach
Netar Mallick
Hugh Markowe
Mark McCarthy
Anna McCormick
Alison Macfarlane
Mike Murphy
Clive Osmond
Stephen Palmer
Mike Quinn
Roberto Rona
Anthony Seaton
Gerry Shaper
Sally Sheard
Steve Smallwood
Jillian Smith
David Strachen
Rober Waller
Charles Warlow
Jean Weddle

References

Chapter 15 Infection in England and Wales, 1938–1993

Abbott JD, Jones DM, Painter MJ and Young SEJ (1985), The epidemiology of meningococcal infections in England and Wales, 1912–1983, *Journal of Infection*, 11: 241–57.

Anderson ES, Galbraith NS and Taylor CED (1961), An outbreak of human infection due to Salmonella typhimurium phage-type 20a associated with infection in calves, *Lancet*, 1: 854–58.

Anonymous (1950), Food poisoning in England and Wales, 1941–48, *Monthly Bulletin of the Ministry of Health and the Public Health Laboratory Service*, 9, pp.148–58.

Anonymous (1994), Of mice and milkmaids, cats and cowpox, *Lancet*, 1: 67.

Bannister BA (1990), Infection and the traveller, *Reviews in Medical Microbiology*, 1: 185–95.

Begg N and Nicoll A (1994), Immunisation, *British Medical Journal*, 309: 1073–5.

Beveridge WJB (1977), *Influenza: the Last Great Plague: An unfinished story of discovery*, New York.

Bisno AL (1991), Group A streptococcal infections and acute rheumatic fever, *New England Journal of Medicine*, 325: 783–93.

Blacklow NR and Greenberg HB (1991), Viral gastroenteritis. *New England Journal of Medicine*, 325: 252–64.

Bloom BR and Murray CJL (1992), Tuberculosis: commentary on a reemergent killer, *Science*, 257: 1055–64.

Bourke SJ (1993ʃ, Chlamydial respiratory infections, *British Medical Journal*, 306: 1219–20.

Bremner JAG (1994), Hantavirus infections and outbreaks in 1993, *Communicable Disease Report*, 4: R5–9.

Brown DW (1993), Filoviruses and imported non-human primates, *PHLS Microbiology Digest*, 10: 195–7.

Bruce-Chwatt LJ (1977), Jet-borne pestilences: today and tomorrow, *Health and Hygiene*, 1: 61–76.

Campbell H (1965), Changes in mortality trends: England and Wales 1931–1961, in *Vital and Health Statistics*, Washington DC: National Centre for Health Statistics, Series 3,3.

Casemore DP (1990), Epidemiological aspects of human cryptosporidiosis, *Epidemiology and Infection*, 104: 14–28.

Cheasty T and Rowe B (1994), New cholera strains, *PHLS Microbiology Digest*, 11: 73–6.

Citron KM, Southern A and Dixon M (1995), *Out of the shadow*, London: Crisis.

Cockburn TA (1959), The evolution of infectious diseases, *International Record of Medicine*, 172: 493–508.

Cockburn A (1967) (ed.), *Infectious Diseases, their Evolution and Eradication*, Springfield, Illinois: Thomas.

Cook GC (1992), Effect of global warming on the distribution of parasitic and other infectious diseases: a review, *Journal of Royal Soc Med*, 85: 688–91.

Cotterall RD (1981), Biological effects of sexual freedom, *Lancet*, 1: 315–19.

Cover TL and Aber RC (1989), Yersinia enterocolitica, *New England Journal of Medicine*, 321: 16–24.

Cowden J (1992), Campylobacter: epidemiological paradoxes, *British Medical Journal*, 305: 132–3.

Cowden JM, Lynch D, Joseph CA, O'Mahony M, Mawer SL, Rowe B and Bartlett CLR (1989), Case-control study of infections with Salmonella enteritidis phage type 4 in England, *British Medical Journal*, 299: 771–3.

Darbyshire JH (1995), Tuberculosis: old reasons for a new increase? *British Medical Journal*, 310: 954–5.

Farr W (1885), in *Vital Statistics: A memorial volume of selections from the reports and writings of William Farr*, Humphreys (1885), republished Metuchen, New Jersey, 1975: Scarecrow Press.

Galbraith NS (1982), Communicable disease surveillance, in *Recent Advances in Community Medicine* (ed. Smith A), London: Churchill Livingstone, pp.127–41.

Galbraith NS (1985), Infectious disease and human travel, in *Recent Advances in Community Medicine* (ed. Smith A), London: Churchill Livingstone, pp.181–203.

Gale AH (1959), *Epidemic Diseases*, London: Spottiswoode.

Gilbert RJ and Roberts D (1990), Foodborne gastroenteritis, in *Topley and Wilson's Principles of Bacteriology, Virology and Immunity*, 8th edn, (eds Parker MT, Deurden BI), 3, Chapter 78, London: Edward Arnold.

Gilbert RJ, McLauchlin J and Velani SK (1993), The contamination of paté by Listeria monocytogenes in England and Wales in 1989 and 1990, *Epidemiology and Infection*, 110: 543–51.

Glover JA (1920), *Special Report Series, Meningococcal Meningitis*, Medical Research Council, 50, London: HMSO.

Glover JA (1947), The enigma of notified dysentery, *Monthly Bulletin of the Ministry of Health and Public Health Laboratory Service*, 6: 46–53.

Hayward AC and Watson JM (1995), Tuberculosis in England and Wales 1982–1993:notifications exceeded predictions, *Communicable Disease Report*, 5: R29–33.

Healing TD, Greenwood MH and Pearson AD (1992), Campylobacters and enteritis, *Reviews in Medical Microbiology*, 3: 159–67.

Hutchinson RI (1956), Some observations on the method of spread of Sonne dysentery, *Monthly Bulletin of the Ministry of Health and Public Health Laboratory Service*, 15: 110–18.

Ispahani P, Donald FE and Aveline AJD (1988), Streptococcus pyogenes bacteraemia: an old enemy subdued, but not defeated, *Journal of Infection*, 16: 37–46.

Lederberg J, Shope RE and Oaks SC (1992), *Emerging infections, Microbial threats to Health in the United States*, Washington DC: National Academic Press.

Logan WPD (1950), Mortality in England and Wales from 1848 to 1947, *Population Studies*, 4: 132–78.

Loudon I (1987), Puerperal fever, the streptococcus, and the sulphonamides, 1911–1945, *British Medical Journal*, 295: 485–90.

Ma P, Govinda S, Visvesara AJ, Theodore FH, Daggett PM and Sawyer TK (1990), Neaglaria and acanthamoeba infections: Review, *Reviews of Infectious Diseases*, 12: 490–513.

Martini GA (1973), Marburg virus disease, *Postgrad Med J*, 49: 542–46.

McCoy JH (1975), Trends in salmonella food poisoning in England and Wales 1941–72, *Journal of Hygiene, Cambridge*, 74: 271–82.

McKeown T and Lowe CR (1974), *An Introduction to Social Medicine*, Oxford: Blackwell, pp.3–22.

Meers PD, Ayliffe GAJ, Emmerson AM, Leigh DA, Mayon-White RT, Mackintosh CA and Strange JL (1981), Report on the National Survey of Infection in Hospitals, 1980, *Journal of Hospital Infection*, 2, (Suppl): 1–51.

Moro ML and McCormick A (1988), Surveillance for communicable disease, in *Surveillance in Health and Disease* (eds Eylenbosch WJ, Noah ND), Oxford: Oxford University Press, pp.166–82.

Mortimer PP (1995), Arsphenamine jaundice and the recognition of instrument-borne virus infection, *Genitourinary Medicine*, 71: 109–19.

Murphy FA (1994), New, emerging, and reemerging infectious diseases, *Advances in Virus Research*, 43: 1–52.

Nieman RE and Lorber B (1980), Listeriosis in adults: a changing pattern. Report of eight cases and review of the literature, 1968–1978, *Review of Infectious Diseases*, 2: 207–27.

Nissel M (1987), *People Count: A history of the General Register Office*, London: HMSO, pp. 120–22.

O'Connell S (1993), Lyme disease: a review, *Communicable Disease Report*, 3: R111–115.

O'Mahony M, Mitchell E, Gilbert RJ, Hutchinson DN, Begg NT, Rodhouse JC and Morris JE (1990), An outbreak of foodborne botulism associated with contaminated hazelnut yoghurt, *Epidemiology and Infection*, 104: 389–95.

OPCS (1992), *Mortality Statistics, Serial tables. Review of the Registrar General on deaths in England and Wales, 1841-1990*, OPCS series DH1 no. 25, London: HMSO.

Orton WT and Henderson WG (1972), The infected terrapin, *Community Medicine*, 127: 89–92.

Palmer SR and Rowe B (1986), Trends in salmonella infection, *PHLS Microbiology Digest*, 3: 18–21.

Pattison JR (1994), Human parvovirus B19, *British Medical Journal*, 308: 149–50.

Pelling M (1978), *Cholera, Fever and English Medicine, 1825–1865*, Oxford: Oxford University Press, pp.1–33.

PHLS Communicable Disease Surveillance Centre (1991), Communicable disease report, *J Public Health Med*, 13: 127–34.

PHLS Communicable Disease Surveillance Centre (1993), Quarterly communicable disease review, *J Public Health Med*, 15: 358–66.

Poolman JT, Lind I, Jonsdottir K, Froholm LO, Jones DM and Zanen HC (1986), Meningococcal serotypes and serogroup B disease in north-west Europe, *Lancet*, 2: 555–8.

Rao VR, Joannes RF, Kilbane P and Galbraith NS (1980), Outbreak of tuberculosis after minimal exposure to infection, *British Medical Journal*, 2: 187–9.

Report (1904), *Report of the Committee on Physical Deterioration*, Cmd 2175, London: HMSO.

Report (1994), Joint Tuberculosis Committee of the British Thoracic Society. Control and prevention of tuberculosis in the United Kingdom: Code of Practice 1994, *Thorax*, 49: 1193–1200.

Sandwith FM (1914), Dysentery, *Lancet*, 2: 638–42.

Savage WG (1913), *Report to the Local Government Board on Bacterial Food Poisoning and Food Infections, Report to the Local Government Board on Public Health and Medical Subjects*, New Series no. 77.

Selwyn S (1991), Hospital infection: the first 250 years, *Journal of Hospital Infection*, 18 (Suppl A): 5–64.

Shortridge KF and Stuart-Harris CH (1982), An influenza epicentre? *Lancet*, 2: 812–13.

Simpson J (1871), *Anaesthesia, Hospitalism, Hermaphroditism, and Proposals to stamp out Smallpox and other Contagious Diseases*, Edinburgh: Adam & Charles Black, p.291.

Small PM, Hopewell PC, Singh SP, Paz A, Parsonnet J, Ruston DC, Schecter GF, Daley CL and Schoolnik GK (1994), The epidemiology of tuberculosis in San Francisco. A population-based study using conventional and molecular methods, *N Engl J Med*, 330: 1703–9.

Stersky A, Todd E and Pivnik H (1980), Food poisoning associated with post-process leakage (PPL) in canned foods, *Journal of Food Protection*, 43: 465–76.

Teo CG (1992), The virology and serology of hepatitis: an overview, *Communicable Disease Report*, 2: R109–114.

Thomas A, Chart H, Cheasty T, Smith HR, Frost JA and Rowe R (1993), Vero cytotoxin-producing Escherichia coli, particularly serogroup O157, associated with human infections in the United Kingdom, *Epidemiology and Infection*, 110: 591–600.

Turnbull PCB (1979), Food poisoning with special reference to salmonella - Its epidemiology, pathogenesis and control, *Clinics in Gastroenterology*, 8: 663–714.

Underwood EA (1947), The history of cholera in Great Britain, *Proceedings of R Soc Med*, 41: 165–73.

Warburton ARE, Jenkins PA, Waight PA and Watson JM (1993), Drug resistance in initial isolates of Mycobacterium tuberculosis in England and Wales, 1982–1991, *Communicable Disease Report*, 3: R175–179.

Watson JM, Meredith SK, Whitmore-Overton E, Bannister R and Darbyshire JH (1993), Tuberculosis and HIV: estimates of the overlap in England and Wales, *Thorax*, 48: 199–203.

Webster RG (1994), While awaiting the next pandemic of influenza A, *British Medical Journal*, 309: 1179–80.

Williams REO, Blowers R, Garrod LP and Shooter R (1960), *Hospital Infection: Causes and Prevention*, London: Lloyd-Luke.

Winner SJ, Eglin RP, Moore VIM and Mayon-White RT (1987), An outbreak of Q fever affecting postal workers in Oxfordshire, *Journal of Infection*, 14: 255–61.

Chapter 16 Communicable diseases: sexually transmitted diseases, including AIDS

Adler MW (1980a), The terrible peril: a historical perspective on the venereal diseases, *British Medical Journal*, 281: 206–11.

Adler MW (1980b), Trends for gonorrhoea and pelvic inflammatory disease in England and Wales and for gonorrhoea in a defined population, *Am J Obstet Gynecol*, 138: 901–4.

Adler MW, Belsey EN and Rogers J (1981), Sexually transmitted diseases in a defined population for women, *British Medical Journal*, 283: 20–33.

Centers for Disease Control (1981), Pneumocystis pneumonia – Los Angeles, *Morbid Mortal Weekly Rep*, 30: 250–2.

Communicable Diseases (Scotland) Unit (1993), *Acquired Immune Deficiency Syndrome and HIV-related Disease in Scotland. Report of a working group convened by the Chief Medical Officer*, The Scottish Office, Home and Health Department (Chairman Dr D Reid), CD(S)U, Glasgow.

Concorde Co-ordinating Committee (1994), Concorde: MRC/ANRS randomised double-blind controlled trial of immediate and deferred zidovudine in symptom-free HIV infection, *Lancet*, 343: 871–80.

Evans B, Catchpole M, Heptonstall J, Mortimer P, McGarigle and Nicoll A (1993), *British Medical Journal*, 306: 426–8.

Eyster E, Gail MH, Ballard JO, Al-Mondhiry H and Goedert JJ (1987), Natural history of human immunodeficiency virus infections in haemophiliacs: effects of T-cell subsets, platelet counts, and age. *Ann Intern Med*, 107: 1–6.

Giesecke J, Johnson AM, Hawkins A, Noone A, Nicoll A, Wadsworth J, Wellings K and Field J (1994), An estimate of the prevalence of human immunodeficiency virus infection in England and Wales by using a direct method, *J R Stat Soc A*, 157: 89–103.

Jacobson L and Westrom L (1969), Objectivised diagnosis of pelvic inflammatory disease, *Am J Obstet Gynecol*, 105: 1088.

Johnson AM and Gill ON (1989), Evidence for recent changes in sexual behaviour in homosexual men in England and Wales, *Phil Trans R Soc Lond B*, 325: 153–61.

Johnson AM, Wadsworth J, Wellings K, Bradshaw S and Field J (1992), Sexual lifestyles and HIV risk, *Nature*, 360: 410–12.

Johnson A, Wadsworth J, Wellings K and Field J (1994), *Sexual Attitudes and Lifestyles*, Oxford: Blackwell Scientific Press.

Lundgren JD, Pederson C, Clumeck N *et al.* (1994a), Survival differences in European patients with AIDS, 1979–1989, *British Medical Journal*, 308: 1068–73.

Lundgren JD, Phillips AN, Pedersen C, Clumeck N, Gatell JM, Johnson AM *et al.* (1994b), Comparison of long-term prognosis of patients with AIDS treated and not treated with zidovudine, *JAMA*, 271: 1088–92.

McCormick A (1994), The impact of human immunodeficiency virus on the population of England and Wales, *Population Trends*, 76: 40–5.

Morris M (1917), *The Nation's Health*, London: Cassel.

Osler W (1917), The campaign against venereal disease. *British Medical Journal*, i: 694–6.

Report of a Working Group (Chairman: Professor NE Day) (1993), The incidence and prevalence of AIDS and other severe HIV disease in England and Wales for 1992-1997: projection using data to the end of June 1992, *Commun Dis Rep*, 3 (suppl 1): S1–17.

Report of a Working Group (Chairman: Professor NE Day) (1996), The incidence and prevalence of AIDS and other severe HIV disease in England and Wales for 1995–1999: projection using data to the end of June 1994. *Commun Dis Rep*, January 1996, vol 6, no 1.

Royal Commission on Venereal Diseases (1916), *Final Report of the Commissioners*, Cmnd 8189, London: HMSO.

Unlinked Anonymous HIV Surveys Steering Group (1995), *Unlinked Anonymous HIV Prevalence Monitoring Programme: England and Wales*, Department of Health.

World Health Organization (1994), *Weekly Epidemiol Rec*, 69: 5–8.

Chapter 17 Time trends in cancer incidence and mortality in England and Wales

Barnes N, Cartwright RA, O'Brien C, Richards IDG, Roberts B and Bird CC (1986), Rising incidence of lymphoid malignancies – true or false? *Br J Cancer*, 53: 393–8.

Beral V (1974), Cancer of the cervix: a sexually transmitted infection? *Lancet*, i: 1037–40.

Beral V, Fraser P and Chilvers C (1978), Does pregnancy protect against ovarian cancer? *Lancet*, i: 1083–7.

Beral V, Hermon C, Reeves G and Peto R (1995), Sudden fall in breast cancer death rates in England and Wales, *Lancet*, 345: 1642–3.

Berrino F, Sant M, Verdecchia A, Capocaccia R, Hakulinen T and Estève J (1995), *Survival of Cancer Patients in Europe: The EUROCARE study*, IARC Scientific Publications no. 132, Lyon: IARC.

Coleman MP, Estève J, Damiecki P, Arsalan A and Renard H (1993), *Trends in Cancer Incidence and Mortality*, IARC Scientific Publications no. 121, Lyon: IARC.

Cuzick J (1994), 'Multiple myeloma', in Trends in Cancer Incidence and Mortality (eds Doll R, Fraumeni JF Jr and Muir CS), *Cancer Surveys*, 19: 455–74.

Dann TC and Roberts DF (1993), Menarcheal age in University of Warwick young women, *J Biosoc Sci*, 25: 531–8.

Davies JM (1981), Testicular cancer in England and Wales: some epidemiological aspects, *Lancet*, i: 928–32.

Doll R (1990), Are we winning the fight against cancer? An epidemiological assessment, EACR – Mühlbock Memorial lecture, *Eur J Cancer*, 26: 500–8.

dos Santos Silva I and Swerdlow AJ (1995), Recent trends in incidence and mortality from breast, ovarian and endometrial cancers in England and Wales and their relation to changing fertility and oral contraceptive use, *Br J Cancer*, 72: 485–92.

Early Breast Cancer Trialists' Collaborative Group (1992), Systemic treatment of early breast cancer by hormonal, cytotoxic, or immune therapy: 133 randomised trials involving 31,000 recurrences and 24,000 deaths among 75,000 women, *Lancet*, 339: 1–15, 71–85.

Forman D, Pike MC, Davey G, Dawson S, Baker K, Chilvers CED, Oliver RTD and Coupland CAC (1994), Aetiology of testicular cancer: association with congenital abnormalities, age at puberty, infertility, and exercise, *Br Med J*, 308: 1393–9.

Grulich AE, Swerdlow AJ, dos Santos Silva I and Beral V (in press), Is the apparent rise in cancer mortality in the elderly real? *Int J Cancer*.

Henderson BE, Depue RH and Pike MC (1983), Estrogen exposure during gestation and risk of testicular cancer, *J Natl Cancer Inst*, 71: 1151–5.

MAFF (1991), *Household Food Consumption and Expenditure 1990: Annual Report of the National Food Survey Committee*, London: HMSO.

OPCS (1983), *Mortality Statistics: Comparison of 8th and 9th Revisions of the International Classification of Diseases, 1978 (sample)*, OPCS series DHI no. 10, London: HMSO.

OPCS (1986), *Cancer Survival 1979–81, Registrations*, OPCS Monitor MB1 86/2, London: HMSO.

Potosky AL, Kessler L, Gridley G, Brown CB and Horm JW (1990), Rise in prostatic cancer incidence associated with increased use of transurethral resection, *J Natl Cancer Inst*, 82: 1624–8.

Spring JA and Buss DH (1977), Three centuries of alcohol in the British diet, *Nature*, 270: 567–72.

Swerdlow AJ (1986), Cancer registration in England and Wales: some aspects relevant to interpretation of the data, *J Royal Stat Soc A*, 149: 146–60.

Swerdlow AJ, Douglas AJ, Vaughan Hudson G and Vaughan Hudson B (1993), Completeness of cancer registration in England and Wales: an assessment based on 2,145 patients with Hodgkin's disease independently registered by the British National Lymphoma Investigation, *Br J Cancer*, 67: 326–9.

Swerdlow A and dos Santos Silva I (1993), *Atlas of Cancer Incidence in England & Wales 1968–85*, Oxford: Oxford University Press.

The Brewer's and Licensed Retailers Association (1994), *Statistical Handbook,* London: Brewing Publications Ltd.

Wald N, Kiryluk S, Darby S, Doll R, Pike M and Peto R (eds) (1988), *UK Smoking Statistics*, Oxford: Oxford University Press.

World Health Organization (1967), *Manual of the International Statistical Classification of Diseases, Injuries, and Causes of Death*, Eighth Revision, Geneva: WHO.

World Health Organization (1978), *Manual of the International Statistical Classification of Diseases, Injuries, and Causes of Death,* Ninth Revision, Geneva: WHO.

Chapter 18 Cardiovascular diseases

Acheson R and Sanderson C (1978), Strokes: social class and geography, *Population Trends*, 12: 13–17.

Acheson RM and Williams DRR (1983), Does the consumption of fruit and vegetables protect against stroke?, *Lancet*, i: 1191–3.

Acierno LJ (1994), *The History of Cardiology*, London: Parthenon.

Anderson R (1992), *The Aftermath of Stroke: the Experiences of Patients and their Families*, Cambridge: University Press, Cambridge.

Anderson TW and Le Riche WH (1970), Ischaemic heart disease and sudden death 1901–1961, *British Journal of Preventive and Social Medicine*, 24: 1–9.

Antonovsky (1968), Social class and the major cardiovascular diseases, *Journal of Chronic Diseases*, 21: 65–106.

Alpha-Tocopherol Beta Carotene Cancer Prevention Study Group (1994), The effect of Vitamin E and beta carotene on the incidence of lung cancer and other cancers in male smokers, *New England Journal of Medicine*, 330: 1029–35.

Balarajan K (1991), Ethnic differences in mortality from ischaemic heart disease and cerebrovascular disease in England and Wales, *British Medical Journal*, 302: 560–4.

Barker DJP and Osmond C (1986), Diet and coronary heart disease in England and Wales during and after the second world war, *Journal of Epidemiology and Community Health*, 40: 37–44.

Barker DJP (1992), *Fetal and infant origins of disease in adult life*, London: British Medical Association.

Baum HM and Goldstein M (1982), Cerebrovascular diseases type specific mortality: 1968–1977, *Stroke*, 13: 810–17.

Beaglehole R (1986), Medical management and the decline in mortality from coronary heart disease, *British Medical Journal*, 92: 33–35.

Ben-Shlomo Y, Davey Smith G, Shipley M and Marmot MG (1994), What determines mortality risk in male former cigarette smokers?, *American Journal of Public Health*, 84: 1235–42.

Bonita R, Scragg R, Stewart A, Jackson R and Beaglehole R (1986), Cigarette smoking and risk of premature stroke in men and women, *British Medical Journal*, 293: 6–8.

Bonita R and Beaglehole R (1989), Increased treatment of hypertension does not explain the decline in stroke mortality in the United States, 1970–1980, *Hypertension* 13: I 69–73.

Bonita R, Stewart A and Beaglehole R (1990), International trends in stroke mortality: 1970–1985, *Stroke*, 21: 989–92.

Bordia AK (1980), The effect of vitamin C on blood lipids, fibrinolytic activity and platelet adhesiveness in patients with coronary artery disease, *Atherosclerosis*, 35: 181–7.

Britton M (1990), *Mortality and Geography – a Review in the mid–1980s*, OPCS series DS no. 9, London: HMSO.

Brown BG, Zha O, X-Q, Sacco DE and Albers JJ (1993), Lipid lowering and plaque regression: new insights into prevention of plaque disruption and clinical events in coronary disease?, *Circulation*, 87: 1781–91.

Brunner E, Davey Smith G, Marmot M, Canner R, Beksinska M and O'Brien J (1996), Childhood social circumstances and psychological and behavioural factors as determinants of plasma fibrinogen, *Lancet*, 347: 1008–13.

Burnand B and Feinstein AR (1992), The role of diagnostic in consistency in changing rates of occurrence for coronary heart disease, *Journal of Clinical and Epidemiology*, 45: 929–40.

Burke GL, Sprafka JM, Folsom AR, Hahn LP, Leupker RV and Blackburn H (1991), Trends in serum cholesterol levels from 1980 to 1987, *New England Journal of Medicine*, 324: 941–6.

Campbell H (1963a), Death rate from disease of the heart: 1876–1959, *British Medical Journal*, ii: 528–35.

Campbell H (1963b), The main cause of increased death rate from disease of the heart: 1920–1959, *British Medical Journal*, ii: 712–17.

Campbell H (1965), *Changes in Mortality Trends: England and Wales*, Vital and health statistics USDHEW NCHS series 3 no. 3, Washington DC.

Charlton JRH (1996), Which areas are healthiest?, *Population Trends*, 83: 17–24.

Clayton DG, Taylor D and Shaper AG (1977), Trends in heart disease in England and Wales 1950–73, *Health Trends*, 9: 1–6.

Clayton DG and Schifflers E (1987), Models for temporal variation in cancer rates I: age-period and age-cohort models, *Statistics in Medicine*, 6: 449–67.

Collins R, Peto R, MacMahon S, Herbert P, Fiebach NH, Eberlein KA, Godwin J, Qizilbash N, Taylor JO and Hennekens CH (1990), Blood pressure, stroke and coronary heart disease: part 2, short term reductions in blood pressure: an overview of randomised drug trials in the epidemiological context, *Lancet*, 335: 827–38.

Cox C, Mann J, Sutherland W and Ball M (1995), Individual variation in plasma cholesterol response to dietary saturated fat, *British Medical Journal*, 311: 1260–4.

Davey Smith G, Shipley MJ and Rose G (1990), The magnitude and causes of socio-economic differentials in mortality: further evidence from the Whitehall study, *Journal of Epidemiology and Community Health*, 44: 260–5.

Davey Smith G and Marmot M (1991), Trends in mortality in Britain 1920–86, *Annals of Nutrition and Metabolism*, 35 (suppl 1): 53–63.

Davey Smith G, Shipley M, Marmot MG and Rose G (1992), Plasma cholesterol concentration and mortality: The Whitehall Study, *Journal of the American Medical Association*, 267: 70–6.

Davey Smith G and Ben-Shlomo Y (1996), Flavanoids intake and coronary mortality; objective data trials are needed, *British Medical Journal*, 312: 1479–80.

Davey Smith G (1997), Socioeconomic differentials, in *Lifecourse Influences on Adult Disease* (eds Kuh D, Ben-Schlomo Y,) Oxford: Oxford University Press (in press).

De Bouver E, De Bacquer D, Braeckman L, Bael G, Rosseneu M and De Backer G (1995), Relation of fibrinogen to lifestyles and to cardiovascular risk factors in a working population, *International Journal of Epidemiology*, 24(5): 915–21.

Devis T (1993), Measuring mortality differences by cause of death and social class defined by occupation, *Population Trends*, 73: 32–5.

DeWood MA, Spores J, Notske R, Mouser LT, Burroughs R, Golden MS and Lang HT (1980), Prevalence of total coronary occlusion during the early hours of transmural myocardial infarction, *New England Journal of Medicine*, 303: 897–902.

DH (1992), *Health of the Nation, Specification of National Indicators*, London: HMSO.

DH (1995), Department of Health Physical Activity Task Force, *More People, More Active, More Often*, DH.

Editorial (1988), Infant nutrition and cardiovascular disease, *Lancet*, i: 568–9.

Enriquez-Sarano M, Klodas E, Garratt KN, Bailey KR, Tajik AJ and Holmes DR (1996), Secular trends in coronary atherosclerosis – analysis in patients with valvular regurgitation, *New England Journal of Medicine*, 335: 316–22.

Epstein F (1989), The relationship of lifestyle to international trends in CHD, *International Journal of Epidemiology*, 18: S203–9.

Ernst E and Res KL (1993), Fibrinogen as a cardiovascular risk factor: meta analysis and review of the literature, *Annals of Internal Medicine*, 118: 956–63

European Secondary Prevention Study Group (1996), Translation of clinical trials into practice: a European population-based study of the use of thrombolysis for acute myocardial infarction, *Lancet*, 347: 1203–7.

Finlayson R (1985), Ischaemic heart disease, aortic aneurysms, and atherosclerosis in the City of London, *Medical History*, suppl 5: 151–68.

Fox SM and Naughton JP (1972), Physical activity and the prevention of coronary heart disease, *Preventive Medicine*, 1: 92–120.

Francis B, Green M and Payne C (1993), *The GLIM system: generalised linear interactive modelling*, Oxford: OUP.

Frankel S, Elwood P, Sweetnam P, Yarnell J and Davey Smith G (1996), Birthweight, body mass index in middle age and incident coronary heart disease, *Lancet* (in press).

Friedberg CK and Horn H (1939), Acute myocardial infarction not due to coronary artery occlusion, *Journal of the American Medical Association*, 112: 1675–9.

Friend G, Page L and Marston R (1979), Food consumption patterns in the US: 1903–13 to 1976, in *Nutrition, Lipids and Coronary Heart Disease* (eds Levy R, Rifkind B, Dennis B, Ernst N) p.489, New York: Raven Press.

Fye WB (1985), The delayed diagnosis of myocardial infarction: it took half a century! *Circulation*, 72: 262–71.

Gale CR, Martyn CN, Winter PD and Cooper C (1995), Vitamin C and risk of death from stroke and coronary heart disease in a cohort of elderly people, *British Medical Journal*, 310: 1563–6.

Garraway WM, Whisnant JP and Drury I (1983), The changing pattern of survival following stroke, *Stroke*, 14: 699–703.

Greenberg ER, Baron JA, Karagas MR, Stukel TA, Nierenberg DW, Stevens MM, Mandel JS and Haile R (1996), Mortality associated with plasma concentration of beta carotene and the effect of oral supplementation, *Journal of the American Medical Association*, 275: 699–703.

Gregory J, Foster K, Tyler H and Wiseman M (1990), *The Dietary and Nutritional Survey of British Adults*, London: HMSO.

Gronbaek M, Deis A, Sorensen TIA, Becker U, Borch-Johnson K, Mueller C, Schnohr P and Jensen G (1994), Influence of sex, age, body mass index and smoking on alcohol intake and mortality, *British Medical Journal*, 308: 302–6.

Guralnick L (1963), Mortality by occupation level and cause of death among men 20–64 years of age, United States, 1950, *Vital Statistics: Special Reports*, 53: 452.

Haberman S, Capildeo R and Rose FC (1978), The changing mortality of cerebrovascular disease, *Quarterly Journal of Medicine*, New Series, XLVII:71–88.

Halliday MK and Anderson TW (1979), The sex differential in ischaemic heart disease: trends by social class 1931–71, *Journal of Epidemiology and Community Health*, 33: 74–7.

Harding S (1995), Social class differences in mortality of men: recent evidence from the OPCS longitudinal study, *Population Trends*, 80: 31–7.

Health Education Authority (1991), *The Smoking Epidemic*, London: HEA.

Heasman MA and Lipworth L (1966), *Accuracy of certification of cause of death*, Studies on Medical and Population Subjects, 20, 23–4, London: HMSO.

Heller RF, Hayward D and Hobbs MST (1983), Decline in rate of death from ischaemic heart disease in the United Kingdom, *British Medical Journal*, 286: 260–2.

Hunninghake DB, Stein EA, Dujovne CA, Harris WS, Feldman EB, Miller VT, Tobert JA, Laskarzewski PM, Quiter E, Held J, Taylor AM, Hopper S, Leonard SB and Brewer BK (1993), The effect of intensive dietary therapy alone or combined with low vastatine in outpatients with hypercholesterolaemia, *New England Journal of Medicine*, 328: 1213–19.

Intersalt Co-operative Research Group (1988), Intersalt: an international study of electrolyte excretion and blood pressure. Results for 24 hour urinary sodium and potassium excretion, *British Medical Journal*, 297: 319–28.

Jackson R and Beaglehole R (1987), Trends in dietary fat and cigarette smoking and the decline in coronary heart disease in New Zealand, *International Journal of Epidemiology*, 16: 377–82.

Jones DR (1987), Heart disease following widowhood, *Journal of Psychosomatic Research*, 31: 325–33.

Joosens JV, Kestelloot H and Amery A (1979), Salt intake and mortality from stroke, *New England Journal of Medicine*, 300: 1396–8.

Kaplan GA, Colin BA, Cohen RD and Guralnik J (1988), The decline in ischaemic heart disease mortality: prospective evidence from the Alameda County Study, *American Journal of Epidemiology*, 127: 1131–42.

Kaplan GA and Keil JE (1993), Socio-economic factors and cardiovascular disease: a review of the literature, *Circulation*, 88: 1973–98

Khaw KT and Barrett-Connor E (1987), Dietary potassium and stroke associated mortality, a 12-year prospective population study, *New England Journal of Medicine*, 16: 235–40.

Khaw KT and Woodhouse P (1995), Interrelation of vitamin C, infection, haemostatic factors, and cardiovascular disease, *British Medical Journal*, 310: 1559–63.

Klag MJ, Whelton PK and Seidler AJ (1989), Decline in US stroke mortality; demographic trends and antihypertensive treatment, *Stroke*, 20: 14–21.

Knox EG (1981), Meterological associations of cerebrovascular disease mortality in England and Wales, *Journal of Epidemiology and Community Health*, 35: 220–3.

Krikler DM (1987), The search for Samojloff: a Russian physiologist in times of change, *British Medical Journal*, 295: 1624–7.

Kuller LH, Ockene JK, Meilahn E, Wentworth DN, Svendsen KH and Neaton JD (1991), Cigarette smoking and mortality, MRFIT Research Group, *Preventive Medicine*, 20: 638–54.

Law MR, Wald NJ, Wu T, Hackshaw A and Bailey A (1994a), Systematic underestimation of association between serum cholesterol concentration and ischaemic heart disease in observational studies: data from the BUPA study, *British Medical Journal*, 308: 363–6.

Law MR, Wald NJ and Thompson SG (1994b), By how much and how quickly does reduction in serum cholestrol concentration lower risk of ischaemic heart disease? *British Medical Journal*, 308: 367–72.

Law MR, Thompson SG and Wald NJ (1994c), Assessing possible hazards of reducing serum cholestrol, *British Medical Journal*, 308: 373–9.

Lawrence C (1992), 'Definite and material': coronary thrombosis and cardiologists in the 1920s, in *Framing Disease: Studies in Cultural History* (eds Rosenberg CE, Golden J) New Brunswick: Rutgers University Press.

Leon DA , Koupilova I, Lithell HO, Berglund L, Mohsen R, Vagero D, Lithell U-B and McKeigue PM (1996), Failure to realise growth potential in utero and adult obesity in relation to blood pressure in 50–year old Swedish men, *British Medical Journal*, 312: 401–6.

Leor J, Poole WK and Kloner RA (1996), Sudden cardiac death triggered by an earthquake, *New England Journal of Medicine*, 334: 413–19.

Lilienfeld AN (1956), Variations in mortality from heart disease, *Public Health Reports*, 71: 545.

MAFF (1990), *Household Food Consumption and Expenditure 1990*, London: HMSO.

MAFF (1993), *National Food Survey 1993*, London: HMSO.

Martin MJ, Hulley SB, Browner WS, Kuller LH and Wentworth D (1986), Serum cholestrol, blood pressure and mortality: implications from a cohort of 363,662 men, *Lancet*, ii: 933–6.

Martin WJ (1956), The distribution in England and Wales of mortality from coronary disease, *British Medical Journal*, i: 1523–5.

McGovern PG, Pankow JS, Shahar E, Doliszny KM, Folsom AR, Blackburn H and Luepker RV (1996), Recent trends in acute coronary heart disease, *New England Journal of Medicine*, 334: 884–90.

McKeigue PM, Mller GJ and Marmot MG (1989), Coronary artery disease in South Asians overseas – a review, *Journal of Clinical Epidemiology*, 42: 597–609.

McKeown T, Record RG and Turner RD (1975), An interpretation of the decline in mortality in England and Wales during the 20th century, *Population Studies*, 29: 391–422.

McLoone P and Boddy FA (1994), Deprivation and mortality in Scotland, 1981 and 1991, *British Medical Journal*, 309: 1465–70.

MacMahon S, Peto R, Cutler J, Collins R, Sorlie P, Neaton J, Abbott R, Godwin J, Dyer A and Stamler J (1990), Blood pressure, stroke and coronary heart disease. Part I, prolonged differences in blood pressure: prospective observation studies corrected for the regression dilution bias, *Lancet*, 335: 765–74.

Meydani M (1995), Vitamin E, *Lancet*, 345: 170–5.

Midgley JP, Matthew AG, Greenwood CMT and Logan AG (1996), Effect of reduced dietary sodium on blood pressure: a meta-analysis of randomised controlled trials, *JAMA*, 275: 1590–7.

Morgan AD (1968), Some forms of undiagnosed coronary disease in 19th century England, *Medical History*, 12: 344–58.

Morgan M, Heller RF and Swerdlow A (1989), Changes in diet and coronary heart disease among social classes in Great Britain, *Journal of Epidemiology and Community Health*, 43: 162–7.

Morris JN (1951), Recent history of coronary heart disease, *Lancet*, i: 1–7 and 69–73.

Morris JN and Crawford MD (1958), Coronary heart disease and physical activity of work: evidence of a national necropsy survey, *British Medical Journal*, ii: 1485–96.

Morris JN (1960), *Epidemiology and Cardiovascular Disease of middle age,* Part 1, Modern Concepts in Cardiovascular Disease, 29: 625–32.

Moser KA, Fox AJ, Jones DR and Goldblatt PO (1986), Evidence of association between unemployment and heart disease from the OPCS Longitudinal Study, *Postgraduate Medical Journal*, 62: 797–9.

Muller JE and Verrier RL (1996), Triggering of sudden death – lessons from an earthquake, *New England Journal of Medicine*, 334: 460–1.

Mulrow CD, Cornell JA, Herrera CR, Kadri A, Farnett L and Aguilar C (1995), Hypertension in the elderly: implications and generalisability of randomised trials, *Journal of the American Medical Association*, 272: 1932–8.

NCHS (1987), Trends in serum cholesterol levels among US adult aged 20–74 years. Data from the National Health and Nutrition Examination Surveys, 1960 to 1980, *Journal of the American Medical Association*, 257 7: 937–42.

Neil HAW, Roe L, Godlee RJP, Moore JW, Clark GMG, Mant D, Brown J, Thorogood M, Stratton IM, Lancaster T and Fowler GH (1995), Randomised trial of lipid lowering dietary advice in general practice: the effects of serum lipids, lioproteins, and antioxidants, *British Medical Journal*, 310: 567–73.

Nicholls ES and Johansen HL (1983), Implications of the changing trends in cerebrovascular disease and ischaemic heart disease mortality, *Stroke*, 14: 153–5.

OPCS (1983), *Mortality Statistics: Comparisons of the Eighth and Ninth Revisions of the ICD, 1978 (sample)*, OPCS series DH1 no. 10, London: HMSO.

OPCS (1990), *The Dietary and Nutritional Survey of British Adults*, London: HMSO (SS1241).

OPCS (1994), *General Household Survey* (and previous editions from 1972), London: HMSO.

OPCS (1995a), *Mortality Statistics: Cause*, series DH2 no. 20, London: HMSO.

OPCS (1995b), *Health Survey for England 1993*, London: HMSO.

Osmond C (1995), Coronary heart disease mortality trends in England and Wales, 1952–1991, *Journal of Public Health and Medicine*, 17: 404–10.

Ostfeld AM (1980), A review of stroke epidemiology, *Epidemiological Reviews*, 2: 136–52.

Prospective Studies Collaboration (1995), Cholesterol, diastolic blood pressure, and stroke: 13,000 strokes in 450,000 people in 45 prospective cohorts, *Lancet*, 346: 1647–53.

Proudfit WL (1983), Origin of concept of ischaemic heart disease, *British Heart Journal*, 50: 209–12.

Rapola JM, Virtamo J, Haukka JK, Heinonen OP, Albanes D, Taylor PR and Huttunen JK (1996), Effect of vitamin E and beta carotene on the incidence of angina pectoris, *Journal of the American Medical Association*, 275: 693–8.

Rawles J (1996), Magnitude of benefit from earlier thrombolitic treatment in acute myocardial infarction: new evidence from Grampian region early anistreplase trial (GREAT), *British Medical Journal*, 312: 212–16.

RCGP (1993), Royal College of General Practitioners, *Weekly Returns Service*.

Record RG and Whitfield AGW (1964), Prevalence of and mortality from coronary artery disease in men, *British Journal of Preventive and Social Medicine*, 18: 202–9.

Rose G and Marmot MG (1981), Social class and coronary heart disease, *British Heart Journal*, 45: 13–19.

Rose G (1991), Cardiovascular diseases. In Holland WW, Detels R, Knox G (eds). *Oxford Textbook of Public Health*, vol. III: pp.175–87, Oxford: OUP.

Ryle JA and Russell WT (1949), The natural history of coronary heart disease, *British Heart Journal*, II: 370–389.

Shepherd J, Cobbe SM, Ford I, Isles CG, Lorimer AR, Macfarlane PW, McKillop JH and Packard CJ (1995), Prevention of coronary heart disease with pravastatin in men with hypercholestremia, *New England Journal of Medicine*, 333: 1301–7.

Stehbens WE (1987a), An appraisal of the epidemic rise of coronary heart disease and its decline, *Lancet*, I: 606–11.

Stehbens WE (1987b), Coronary heart disease mortality rates, *Lancet*, i: 1483 (letter).

Stephen AM and Sieber GM (1994), Trends in individual fat consumption in the UK 1900–1985, *British Journal of Nutrition*, 71: 775–88.

Stephens NG, Parsons A, Schofield PM, Kelly F, Cheeseman K, Mitchison J and Brown MJ (1996), Randomised controlled trial of vitamin E in patients with coronary disease: Cambridge Heart Antioxidant Study (CHAOS), *Lancet*, 347: 781–6.

Sytkowski PA, Agostino RB, Belanger A and Kannel WB (1996), Sex and time trends in cardiovascular disease incidence and mortality: the Framingham Study, 1950–1989, *American Journal of Epidemiology*, 143 (4): 338–50.

Tanaka H, Udea Y, Date C et al (1981), Incidence of stroke in Shibata, Japan: 1976–1978, *Stroke*, 12: 460–6.

Taylor W and Dauncey M (1955), Changing patterns of mortality in England and Wales III. Mortality in old age, *British Journal of Preventive and Social Medicine*, 9: 162–8.

Traven ND, Kuller LH, Ives DG, Ruytan GH and Perper JA (1995), Coronary heart disease mortality and sudden death: Trends and patterns in 35 to 44 year old white males: 1970–1990, *American Journal of Epidemiology*, 142: 53–63.

Tuomilehto J, Nissinen A, Wolf E, Geboers J, Piha T and Puska P (1985), Effectiveness of treatment with antihypertensive drugs and trends in mortality from stroke in the community, *British Medical Journal*, 291: 857–60.

Wannamethee SG, Shaper AG, Whincup PH and Walker M (1995), Smoking cessation and the risk of stroke in middle–aged men, *Journal of the American Medical Association*, 274: 155–60.

Wannamethee G and Shaper AG (1992), Physical activity and stroke in British middle-aged men, *British Medical Journal*, 304: 597–601.

Waterhouse J, Muir C, Correa P and Powell J (1976), *Cancer Incidence in Five Continents*, vol.III, p.456, IARC Scientific Publications No.15, Lyon: International Agency for Research on Cancer.

Whisnant JP (1984), The decline of stroke, *Stroke*, 15: 160–8.

Wolfe CDA and Burney PGJ (1992), Is stroke mortality on the decline in England? *American Journal of Epidemiology*, 136: 558–65.

Yates PO (1964), A change in the pattern of cerebrovascular disease, *Lancet*, i: 65–9.

Zarate AO (1994), *International Mortality Chartbook, Levels and trends, 1955–1991*, Hyattsville: US DHHS.

Chapter 19 Neurological diseases

Alter M, Zhen-Xin Z, Davanipour Z, Sobel E, Zibulewski J, Schwartz G and Friday G (1986), Multiple sclerosis and childhood infection, *Neurology*, 36: 1386–9.

Armstrong M, Daly AK, Cholerton S, Bateman DN and Idle JR (1992), Mutant debrisoquine hydroxylation genes in Parkinson's disease, *Lancet*, 339: 1017–8.

Breteler MB, Claus JJ, van Duijn CM, Launer LJ and Hofman A (1992), Epidemiology of Alzheimer's disease, *Epidemiological Review*, 14: 59–82.

Brown RH (1995), Amyotrophic lateral sclerosis: recent insights from genetics and transgenic mice, *Cell*, 80: 687–92.

Brown EL and Knox EG (1972), Epidemiological approach to Parkinson's disease, *Lancet*, i: 974–6.

Chancellor A, Slattery J, Holloway SM and Warlow CP (1993), The prognosis of adult-onset motorneurone disease: a prospective study based on the Scottish Motor Neurone Disease Register, *Journal of Neurology*, 240: 339–46.

Chancellor A, Swingler RJ, Carstairs V and Elton RA (1992), Affluence, age and motorneurone disease, (letter), *Journal of Epidemiology and Community Health*, 46: 172–3.

Chancellor AM and Warlow CP (1992), Adult onset motorneurone disease: worldwide mortality, incidence and distribution since 1950, *Journal of Neurology, Neurosurgery and Psychiatry*, 55: 1106–15.

Cockerell OC, Johnson AL, Sonder JWAS, Hart YM, Goodridge DME and Shorvon SD (1994a), Mortality from epilepsy: results from a prospective population-based study, *Lancet*, 344: 918–21.

Cockerell OC, Hart YM, Sander JWAS and Shorvon SD (1994b), The cost of epilepsy in the United Kingdom: an estimation based on the results of two population-based studies, *Epilepsy Research*, 18: 249–60.

Compston DAS (1990), The dissemination of multiple sclerosis, *Journal of the Royal College of Physicians of London*, 24: 207–18.

Compston DAS, Kellar-Wood H and Wood N (1994), Multiple sclerosis, in *Genetics of Neurology, Bailliere's Clinical Neurology* (ed. Harding AE), vol. 3: 353–71, London: Bailliere Tindall.

Compston DAS, Vakarelis BN, Paul E, McDonald WI, Batchelor JR and Mims CA (1986), Viral infection in patients with multiple sclerosis and HLA-DR matched controls, *Brain*, 109: 325–44.

Duvoisin RC, Gearling FR, Schweizer MD and Yahr MD (1969), A family study of parkinsonism, in *Progress in neurogenetics* (eds Barbeau A and Brunetti JR), Amsterdam: Excerpta Medica 492–6.

Elian M, Dean G and Nightingale S (1990), Multiple sclerosis among United Kingdom born children of immigrants from the Indian subcontinent, Africa and the West Indies, *Journal of Neurology, Neurosurgery and Psychiatry*, 53: 906–11.

Francis DA, Batchelor JR, McDonald WI, Hing SN, Dodi IA, Fielder AH, Hern JE and Downie AW (1987), Multiple sclerosis in north-east Scotland: an association with HLA-DQw1, *Brain*, 110: 181–6.

Gomez JG, Arciniegas E and Torres J (1978), Prevalence of epilepsy in Bogota, Colombia, *Neurology*, 28: 90–4.

Goodridge DMG and Shorvon SD (1983), Epileptic seizures in a population of 6000: demography, diagnosis and classification, *British Medical Journal*, 287: 641–7.

Gunnarsson LG, Lindberg G, Soderfelt B and Axelson O (1990), The mortality of motorneurone disease in Sweden 1961–1985, *Arch Neurol*, 47: 42–6.

Haerer AF, Anderson DW and Schoenberg BS (1986), Prevalence and clinical features of epilepsy in a bi-racial United States population, *Epilepsia*, 27: 66–75.

Hammond SR, McLeod JG, Millingen KS, Stewart-Wynne EG, English D, Holland JT and McCall MG (1988), The epidemiology of multiple sclerosis in three Australian cities: Perth, Newcastle and Hobart, *Brain*, 111: 1–25.

Hofman A, Rocca WA, Brayne C, Breteler MMB, Clarke M, Cooper B, Copeland JR, Dartigues JF, da Silva Droux A and Hagnell O, Heeren TJ, Engedal K, Jonker D, Lindesay J, Lobo A, Mann AH, Mölsä PK, Morgan K, O'Connor DW, Sulkava R, Kay DWK, and Amaducci L (1991), The prevalence of dementia in Europe: a collaborative study of the 1980–1990 findings, *International Journal of Epidemiology*, 20: 736–48.

Hopkins A (1989), Lessons for neurologists from the United Kingdom Third National Morbidity Survey, *Journal of Neurology, Neurosurgery and Psychiatry*, 52: 430–3.

Jones CT, Swingler RJ, Simpson SA and Brock DJ (1995), Superoxide dismutase mutations in a cohort of Scottish amyotrophic lateral sclerosis patients, *Journal of Medical Genetics*, 32: 290–2.

Kessler II (1972a), Epidemiologic studies of Parkinson's disease: II: A hospital-based survey, *American Journal of Epidemiology*, 95: 308–18.

Kessler II (1972b), Epidemiologic studies of Parkinson's disease: III: A community-based survey, *American Journal of Epidemiology*, 96: 242–54.

Kurland LT, Radhakrishnan K, Smith GE, Armon C and Nemetz PN (1992), Mechanical trauma as a risk factor in classic amyotrophic lateral sclerosis: lack of epidemiological evidence, *Journal of Neurological Science*, 113: 133–43.

Kurtzke JF, Beebe GW and Norman JE (1979), Epidemiology of multiple sclerosis in Veterans 1: Race, sex and geographical distribution, *Neurology*, 29: 1228–35.

Leigh PN and Ray-Chaudhuri K (1994), Motorneurone disease, *Journal of Neurology, Neurosurgery and Psychiatry*, 57: 886–96.

Li T, Swash M, and Alberman E (1985), Morbidity and mortality in motorneurone disease: comparison with multiple sclerosis and Parkinson's disease: age and sex specific rates and cohort analyses, *Journal of Neurology, Neurosurgery and Psychiatry*, 48: 320–7.

Marmot MG (1980), Parkinson's disease and encephalitis: the cohort hypothesis re-examined, in *Clinical Neuroepidemiology* (ed. Rose FC), pp.391–401: Tunbridge Wells: Pitman Medical.

Martyn CN (1991), The epidemiology of multiple sclerosis, in *McAlpine's Multiple Sclerosis* (ed. Matthews WB), pp.3–42, Edinburgh: Churchill Livingstone.

Martyn CN (1994), Epidemiology, in *Motor Neurone Disease* (ed. Williams AC), pp.393–426, London: Chapman Hall.

Martyn CN, Barker DJP, and Osmond C (1988), Motoneurone disease and past poliomyelitis in England and Wales, *Lancet*, i: 1319–22.

Martyn CN, Cruddas M and Compston DAS (1993), Symptomatic Epstein-Barr virus infection in multiple sclerosis, *Journal of Neurology, Neurosurgery and Psychiatry*, 56: 167–8.

Martyn CN and Pippard EC (1988), Usefulness of mortality data in determining the geography and time trends of dementia, *Journal of Epidemiology and Community Health*, 42: 134–7.

Matthew WB (ed.) (1991), *McAlpine's Multiple Sclerosis*, Edinburgh: Churchill Livingstone.

Miller DH, Hammond SR, McLeod JG, Purdie G and Skegg DC (1990), Multiple sclerosis in Australia and New Zealand: are the determinants genetic or environmental? *Journal of Neurology, Neurosurgery and Psychiatry*, 53: 903–5.

Morrow JI and Patterson VH (1987), The neurological practice of a district general hospital, *Journal of Neurology, Neurosurgery and Psychiatry*, 50: 1397–401.

Neilson S, Robinson I and Hunter M (1992), Longitudinal Gompertzian analysis of ALS mortality in England and Wales 1963–1989: Estimates of susceptibility in the general population, *Mechanisms of Ageing and Development*, 64: 201–16.

Osmond C and Gardner MJ (1982), Age, period and cohort models applied to cancer mortality rates, *Statistics in Medicine*, 1: 245–59.

Osuntokun BO, Ogunniyi LIG, Lekwaumwa TA *et al.* (1990), Epidemiology of dementia in Nigerian Africans, in *Advances in Neurology* (eds Chopra JS, Jagannanthan K and Sawney IMS), pp.331–42, Amsterdam: Elsevier.

Poskanzer DC and Schwab RS (1963), Cohort analysis of Parkinson's syndrome: evidence for a single etiology related to subclinical infection about 1920, *Journal of Chronic Disability*, 16: 961–73.

Poskanzer DC, Shapira K and Miller H (1963), Multiple sclerosis and poliomyelitis, *Lancet*, ii: 917–21.

Ritchie K and Kildea D (1995), Is senile dementia age-related or ageing-related? Evidence from a meta-analysis of dementia prevalence in the oldest old, *Lancet*, 34: 931–4.

Robertson N and Compston DAS (1995), Surveying multiple sclerosis in the United Kingdom, *Journal of Neurology, Neurosurgery and Psychiatry*, 58: 2–6.

Rodgers-Johnson P, Garruto RM, Yanagihara R, Chen KM, Gajdusek DC and Gibbs CJ Jr (1986), Amyotrophic lateral sclerosis and parkinsonism-dementia on Guam: a 30 year evaluation and neuropathological trends, *Neurology*, 36: 7–13.

Rosen DR, Siddique T, Patterson D, Figlewicz DA, Sapp P, Hentati A, Donaldson D, Goto J, O'Regan JP, Deng H-X, Rahmani Z, Krizus A, McKenna-Yasek D, Cayabyab A, Gaston SM, Berger R, Tanzi RE, Halperin JJ, Herzfeldt B, Van den Bergh R, Hung W-Y, Bird T, Deng G, Mulder DW, Smyth C, Laing NG, Soriano E, Pericak-Vance MA, Haines J, Rouleau GA, Gusella JS, Horvitz HR and Brown RH jr (1993), Mutations in Cu/Zn superoxide dismutase gene are associated with familial amyotrophic lateral sclerosis, *Nature*, 362: 59–62.

Rothstein JD, Martin IJ and Kuncl RW (1994), Decreased glutamate transport by the brain and spinal cord in amyotrophic lateral sclerosis, *New England Journal of Medicine*, 330: 585–91.

Sadovnick AD, Armstrong H, Rice GPA, Bulman D, Hashimoto L, Paty DW, Hashimoto SA, Warren S, Hader W, Murray TJ, Seland TP, Metz L, Bell R, Duquette P, Gray T, Nelson R, Weinshenker B, Brunet D and Ebers GC (1993), A population based study of multiple sclerosis in twins: update, *Annals of Neurology*, 33: 281–5.

Sander JWAS, Cockerell OC, Hart YM and Shorvon SD (1993), Is the incidence of epilepsy falling in the United Kingdom?, *Lancet*, 342: 874.

Sander JWAS, Hart YM, Johnson AL and Shorvon SD (1990), National General Practice Study of Epilepsy: newly diagnosed epilepsy seizures in the general population, *Lancet*, 336: 1267–71.

Sutherland JM (1956), Observations on the prevalence of multiple sclerosis in northern Scotland, *Brain*, 79: 635–54.

Swingler RJ and Compston DAS (1986), The distribution of multiple sclerosis in the United Kingdom, *Journal of Neurology, Neurosurgery and Psychiatry*, 49: 1115–24.

Swingler RJ, Davidson DLW, Roberts RC, and Moulding FC (1994), The costs of epilepsy in patients attending an out-patient clinic, *Seizure*, 3: 115–20.

Swingler RJ, Fraser H, and Warlow CP (1992), Motorneurone disease and polio in Scotland, *Journal of Neurology, Neurosurgery and Psychiatry*, 55: 1116–20.

Tanner CM (1992), Epidemiology of Parkinson's disease, *Neurological Clinics*, 10: 317–29.

Wade DT and Langton-Hewer R (1987), The epidemiology of some neurological diseases, *International Rehabilitation Medicine*, 8: 129–37.

Ward CD, Duvoisin RC, Ince SE, Nutt JD, Eldridge R and Calne DB (1983), Parkinson's disease in 65 pairs of twins and in a set of quadruplets, *Neurology*, 33: 815–23.

Williams GR (1966), Morbidity and mortality with parkinsonism, *Journal of Neurosurgery*, 24: 138–43.

Williams ES and McKeran RO (1986), Prevalence of multiple sclerosis in a south London borough, *British Medical Journal*, 293: 237–9.

Yoshida S, Mulder DW, Kurland LT, Chu CP and Okazaki H (1986), Follow-up study on amyotrophic lateral sclerosis in Rochester, Minnesota, 1925–1984, *Neuroepidemiology*, 5: 61–70.

Chapter 20 Diseases of the respiratory system

Air Monitoring Group (1994), *Air Pollution in the UK: 1992/3*, Stevenage: Warren Springs Laboratory.

Allchin WH (1902), *A Manual of Medicine*, vol IV. *Diseases of the Respiratory and Circulatory Systems*, London: Macmillan & Co.

Anonymous (1964), *Colliery Year Book and Coal Trades Directory*, London: Colliery Guardian, p.336.

Anonymous (1971), Cromoglycate in asthma and hayfever, *Lancet*, ii (7736): 1243–4.

Anonymous (1972), Beclomethasone dipropionate aerosol in asthma, *Lancet*, ii: 1239–40.

Arshad SH, Matthews S, Gant C and Hide DW (1992), Effect of allergen avoidance on development of allergic disorders in infancy, *Lancet*, 339: 1493–7.

Attfield MD (1985), Longitudinal decline in FEV1 in United States coalminers, *Thorax*, 40: 132–7.

Barbee RA, Halonen M, Kaltenborn WT and Burrows B (1991), A longitudinal study of respiratory symptoms in a community population sample. Correlations with smoking, allergen skin-test reactivity and serum IgE, *Chest*, 99: 20–6.

Barker DJP and Osmond C (1986), Childhood respiratory infection and adult chronic bronchitis in England and Wales, *British Medical Journal*, 293: 1271–5.

Barker DJP, Osmond C and Law CM (1989), The intrauterine and early postnatal origins of cardiovascular disease and chronic bronchitis, *J Epidemiol Commun Health*, 43: 237–40.

Barker DJP, Godfrey KM, Fall C, Osmond C, Winter PD, Shaheen SO (1991), Relation of birth weight and childhood respiratory infection to adult lung function and death from chronic obstructive airways disease, *British Medical Journal*, 303: 671–5.

Bates DV, Baker-Anderson M and Sitzo R (1990), Asthma attack periodicity: a study of hospital emergency visits in Vancouver, *Environ Res*, 51: 51–70.

Beaumont GE (1932), *Medicine, Essentials for Practitioners and Students*, London: J & A Churchill.

Beaumont GE (1942), *Medicine, Essentials for Practitioners and Students*, London: J & A Churchill.

Beaumont GE (1948), *Medicine, Essentials for Practitioners and Students*, London: J & A Churchill.

Beaumont GE (1953), *Medicine, Essentials for Practitioners and Students*, London: J & A Churchill.

Bellomo R, Gigliotti P, Treloar A, Holmes P, Suphioglu C, Singh M and Knox B (1992), Two consecutive thunderstorm associated epidemics of asthma in the city of Melbourne. The possible role of rye grass pollen, *Med J Aust*, 156: 834–7.

Blanc P (1987), Occupational asthma in a national disability survey, *Chest*, 92: 613–17.

Bradley WH, Logan WPD and Martin AE (1958), The London Fog of December 2nd-5th, 1957, *Mon Bull Minist Hlth Lab Serv*, 17: 156–66.

Brimblecombe P (1987), *The Big Smoke. A History of Air Pollution in London since Medieval Times*, London: Methuen.

British Coal Corporation (1992), *British Coal Annual Report 1991–92*, pp.30–1.

Broughton GFJ (1987), *Ozone in the UK – a Summary of Results from Instrumented Air Pollution Monitoring Networks, 1972–1986*.

Burney PGJ (1989), The effect of death certification practice on recorded national asthma mortality rates, *Rev Epidem et Santé Publ*, 37: 385–9.

Burney PGJ (1992), Epidemiology, in *Asthma* (eds Clark T, Godfrey S and Lee T), London: Chapman & Hall, pp.254-307.

Burney PGJ (1993), Asthma: evidence for a rising prevalence, *Proc R Coll Physicians Edin*, 23: 595–600.

Burney PGJ, Chinn S and Rona RJ (1990), Has the prevalence of asthma increased in children? Evidence from the national study of health and growth 1973–86, *British Medical Journal*, 300: 1306–10.

Burr ML, Butland BK, King S and Vaughan-Williams E (1989), Changes in asthma prevalence: two surveys 15 years apart, *Arch Dis Child*, 64: 1452–6.

Burrows B, Knudson RJ, Camilli AE, Lyle SK and Lebowitz MD (1987), The 'horse-racing effect' and predicting decline in forced expiratory volume in one second from screening spirometry, *Am Rev Respir Dis*, 135: 788–93.

Burrows B, Knudson RJ, Cline MG and Lebowitz MD (1988), A reexamination of risk factors for ventilatory impairment, *Am Rev Respir Dis*, 138: 829–36.

Cameron N (1979), The growth of London schoolchildren 1904–1966: an analysis of secular trend and intra-county variation, *Ann Human Biol*, 6: 505–25.

Camilli AE, Burrows B, Knudson B, Lyle SK and Lebowitz MD (1987), Longitudinal changes in forced expiratory volume in one second in adults. Effects of smoking and smoking cessation, *Am Rev Respir Dis*, 135: 794–9.

Camilli AE, Robbins DR and Lebowitz MD (1991), Death certificate reporting of confirmed airways obstructive disease, *Am J Epidemiol*, 133: 795–800.

Chakraverty P, Cunningham P, Shen GZ, and Pereira MS (1986), Influenza in the United Kingdom 1982–85, *J Hygiene*, 97: 347–58.

Chan-Yeung M and Lam S (1986), State of Art. Occupational asthma, *Am Rev Respir Dis*, 133: 686–703.

Charpin D, Birnbaum J, Haddi E, Lanteaume A, Toumi M, Faraj F, Van der Brempt X and Vervloet D (1991), Altitude and allergy to house-dust mites, *Am Rev Respir Dis*, 143: 983–6.

Chinn S, Florey C du V, Baldwin IG and Gorgol M (1981), The relation of mortality in England and Wales 1969–73 to measurements of air pollution, *J Epidemiol Commun Health*, 35: 174–9.

Choo-Kang YF, Simpson WT and Grant IW (1969), Controlled comparison of the bronchodilator effects of three beta-adrenergic stimulant drugs administered by inhalation to patients with asthma, *British Medical Journal*, 2: 287–9.

Christian HA (1947), *The Principles and Practice of Medicine*, London, New York: D Appleton Century Co.

Clark TJH (1972), Effect of beclomethasone dipropionate delivered by aerosol in patients with asthma, *Lancet*, i: 1361–4.

Clayton D and Schifflers E (1987), Models for temporal variation in cancer rates. II: Age-period-cohort models, *Stat Med*, 6: 469–81.

Colley JRT, Douglas JWB and Reid DD (1973), Respiratory disease in young adults: influence of early childhood lower respiratory tract illness, social class, air pollution, and smoking, *British Medical Journal*, 3: 195–8.

COMEAP (1995), *Air Pollution and Asthma*, Department of Health, London: HMSO.

Crimi E, Voltolini S, Gianiorio P, Orengo G, Troise C, Brusasco V, Crimi P and Negrini A (1990), Effect of seasonal exposure to pollen on specific bronchial sensitivity in allergic patients, *J Allergy Clin Immunol*, 85: 1014–19.

Davis JB and Bulpitt CJ (1981), Atopy and wheeze in children according to parental atopy and family size, *Thorax*, 36: 185–9.

DHSS (1963-1994), *Social Security Statistics* (various years), London: HMSO.

DHSS (1984), *Social Security Statistics*, London: HMSO.

Devalia JL, Rusznak C, Herdman MJ, Trigg CJ, Tarraf H and Davies RJ (1994), Effect of nitrogen dioxide and sulphur dioxide on airway response of mild asthmatic patients to allergen inhalation, *Lancet*, 344: 1668–71.

Dockery DW, Speizer FE, Ferris BG, Ware JH, Louis TA and Spiro A (1988), Cumulative and reversible effects of lifetime smoking on simple tests of lung function in adults, *Am Rev Respir Dis*, 137: 286–92.

Dockery DW, Pope AC, Xu X, Spengler J, Ware J, Ferris B and Speizer F (1993), An association between air pollution and mortality in six US cities, *N Engl J Med*, 329: 1753–9.

Doll R and Peto R (1976), Mortality in relation to smoking: 20 years' observations on male British doctors, *British Medical Journal*, 2: 1525–36.

Doll R, Gray R, Hafner B and Peto R (1980), Mortality in relation to smoking: 22 years' observations in female British doctors, *British Medical Journal*, 1: 967–71.

Easton AJ and Eglin RP (1989), Epidemiology of parainfluenza virus type 3 in England and Wales over a ten-year period, *Epidemiol Infect*, 102: 531–5.

Farebrother MJB, Kelson MC and Heller RF on behalf of the EEC working party (1985), Death certification of farmer's lung and chronic airways diseases in different countries of the EEC, *Br J Dis Chest*, 79: 352–60.

Fletcher C and Peto R (1970), The natural history of chronic airflow obstruction, *British Medical Journal*, 1: 1645–8.

Fletcher C, Peto R, Tinker C and Speizer FE (1976), *The Natural History of Chronic Bronchitis and Emphysema*, Oxford: Oxford University Press.

Florey H (1946), Penicillin progress. *The British Encyclopaedia of Medical Practice. Medical Progress*, London: Butterworth & Co.

Floud R, Wachter K and Gregory A (1990), *Height, Health and History. Nutritional Status in the United Kingdom, 1750–1980*, Cambridge: Cambridge University Press.

Forsberg B, Stjemberg N, Falk M, Lundback B, and Wall S (1993), Air pollution levels, meterological conditions and asthma symptoms, *Eur Respir J*, 6: 1109–15.

Gaddie J, Petrie GR, Reid IW, Sinclair DJM, Skinner C and Palmer KNV (1973), Aerosol beclomethasone dipropionate in chronic bronchial asthma, *Lancet*, 1: 691–3.

Gau DW and Diehl AK (1982), Disagreement among general practitioners regarding cause of death, *British Medical Journal*, 284: 239–41.

Gillham CA, Leech PK and Eggleston HS (1992), *UK Emissions of Air Pollutants 1970–1990*, Stevenage: Warren Spring Laboratory.

Gold DR, Tager IB, Weiss ST, Tosteson TD and Speizer FE (1989), Acute lower respiratory illness in childhood as a predictor of lung function and chronic respiratory symptoms, *Am Rev Respir Dis*, 140: 877–84.

Green WF, Nicholas NR, Salome CM and Woolcock AJ (1989), Reduction of house dust mites and mite allergens: effects of spraying carpets and blankets with Allersearch DMS, an acaracide combined with an allergen denaturing agent, *Clin Expl Allergy*, 19: 203–7.

Hilberman M (1975), The evolution of intensive care units, *Crit Care Med*, 3: 159–65.

Hnizdo E (1992), Health risks among white South African goldminers - dust, smoking and chronic obstructive pulmonary disease, *S Afr Med J*, 81: 512–17.

Hogg JC (1971), *The Effect of Lung Growth on the Distribution of Airways Resistance*, Ciba Foundation Study Group, 38: 47–62.

Holland WW, Halil T, Bennett AE and Elliott A (1969), Factors influencing the onset of chronic respiratory disease, *British Medical Journal*, 2: 205–8.

Holland WW, Bennett AE, Cameron IR, Florey CdV, Leeder S, Schilling R, Swan A and Waller R (1979), Health effects of particulate pollution: reappraising the evidence, *Am J Epidemiol*, 110: 525–659.

Howell JB and Altounyan RE (1967), A double-blind trial of disodium cromoglycate in the treatment of allergic bronchial asthma, *Lancet*, ii(515), 539–42.

Inman WHW and Adelstein AM (1969), Rise and fall of asthma mortality in England and Wales in relation to use of pressurised aerosols, *Lancet*, ii: 279–84.

Johnston SL, Pattemore PK, Sanderson G, Smith S, Lampe F, Joseph L, Symington P, O'Toole S, Myint S, Tyrell D and Holgate S (1995), Community study of the role of viral infections in exacerbations of asthma in 9-11 year old children, *British Medical Journal*, 310: 1225–8.

Kalra S, Crank P, Hepworth J, Pickering CAC and Woodcock AA (1992), Absence of seasonal variation in concentrations of the house dust mite allergen Der p I in South Manchester homes, *Thorax*, 47: 928–31.

Karjalainen J, Lindqvist A and Laitinen LA (1989), Seasonal variability of exercise-induced asthma especially outdoors. Effect of birch pollen allergy, *Clin Expl Allergy*, 19: 273–8.

Kauffmann F, Drouet D, Lellouch J and Brille D (1982), Occupational exposure and 12-year spirometric changes among Paris area workers, *Br J Ind Med*, 39: 221–32.

Korsgaard J (1983), Mite asthma and residency. A case-control study on the impact of exposure to house-dust mites in dwellings, *Am Rev Respir Dis*, 128: 231–5.

Krzyzanowski M and Kauffmann F (1988), The relation of respiratory symptoms and ventilatory function to moderate occupational exposure in a general population. Results from the French PAARC study of 16,000 adults, *Int J Epidemiol*, 17: 397–406.

Kuller LH, Ockene JK, Townsend M, Browner W, Meilahn E and Wentworth DN (1989), The epidemiology of pulmonary function and COPD mortality in the Multiple Risk Factor Intervention Trial, *Am Rev Respir Dis*, 140: S76–81.

La Croix AZ, Lipson S, Miles TP and White L (1989), Prospective study of pneumonia hospitalizations and mortality of U.S. older people: the role of chronic conditions, health behaviours, and nutritional status, *Public Health Reports*, 104: 350–60.

Lau S, Falkenhorst G, Weber A, Werthmann I, Lind P, Buettner-Goetz P and Wahn U (1989), High mite-allergen exposure increases the risk of sensitisation in atopic children and young adults, *J Allergy Clin Immunol*, 84: 718–25.

Lebowitz MD (1981), Multivariate analysis of smoking and other risk factors for obstructive lung diseases and related symptoms, *J Chron Dis*, 35: 751–8.

Lebowitz MD, Holberg CJ, Knudson RJ and Burrows B (1987), Longitudinal study of pulmonary function development in childhood, adolescence, and early adulthood, *Am Rev Respir Dis*, 136: 69–75.

Logan WPD (1949), Fog and mortality, *Lancet*, i: 78.

Logan WPD (1953), Mortality in the London fog incident, 1952, *Lancet*, i: 336–8.

Logan WPD (1956), Mortality from fog in London, January, 1956, *British Medical Journal*, i: 722–5.

Loughlin GM and Taussig LM (1979), Pulmonary function in children with a history of laryngotracheobronchitis, *J Pediatr*, 94: 365–9.

Love RG and Miller BG (1982), Longitudinal study of lung function in coal-miners, *Thorax*, 37: 193–7.

Madonini E, Briatico-Vangosa G, Pappacoda A, Maccagni G, Cardani A and Saporiti F (1987), Seasonal increase of bronchial reactivity in allergic rhinitis, *J Allergy Clin Immunol*, 79: 358–63.

Mao Y, Semenciw R, Morrison H and Wigle DT (1990), Seasonality in epidemics of asthma mortality and hospital admission rates, Ontario, 1979–86, *Can J Public Health*, 81: 226–8.

Martin AE (1964), Mortality and morbidity statistics and air pollution, *Proc R Soc Med*, 57: 969–75.

Martin AE and Bradley WH (1960), Mortality fog and atmospheric pollution – an investigation during the winter of 1958–59, *Monthly Bull Minist Health (Lond)*, 19–56.

Martin AE (1961), Epidemiologic studies of atmospheric pollution, *Monthly Bull Minist Health (Lond)*, 20: 42–50.

Martinez FD, Morgan WJ, Wright AL, Holberg CJ and Taussig LM (1988), Diminished lung function as a predisposing factor for wheezing respiratory illness in infants, *N Engl J Med*, 319: 1112–17.

Mitchell RS, Maisel JC, Dart GA and Silvers GW (1971), The accuracy of the death certificate in reporting cause of death in adults. With special reference to chronic bronchitis and emphysema, *Am Rev Respir Dis*, 104: 844–50.

Morrison Smith J (1976), The prevalence of asthma and wheezing in children, *Br J Dis Chest*, 70: 73–7.

Morrow Brown H, Storey G and George WHS (1972), Beclomethasone dipropionate: a new steroid aerosol for the treatment of allergic asthma, *British Medical Journal*, 1: 585–90.

Ninan TK and Russell G (1992), Respiratory symptoms and atopy in Aberdeen school children: evidence from two surveys 25 years apart, *British Medical Journal*, 304: 873–5.

Noah ND (1974), Mycoplasma pneumonia infection in the United Kingdom – 1967–73, *British Medical Journal*, 2: 544–6.

O'Halloran MT, Yunginger JW, Offord KP, Somers M, O'Connell E, Ballard D and Sachs M (1991), Exposure to an aeroallergen as a possible precipitating factor in respiratory arrest in young patients with asthma, *N Engl J Med*, 324: 359–63.

OPCS (1981), *Census for England and Wales 1981*, London: HMSO.

OPCS (1987), *Birth Statistics*, OPCS series FM1 no. 13, London: HMSO.

Osler W (1892), *The Principles and Practice of Medicine*, Edinburgh & London: Young J. Pentland.

Osler W and McCrea T (1920), *The Principles and Practice of Medicine*, London & New York: D Appleton & Co.

Osler W, Christian HA and McCrea T (1938), *The Principles and Practice of Medicine*, London & New York: D Appleton & Co.

Ozkaynak H and Spengler JD (1985), Analysis of health effects resulting from population exposures to acid precipitation precursors, *Environ Health Perspect*, 63: 45–55.

Parker DR, O'Connor GT, Sparrow D, Segal MR and Weiss ST (1990), The relationship of nonspecific airway responsiveness and atopy to the rate of decline of lung function. The normative aging study, *Am Rev Respir Dis*, 141: 589–94.

Platts-Mills TAE, Hayden M, Chapman MD, and Wilkins SR (1987), Seasonal variation in dust mite and grass-pollen allergens in dust from the houses of patients with asthma, *J Allergy Clin Immunol*, 79: 781–91.

Plotkowski MC, Puchelle E, Beck G and Jacquot J (1986), Adherence of Type I Streptococcus pneumoniae to tracheal epithelium of mice infected with Influenza A/PR8 virus, *Am Rev Respir Dis*, 134: 1040–4.

Pocock SJ, Cook DG and Beresford SAA (1981), Regression of area mortality rates on explanatory variables: what weighting is appropriate? *Appl Statist*, 30: 286–95.

Pope CA, Schwartz J and Ransom MR (1992), Daily mortality and PM10 pollution in Utah Valley, *Arch Environ Health*, 47: 211–17.

Price FW (1922), *A Textbook of the Practice of Medicine*, London: Henry Frowde and Hodder & Stoughton.

Price JA, Pollock I, Little SA, Longbottom JL and Warner JO (1990), Measurement of airborne mite allergen in homes of asthmatic children, *Lancet*, 336: 895–7.

Pride NB (1969), Asthma – treatment, *British Medical Journal*, 4: 359–61.

Priftis K, Anagnostakis J, Harokopos E, Orfanou I, Petraki Ma and Saxoni-Papageorgiou P (1993), Time trends and seasonal variation in hospital admissions for childhood asthma in the Athens region of Greece: 1978-88, *Thorax*, 48: 1168–9.

Registrar General (1947), *Registrar General's Statistical Review of England and Wales for the years 1938 and 1939*, London: HMSO.

Roebuck MO (1976), Rhinoviruses in Britain 1963–1973, *J Hygiene*, 76: 137–46.

Samet JM, Tager IB and Speizer FE (1983), The relationship between respiratory illness in childhood and chronic air-flow obstruction in adulthood, *Am Rev Respir Dis*, 127: 508–23.

Schwartz J (1991), Particulate air pollution and daily mortality in Detroit, *Environ Res*, 56: 204–13.

Schwartz J and Dockery DW (1992a), Increased mortality in Philadelphia associated with daily air pollution concentrations, *Am Rev Respir Dis*, 145: 600–4.

Schwartz J and Dockery DW (1992b), Particulate air pollution and daily mortality in Steubenville, Ohio, *Am J Epidemiol*, 135: 12–19.

Schwartz J and Marcus A (1990), Mortality and air pollution in London: a time series analysis, *Am J Epidemiol*, 131: 185–94.

Schwartz J, Slater D, Larson TV, Pierson WE and Koenig JQ (1993), Particulate air pollution and hospital emergency room visits for asthma in Seattle, *Am Rev Respir Dis*, 147: 826–31.

Shaheen SO, Barker DJP, Shiell AW, Crocker FJ, Wield GA and Holgate ST (1994), The relationship between pneumonia in early childhood and impaired lung function in late adult life, *Am J Respir Crit Care Med*, 149: 616–19.

Silverman M, Connolly NM, Balfour-Lynn L and Godfrey S (1972), Long-term trial of disodium cromoglycate and isoprenaline in children with asthma, *British Medical Journal*, 3(823): 378–81.

Sotomayor H, Badier M, Vervolet D and Orehek J (1984), Seasonal increase of carbachol airway responsiveness in patients allergic to grass pollen. Reversal by corticosteroids, *Am Rev Respir Dis*, 130: 56–8.

Soutar C, Campbell S, Gurr D, Lloyd M, Love R, Cowie H, Cowie A and Seaton A (1993), Important deficits of lung function in three modern colliery populations. Relations with dust exposure, *Am Rev Respir Dis*, 147: 797–803.

Sporik R, Holgate ST, Platts-Mills TAE and Cogswell JJ (1990), Exposure to house-dust mite allergen (Der p I) and the development of asthma in childhood. A prospective study, *N Engl J Med*, 323: 502–7.

Stewart CJ and Nunn AJ (1985), Are asthma mortality rates changing?, *Br J Dis Chest*, 79: 229–34.

Stolley PD and Schinnar R (1978), Association between asthma mortality and isoproterenol aerosols: a review, *Preventive Med*, 7: 519–38.

Storr J and Lenney W (1989), School holidays and admissions with asthma, *Arch Dis Child*, 64: 103–7.

Strachan DP (1989), Hay fever, hygiene, and family size, *British Medical Journal*, 299: 1259–60.

Strope GL, Stewart PW, Henderson FW, Ivins SS, Stedman HC and Henry MM (1991), Lung function in school-age children who had mild lower respiratory illnesses in early childhood, *Am Rev Respir Dis*, 144: 655–62.

Tager IB, Segal MR, Speizer FE and Weiss ST (1988), The natural history of forced expiratory volumes. Effect of cigarette smoking and respiratory symptoms, *Am Rev Respir Dis*, 138: 837–49.

Tanner JM, Hayashi T, Preece M and Cameron N (1982), Increase in length of leg relative to trunk in Japanese children and adults from 1957 to 1977: comparison with British and with Japanese Americans, *Ann Human Biol*, 9: 411–23.

Viegi G, Prediletto R, Paoletti P, Carrozzi L di Pede F, Vellutini M, di Pede C, Guintini C and Lebowitz M (1991), Respiratory effects of occupational exposure in a general population sample in North Italy, *Am Rev Respir Dis*, 143: 510–15.

Voter KZ, Henry MM, Stewart PW and Henderson FW (1988), Lower respiratory illness in early childhood and lung function and bronchial reactivity in adolescent males, *Am Rev Respir Dis*, 137: 302–7.

Wald N, Kiryluk S, Darby S, Doll R, Pike M and Peto R (1988), *UK Smoking Statistics*, Oxford: Oxford University Press.

Ware JH, Thibodeau LA, Speizer FE, Colome S and Ferris BJ (1981), Assessment of the health effects of atmospheric sulfur oxides and particulate matter: evidence from observational studies, *Environ Health Perspect*, 41: 255–76.

Warren Spring Laboratory (1972), *National Survey of Air Pollution 1961–71*, vol. 1, Department of Trade and Industry.

Weiss KB (1990), Seasonal trends in US asthma hospitalizations and mortality, *JAMA*, 263: 2323–8.

Whincup PH, Cook DG, Strachan DP and Papacosta O (1993), Time trends in respiratory symptoms in childhood over a 24 year period, *Arch Dis Child*, 68: 729–34.

Williams HC, Strachan D and Hay RH (1992), Eczema and family size, *Clin Res*, 40: 464A.

Winter GF and Inglis JM (1987), Respiratory viruses in children admitted to hospital in Edinburgh 1972–1985, *J Infection*, 15: 103–7.

Woodhouse PR, Khaw K-T, Plummer M, Foley A and Meade TW (1994), Seasonal variations of plasma fibrinogen and factor VII activity in the elderly: winter infections and death from cardiovascular disease, *Lancet*, 343: 435–9.

Xu X, Chrstiani DC, Dockery DW and Wang L (1992), Exposure-response relationships between occupational exposures and chronic respiratory illness: a community-based study, *Am Rev Respir Dis*, 146: 413–18.

Yamaguchi S, Kano K, Shimojo N, Sano K, Xu X, Watanabe H, Kameyama M, Santamaria M, Liu S, Wang L, Chen Y, Song W, Ma F, and Lu L (1988), Risk factors in chronic obstructive pulmonary malfunction and 'chronic bronchitis' symptoms in Beijing district: a joint study between Japan and China, *J Epidemiol Commun Health*, 43: 1–6.

Young RA and Beaumont GE (1941), *Lobar Pneumonia. A Textbook of the Practice of Medicine*, London: Humphrey Milford and Oxford University Press.

Young RA and Beaumont GE (1950), *Asthma. A Textbook of the Practice of Medicine*, London: Humphrey Milford and Oxford University Press.

Young RA, Beaumont GE and Boland ER (1956), *Asthma. Price's Textbook of the Practice of Medicine*, London: Oxford University Press.

Chapter 21 Renal diseases

Balarajan R and Bulusu L (1990), Mortality among migrants in England and Wales, 1978–83, in *Mortality and Geography: a Review in the mid–1980s, England Wales* (ed. Britton M) OPCS series DS no. 9, pp.103–121 (see Appendix tables), London: HMSO.

Beech R, Mandalia S, Melia J, Mays N and Swan A (1993), Purchasing services for end stage renal failure: the potential and limitations of existing information sources, *Health Trends*, 25: 60–4.

Burden AC, NcNally P, Feehally J and Walls J (1992), Increased incidence of endstage renal failure secondary to diabetes mellitus in Asian ethnic groups in the United Kingdom, *Diabet Med*, 9: 641–5.

Burton P and Walls J (1987), Selection adjusted comparison of life expectancy of patients on continuous ambulatory peritoneal dialysis haemodialysis and transplantation, *Lancet*, i: 1115–8.

Cameron JS and Challah S (1986), Treatment of endstage renal failure due to diabetes in the United Kingdom 1975–84, *Lancet*, ii: 962–6

Calne RY, White DJ and Thiru S (1978), Cyclosporin A in patients receiving allografts from cadaver donors, *Lancet*, 2: 1323–7.

Catalano C, Goodship T, Tapson J, Venning MK, Taylor RMR, Proud G, Tunbridge WMG, Elliot RN, Ward MK, Albert: KGMM and Wilkinson R (1990), Renal replacement treatment for diabetic patients in Newcastle upon Tyne and the Northern Region 1964–88, *British Medical Journal*, 301: 535–9.

Challah S, Wing AJ, Bauer R, Morris RW and Schroeder SA (1984), Negative selection of patients for dialysis and transplantation in the United Kingdom, *British Medical Journal*, 288: 1119–22.

Charra B, Chazot C, Calemard E and Laurent G (1993), Survival on renal replacement therapy, *Lancet*, 341: 954.

Clark TJ, Richards N, Adu J and Michael J(1993), Increased prevalence of dialysis dependent renal failure in ethnic minorities in the West Midlands, *Nephrol Dial Transplant*, 8: 146–8.

Dalziell M and Garrett C (1987), Interregional variation in treatment of endstage renal failure, *British Medical Journal*, 294: 1382–83.

DH (1994), *Report of the Health Care Strategy Unit Review of Renal Services. Part II: Evidence for the Review*, London: DH.

European Dialysis and Transplant Association (1992), Report on the Management of Renal Failure in Europe 1991, *Nephrol Dial Transplant*, 7: Suppl 2.

Feest TG, Round A and Hamad S (1993), Incidence of severe acute renal failure in adults: results of a community based study, *British Medical Journal*, 306: 431–83.

Feest TG, Mistry CD, Grimes DS and Mallick NP(1990), Incidence of advanced chronic renal failure and the need for endstage renal replacement therapy, *British Medical Journal*, 301: 897–900.

Gokal R (1992), Chapter 10.1 in *Oxford Textbook of Clinical Nephrology*, vol. 2 (eds Cameron, Davison, Grunfeld, Kerr, Ritz), Oxford: Oxford University Press.

Goldacre MJ (1993), Cause specific mortality: underlying uncertain tips of the disease iceberg, *J Epidemiol Comm Hlth*, 47: 491–6.

Joint Working Party on Diabetic Renal Failure of the British Diabetic Association Renal Association and Research unit of the Royal College of Physicians (1989), Treatment of and mortality from diabetic renal failure in patients identified in the 1985 United Kingdom survey, *British Medical Journal*, 299: 1135–6.

Kazuo O (1992), Vascular access, Chapter 10.1 in: *Oxford Textbook of Clinical Nephrology*, vol. 2 (eds Cameron, Davison, Grunfeld, Kerr, Ritz), Oxford: Oxford University Press.

Kessner DM and Florey C du V (1967), Mortality trends for acute and chronic nephritis and infections of the kidney, *Lancet*, ii: 979–83.

Khan IH, Catto G, Edward N, Fleming L, Henderson I and Macleod AM (1993), Influence of coexisting renal disease on survival on renal replacement therapy, *Lancet*, 341: 415–18.

Khan IH, Catto G, Edward N and MacLeod AM (1994), Chronic renal failure: factors influencing nephrology referral, *QJMed*, 87: 559–64.

Klag MJ, Whelton PK, Randall BL, *et al.* (1996), Blood pressure and endstage renal disease in men, *N Engl J Med*, 334: 13: 180.

Lightstone L, Rees AJ, Tomson C, Walls J, Winnearls CJ and Feehally J (1995), High incidence of endstage renal disease in Asians in the UK, *QJMed*, 88(3): 167–73.

London Renal Services Review Group (1993), Report of an independent review of specialist services in London, *Renal,* London: HMSO.

Mather HM and Keen H (1985), The Southall diabetes survey: prevalence of known diabetes in Asians and Europeans, *British Medical Journal*, 291: 1081–4.

McGeown M (1972), Chronic renal failure in Northern Ireland 1968–70. A prospective survey, *Lancet*, I: 307–10.

McGeown M (1990), Prevalence of advanced renal failure in Northern Ireland, *British Medical Journal*, 301: 900–03.

McMillan M, Briggs J and Junor B (1990), Outcome of renal replacement treatment in patients with diabetes mellitus, *British Medical Journal*, 301: 540–4.

NHS Executive (1996), *Renal Purchasing Guidelines*, London: NHS Executive.

Nicolucci A, Cubasso D, Labbrozzi D *et al* (1992), Effect of coexistent diseases on survival of patients undergoing dialysis, *ASAIO*, 38: M291–5.

Nissenson A (1993), Dialysis treatment in the elderly patient, *Kidney International*, 43: supp 40: 51–7.

OPCS (1990), *Tabular list of the Classification of Surgical Operations and Procedures, 4th revision: consolidated version*, London: HMSO.

OPCS (1987), *Hospital In-patient Enquiry*, OPCS series MB4 no. 26, London: HMSO.

OPCS (1986), *Decennial Supplement*, London: HMSO.

Pendreigh DM, Howitt LF and Heasman MA (1972), Survey of chronic renal failure in Scotland, *Lancet*, i: 304–7.

Perneger TV, Brancasti F, Whelton PK and Klag MJ (1995), Studying the causes of kidney disease in humans: a review of methodologic obstacles and possible solutions, *Am J Kid Dis*, 25: 722–31.

Renal Association (1991), *The Provision of Services for Adult Patients with Renal Disease in the United Kingdom,* London: Renal Association.

Richet G (1991), From Brights Disease to modern nephrology - Pierre Rayers innovative method of clinical investigation, *Kidney Int*, 39: 787–92.

Roderick P, Jones I, Raleigh Vs, McGeown M and Mallick N (1994), Population need for renal replacement therapy in the Thames Regions: the ethnic dimension, *British Medical Journal*, 309: 1111–4.

Roderick PJ, Raleigh VS, Hallam L and Mallick NP (1996), The need and demand for renal replacement therapy in ethnic minorities in England, *J Epidemiol Comm Hlth*, 50: 334-9.

Rostand SG, Kirk KA, Rutsky EA and Pate BA (1982), Racial differences in the incidence of treatment for endstage renal disease, *N Engl J Med*, 306: 1276–1279.

Silbiger S and Neugarten J (1995), The impact of gender on the progression of chronic renal disease, *Am J Kid Dis*, 25: 515–33.

United Kingdom Transplant Support Service Authority (UKTSSA) (1993), *Renal Transplant Audit 1981–91*, Bristol: UKTSSA.

USRDS Annual Report (1992), Comorbid conditions and correlations with mortality risk among 3399 incident haemodialysis patients, *Am J Kid Dis*, 20 Supp 2: 32–38.

Waters WE (1968), Trends in mortality from nephritis and infections of the kidney in England and Wales, *Lancet*, i: 241–3.

Williams B, Burton P, Feehally J and Walls J (1989), The changing face of endstage renal disease in a UK renal unit, *J Royal Coll Physicians*, 23: 116–20.

Working group on the Renal Association Subcommittee on Provision of Treatment for Chronic Renal Failure (1992), *Provision of Services for Adult Patients with Renal Disease in the United Kingdom*, London: Royal College of Physicians of London and the Renal Association.

World Health Organization (1977), *International Classification of Diseases, 9th revision*, vol. 1, London: HMSO.

Wood IT, Mallick NP and Wing AJ (1987), Prediction of resources needed to achieve the national target for treatment of renal failure, *British Medical Journal*, 294: 1467–70.

Chapter 22 Digestive diseases

Addiss DG, Shaffer N, Fowler BS and Tauxe RV (1990), The epidemiology of appendicitis and appendectomy in the United States, *Am J Epidemiol*, 132: 10–25.

Corfield AP, Cooper MJ and Williamson RCN (1985), Acute pancreatitis: a lethal disease of increasing incidence, *Gut*, 26: 724–9.

DHSS, OPCS (1987), *Hospital In-patient Enquiry 1985 main tables*, OPCS series MB4 no. 27, London: HMSO.

DSS (1994), *Social Security Statistics*, London: HMSO.

Donnan SPB and Lambert PM (1976), Appendicitis: incidence and mortality, *Population Trends*, 5: 26–8, London: HMSO.

Fellows IW, Freeman JG and Holmes GKT (1990), Crohn's disease in the city of Derby, 1951–85, *Gut*, 31: 1262–5.

Heaton KW, Braddon FEM, Mountford RA, Hughes AO and Emmett PM (1991), Symptomatic and silent gall stones in the community, *Lancet*, 32: 316–20.

Heaton KW, O'Donnell LJD, Braddon FEM, Mountford RA, Hughes AO, and Cripps PJ (1992), Symptoms of irritable bowel syndrome in a British urban community: consulters and nonconsulters, *Gastroenterology*, 102: 1962–7.

Henry DA, Lim LL-Y, Rodriguez LAG, Gutthann SP, Carson JL, Griffin M, Savage R, Logan R, Moride Y, Hawkey C, Hill S, and Fries JT (1996), Variability and risk of gastrointestinal complications with individual nonsteroidal anti-inflammatory drugs, Results of a collaborative meta-analysis, *Br Med J*, 312: 1563–6.

Lam C-M, Murray FE and Cuschieri A (1996), Increased cholecystectomy rate after the introduction of laparoscopic cholecystectomy in Scotland, *Gut*, 38: 282–4.

Langman MJS (1979), Diverticular disease and appendicitis, in *The Epidemiology of Chronic Digestive Disease* (ed Langman MJS), Arnold, pp.103–13.

Langman MJS, Weil J, Wainwright P, Lawson DH, Rawlins MD, Logan RFA, Murphy M, Vessey MP and Colin-Jones DG (1994), Risks of bleeding peptic ulcer associated with individual non-steroidal anti-inflammatory drugs, *Lancet*, 343: 1075–8.

Lee FI and Nguyen-Van-Tam JS (1994), Prospective study of incidence of Crohn's disease in northwest England: no increase since the late 1970s, *Eur J Gastroenterol Hepatol*, 6: 27–31.

McCormick A, Fleming D and Charlton J (1995), *Morbidity Statistics from General Practice: Fourth National Study 1991–1992*, OPCS series MB5 no. 3, London: HMSO.

Miller DS, Keighley AC and Langman MJS (1974), Changing patterns in epidemiology of Crohn's disease, *Lancet*, 2: 691–3.

Panos MZ, Walt RP, Stevenson C and Langman MJS (1995), Rising death rate from non-malignant disease of the oesophagus (NMOD) in England and Wales, *Gut*, 36: 488–91.

Penston JG, Crombie IK, Waugh NR and Wormsley KG (1993), Trends in morbidity and mortality from peptic ulcer disease: Tayside versus Scotland, *Aliment Pharmacol Ther*, 7: 429–42.

Primatesta P and Goldacre MJ (1994), Appendicectomy for acute appendicitis and for other conditions: an epidemiological study, *Int J Epidemiol*, 23: 155–60.

Rockall TA, Logan RFA, Devlin HB and Northfield TC (1995), on behalf of the steering committee and members of the national audit of acute upper gastrointestinal haemorrhage, *British Medical Journal*, 311: 222–6.

RCGP, OPCS and DHSS (1986), *Morbidity Statistics from General Practice: Third National Study 1981–1982*, OPCS series MB5 no. 1, London: HMSO .

Sinclair TS, Brunt PW and Mowat NAG (1983), Nonspecific proctocolitis in Northeastern Scotland: a community study, *Gastroenterology*, 85: 1–11.

Sonnenberg A (1990), Hospital discharges for inflammatory bowel disease: time trends from England and the United States, *Dig Dis Sci*, 35: 375–81.

Sonnenberg A (1995), Temporal trends and geographical variations of peptic ulcer disease, *Aliment Pharmacol Ther*, 9: 3–12.

Srivastava ED, Mayberry JF, Morris TJ, Smith PM, Williams GT, Roberts GM, Newcombe RG and Rhodes J (1992), Incidence of ulcerative colitis in Cardiff over 20 years: 1968–87, *Gut*, 33: 256–8.

Susser M (1982), Period effects, generation effects and age effects in peptic ulcer mortality, *J Chron Dis*, 35: 29–40.

Thomas GAO, Millar-Jones DM, Rhodes J, Roberts GM, Williams GT and Mayberry JF (1995), Incidence of Crohn's disease in Cardiff over 60 years: 1986–1990 an update, *Eur J Gastroenterol Hepatol*, 7: 401–5.

Walt R, Katschinski B, Logan R, Ashley J and Langman M (1986), Rising frequency of ulcer perforation in elderly people in the United Kingdom, *Lancet*, i: 489–92.

Chapter 23 Musculoskeletal diseases

Allan, Waddell (1991), An historical perspective on low back pain and disability, *Acta Orthopaedica Scandinavica* 60, (suppl. 234): 1–23.

Altman R, Asch E, Bloch D, Bole G, Borenstein D, Brandt K, Christy W, Cooke TD, Greenwald R, Hochberg M, Howell D, Kaplan D, Koopman W, Longley S III, Mankin H, McShane DJ, Medsger T Jr, Meenan R, Mikkelsen W, Moskowitz R, Murphy W, Rothschild B, Segal M, Sokoloff L and Wolfe F (1986), Development of criteria for the classification and reporting of osteoarthritis: classification of osteoarthritis of the knee, *Arthritis and Rheumatism* 29 (8): 1039–49.

Altman R, Alarcon G, Appelrouth D, Bloch D, Borenstein D, Brandt K, Brown C, Cook TD, Daniel W, Feldman D, Greenwald R, Hochberg M, Howell D, Ike R, Kapila P, Kaplan D, Koopman W, Marino C, McDonald E, McShane DJ, Medsger T, Michel B, Murphy WA, Osial T, Ramsey-Goldman R, Rothschild B and Wolfe F (1991), The American College of Rheumatology criteria for the classification and reporting of osteoarthritis of the hip, *Arthritis and Rheumatism* 34 (5): 505–13.

Anderson JJ and Felson D (1988), Factors associated with osteoarthritis of the knee in the first National Health and Nutrition Examination Survey (HANES I): Evidence for an association with overweight, race, and physical demands of work, *American Journal of Epidemiology* 128: 179–89.

Anderson GH, Raymakers R and Gregg PJ (1993), The incidence of proximal femoral fractures in an English county, *Journal of Bone and Joint Surgery*, 75B: 441–4.

Ansell BM and Wood PHN (1976), Prognosis in juvenile chronic polyarthritis, *Clinics in Rheumatic Diseases*, 2: 397–412.

Arnett FC, Edworthy SM, Bloch DA, McShane DJ, Fries JF, Cooper NS, Healey, LA, Kaplan SR, Liang MH, Luthra HS, Medsger TA Jr, Mitchell DM, Neustadt DH, Pinals RS, Schaller JG, Sharp JT, Wilder RL and Hunder GG (1988), The American Rheumatism Association 1987 revised criteria for the classification of rheumatoid arthritis, *Arthritis and Rheumatism*, 31(3): 15–24.

Badley EM and Tennant A (1993), Impact of disablement due to rheumatic disorders in a British population: estimates of severity and prevalence from the Calderdale Rheumatic Disablement Survey, *Annals of the Rheumatic Diseases,* 52: 6–13.

Bannatyne GA, Wohlmann AS and Blaxall FR (1896), Rheumatoid arthritis: its clinical history, aetiology and pathology, *Lancet,* i: 1120–5.

Bennett PH and Wood PHN (eds.) (1968), Population studies of the rheumatic diseases, *Proceedings of the Third International Symposium,* International Congress Series No. 148, Amsterdam: Exerpta Medica Foundation.

Blaxter M (1990), *Health and Lifestyles,* London: Tavistock, Routledge.

Boyce WJ and Vessey MP (1985), Rising incidence of fracture of the proximal femur, *Lancet,* i: 150–1.

Brewerton DA, Caffrey M, Hart DF, James DCO, Nicholls A and Sturrock RD (1973), Ankylosing spondylitis and HL-A27, *Lancet,* i: 904–6.

Calin A, Elswood J, Rigg S and Skerington SM (1988), Ankylosing spondylitis - an analytical review of 1500 patients: the changing pattern of disease, *Journal of Rheumatology,* 15: 1234–8.

Carbone LD, Cooper C, Michet CJ, Atkinson EJ, O'Fallon WM and Melton LJ III (1992), Ankylosing spondylitis in Rochester, Minnesota 1935–1989, *Arthritis and Rheumatism,* 35 (12): 1476–82.

Cohen AS, Reynolds WE, Franklin EC, Kulha JP, Ropes MW, Shulman LE and Wallace SL (1971), Preliminary criteria for the classification of systemic lupus erythematosus, *Bulletin of Rheumatic Disorders,* 21: 643–8.

Cooper C and Melton LJ (1992), Vertebral fractures, *British Medical Journal,* 304: 793–4.

Copeman WSC (1964), *A short History of the Gout and the Rheumatic Diseases,* Berkley, Los Angeles: University of California Press.

Croft P, Coggon D, Cruddas M and Cooper C (1992), Osteoarthritis of the hip: an occupational disease in farmers, *British Medical Journal,* 304: 1269–72.

Cummings SR (1991), Epidemiologic studies of osteoporotic fractures: methodologic issues, *Calciferous Tissue International,* 49, (suppl.): 515–20.

Currie WJC (1979), Prevalence and incidence of the diagnosis of gout in Great Britain, *Annals of the Rheumatic Diseases,* 38: 101–6.

Deyo RA and Tsui-Wu Y-J (1987), Functional disability due to back pain, *Arthritis and Rheumatism,* 30(11): 1247–53.

Dillane JB, Fry J and Kalton G (1966), Acute back syndrome - a study from general practice, *British Medical Journal,* ii: 82–4.

Donaldson LJ, Parsons L and Cook AJ (1989), Death certification in fractured neck of femur, *Public Health,* 103: 237–43.

Dugowson CE, Koepsell TD, Voigt LF, Bley L, Nelson JL and Daling JR (1991), Rheumatoid arthritis in women: incidence rates in group health co-operative, Seattle, Washington 1987–1989, *Arthritis and Rheumatism,* 34 (12): 1502–7.

Dunnel K and Cartwright A (1972), *Medicine Takers, Prescribers and Hoarders,* London: Routledge and Keegan.

Duthie JJR, Brown PE, Truelove LH, Baragar FD and Lawrie AJ (1964), Course and prognosis in rheumatoid arthritis: a further report, *Annals of the Rheumatic Diseases,* 23: 193–202.

Fries JF, Gurkirpal S, Bloch DA and Calin A (1989), The natural history of ankylosing spondylitis: is the disease really changing?, *Journal of Rheumatology,* 16: 860–3.

Frymoyer JW and Cats-Baril WL (1991), An overview of the incidence and costs of low back pain, *Orthopedic Clinics of North America,* 22: 263–71.

Glynn RJ, Campion EW and Silbert JE (1982), Trends in serum uric acid levels 1961–1980, *Arthritis and Rheumatism,* 26(1): 87–93.

Grahame R, Lloyd-Jones K, Swannell AJ and Wood PHN (1986), A report on rheumatology manpower 1986, *British Journal of Rheumatology,* 25: 305–12.

Guccione AA, Felson DT and Anderson JJ (1990), Measuring functional status in elders: methodological issues in the study of disease and disability, *American Journal of Public Health,* 80: 945–9.

Hargraves MM, Richmond H and Morton R (1949), Presentation of two bone marrow elements: the 'tart' cell and the 'LE' cell, *Proceedings of the Staff Meetings of the Mayo Clinic,* 24: 234–7.

Hart DJ, Leedham-Green M and Spector TD (1991), The prevalence of knee osteoarthritis in the general population using different clinical criteria, *British Journal of Rheumatology,* 30, (suppl. 2): 72.

Haserick JR (1950), Blood factor in acute disseminated lupus erythematosus, *Archives of Dermatology,* (Chicago) 61: 889–91.

Hochberg MC (1987), Prevalence of systemic lupus erythematosus in England and Wales, 1981–2, *Annals of the Rheumatic Diseases,* 46: 664–6.

Hochberg MC (1985), The incidence of systemic lupus erythematosus in Baltimore, Maryland 1970–7, *Arthritis and Rheumatism,* 28(1): 80–6.

Hopkinson ND, Doherty M, and Powell RJ (1993), The prevalence and incidence of systemic lupus erythematosus in Nottingham, UK 1989–1990, *British Journal of Rheumatism,* 32: 110–5.

Kellgren JH and Lawrence JS (1958), Osteoarthritis and disc degeneration in an urban population, *Annals of the Rheumatic Diseases,* 17: 388–97.

Kellgren JH, Jeffrey MR and Ball J (1963), *The epidemiology of chronic rheumatism,* vol. 2: Atlas of standard radiographs, Oxford: Blackwell Scientific.

Landré-Beauvais A-J (1800), *Doit-on Admettre une Nouvelle Espéce de Goutte sans la Denomination de Goutte Asthénique Primitive?,* Doctoral Thesis, Paris.

Lawrence JS (1961), Prevalence of rheumatoid arthritis, *Annals of the Rheumatic Diseases,* 20: 11–17.

Lawrence JS (1977), *Rheumatism in Populations,* London: Heinemann.

Lawrence JS (1963), The prevalence of ankylosing spondylitis, *British Journal of Clinical Practice,* 17: 699–705.

Lawrence JS, Bremner JM and Bier F (1966), Osteoarthritis: Prevalence in the population and relationship between symptoms and X-ray changes, *Annals of the Rheumatic Diseases,* 25: 1–24.

Lawrence RC, Everett DF, Coroni-Huntley J and Hochberg MC (1987), Excess mortality and decreased survival in females with osteoarthritis, *Arthritis and Rheumatism,* 30 (4), (suppl.): 130.

Lees B, Molleson T, Arnett TR and Stevenson JR (1993), Differences in proximal femur bone density over two centuries, *Lancet,* 341: 673–5.

Lewis P, Hazleman BL, Hanna R and Roberts S (1980), Cause of death in patients with rheumatoid arthritis with particular reference to azathioprine, *Annals of the Rheumatic Diseases,* 39: 457–61.

Liang M and Komaroff AL (1982), Roentgenograms in primary care patients with acute low back pain: a cost-effectiveness analysis, *Archives of Internal Medicine,* 142: 1108–12.

Logan WPO and Cushion AA (1985), *Morbidity Statistics from General Practice,* vol. 1 (General), London: HMSO.

Martin J and White A (1988), *The Prevalence of Disability among Adults: OPCS Surveys of Disability in Great Britain, Report I,* OPCS Social Survey Division, London: HMSO.

Masi AT, Rodnon GP, Medsger TA Jr, Altman RD, D'Angelo WA, Fries JF, LeRoy EC, Kirsner AB, MacKensie AH, McShane DJ, Myers AR and Sharp GC (1980), Preliminary criteria for the classification of systemic sclerosis (scleroderma), *Arthritis and Rheumatism,* 23(5): 581–90.

Melton LJ III, O'Fallon WM and Riggs BL (1987), Secular trends in the incidence of hip fractures, *Calciferous Tissue International,* 41: 57–64.

Melton LJ III, Chrischilles EA and Cooper C et al (1992), How many women have osteoporosis?, *Journal of Bone and Mineral Research,* 7: 1005–10.

Miller SWM and Evans JG (1985), Fractures of the distal forearm in Newcastle: an epidemiological study, *British Medical Journal,* 14: 155–8.

Mixter WJ and Barr JS (1934), Rupture of the intervertebral disc with involvement of the spinal canal, *New England Journal of Medicine,* 211: 210–5.

Monson RR and Hall AP (1976), Mortality among arthritics, *Journal of Chronic Diseases,* 29: 459–67.

Nordin BEC, Peacock M, Aaron J, Crilly RG, Heyburn PJ, Horsman A and Marshall D (1980), Osteoporosis and osteomalacia, *Clinics in Endocrinology and Metabolism*, 9: 177–204.

Nossent JC (1992), Systemic lupus erythematosus on the Caribbean island of Curaçao: an epidemiological investigation, *Annals of the Rheumatic Diseases*, 51: 1197–201.

OPCS (1989), *General Household Survey*, London: HMSO.

Osler W (1904), On the visceral manifestations of the erythema group of skin diseases, *American Journal of Medical Science*, 127: 1–23.

Papageorgiou AC and Rigby AS (1991), Review of UK data on the rheumatic diseases, 7 Low back pain, *British Journal of Rheumatology*, 30: 208–10.

Pedersen PA (1981), Prognostic indicators in low back pain, *Journal of the Royal College of General Practitioners*, 31: 209–16.

Pope MJ, Rosen JC, Wilder DG and Frymoyer JW (1980), The relation between biomechanical and psychological factors in patients with low back pain, *Spine*, 5: 173–8.

Prior P, Symmons DPM, Scott DL, Brown R and Hawkins CF (1984), Cause of death in rheumatoid arthritis, *British Journal of Rheumatology*, 23: 2–9.

Reilly PA, Cosh JA, Maddison PJ, Rasker JJ and Silman AJ (1990), Mortality and survival in rheumatoid arthritis: a 25 year prospective study of 100 patients, *Annals of the Rheumatic Diseases*, 49: 363–9.

Ropes MW, Bennett G, Cobb S, Jacox R and Jessar R (1958), A revision of diagnostic criteria for rheumatoid arthritis, *Bulletin on the Rheumatic Diseases*, 9: 175–6.

Rose HM, Ragan C, Pearce E and Lipman MO (1948), Differential agglutination of normal and sensitized sheep erythrocytes by sera of patients with rheumatoid arthritis, *Proceedings of the Society of Experimental Biology and Medicine*, 68: 1–6.

Rothschild BM and Woods RJ (1990), Symmetrical erosive disease in Archaic Indians: The origin of rheumatoid arthritis in the New World?, *Seminars in Arthritis and Rheumatism*, 19: 278–84.

RCGP, OPCS and DHSS (1979), *Morbidity Statistics from General Practice: Second National Study 1970–71*, London: HMSO.

RCGP, OPCS and DHSS (1988), *Morbidity Statistics from General Practice: Third National Study 1981–82*, London: HMSO.

RCGP, OPCS and DH (1995), *Morbidity Statistics from General Practice: Fourth National Study 1991–92*, London: HMSO.

Samanta A, Feehally J, Roy S, Nichols FE, Sheldon PJ and Wallis J (1991), High prevalence of systemic disease and mortality in Asian subjects with systemic lupus erythematosus, *Annals of the Rheumatic Diseases*, 50: 490–2.

Samanta A, Roy S, Feehally J and Symmons DPM (1992), The prevalence of diagnosed systemic lupus erythematosus in Whites and Indian Asian immigrants in Leicester City, UK, *British Journal of Rheumatism*, 31: 679–82.

Scott DL, Symmons DPM, Coulton BL and Popert AJ (1987), Long-term outcome of treating rheumatoid arthritis: results after 20 years, *Lancet*, i: 1108–11.

Siegel M and Lee SL (1973), The epidemiology of systemic lupus erythematosus, *Seminars in Arthritis and Rheumatism*, 3: 1–54.

Silman AJ, Davies P, Currey HLF and Evans SJW (1983), Is rheumatoid arthritis becoming less severe? *Journal of Chronic Diseases*, 36: 891–7.

Silman AJ (1988), Has the incidence of rheumatoid arthritis declined in the United Kingdom?, *British Journal of Rheumatology*, 27: 77–9.

Silman A, Jannini S, Symmons D and Bacon P (1988), An epidemiological study of scleroderma in the West Midlands, *British Journal of Rheumatology*, 27: 286–90.

Silman AJ (1991), Mortality from scleroderma in England and Wales 1968–1985, *Annals of the Rheumatic Diseases*, 50: 95–6.

Smith PG and Doll R (1982), Mortality of patients with ankylosing spondylitis after a single treatment course of x-rays, *British Medical Journal*, 284: 499–500.

Spector TD, Cooper C and Fenton LA (1990), Trends in admissions for hip fracture in England and Wales 1968–1985, *British Medical Journal*, 300: 1173–4.

Spector TD, Hart DJ and Powell RJ (1993), Prevalence of rheumatoid arthritis and rheumatoid factor in women: evidence for a secular decline, *Annals of the Rheumatic Diseases*, 52: 254–7.

Steen V, Conte C, Santoro D, Casterline GLZ, Oddis CV and Medsger TA Jr (1988), Twenty year incidence survey of systemic sclerosis, *Arthritis and Rheumatism*, 31(4) (suppl.): A117.

Still GF (1897), On a form of chronic joint disease in childhood, *Medico-Chirurgical Transactions*, 80: 47–59.

Symmons DPM, Jones S and Hothersall TE (1991a), Rheumatology manpower in the 1990s, *British Journal of Rheumatology*, 30: 119–22.

Symmons DPM, van Hemert AM, Vandenbroucke JP and Valkenburg HA (1991b), A longitudinal study of back pain and radiological changes in the lumbar spine of middle aged women, I, Clinical findings, *Annals of the Rheumatic Diseases*, 50: 158–61.

Symmons DPM, Barrett EM, Bankhead C, Chakravarty K, Scott DGI and Silman AJ (1994), The incidence of rheumatoid arthritis in the United Kingdom: results from the Norfolk Arthritis Register, *British Journal of Rheumatology*, 33: 275–9.

Tan E, Cohen A, Fries J, Masi AT, McShane DJ, Rothfield NF, Schaller JG, Talal N and Winchester RJ (1982), The 1982 revised criteria for the classification of systemic lupus erythematosus, *Arthritis and Rheumatism*, 25(11): 1271–7.

Vandenbroucke JP, Valkenburg HA, Boersma JW, Festen JJM and Cats A (1982), Oral contraceptives and rheumatoid arthritis: further evidence for a preventive effect, *Lancet*, ii: 830–42.

Waaler E (1940), On the occurrence of a factor in human serum activating the specific agglutination of sheep blood corpuscles, *Acta Pathologica et Microbiologica Scandinavica*, 17: 172–88.

Waddell G (1992), Biopsychosocial analysis of low back pain, *Baillière's Clinical Rheumatology*, 6: 523–57.

Wallace SL, Robinson H, Masi AT, Decker JL, McCarty DJ and Yu T'S-F (1977), Preliminary criteria for the classification of the acute arthritis of primary gout, *Arthritis and Rheumatism*, 20(3): 895–900.

Walsh K, Cruddas M and Coggan D (1992), Low back pain in eight areas of Britain, *Journal of Epidemiology and Community Health*, 46: 227–30.

Wells N (1985), *Back Pain*, London: Office of Health Economics.

Williams M, Frankel S, Nanchahal K, Coast J and Donovan J (1992a), *Total Hip Replacement*, Bristol: Health Care Evaluation Unit.

Williams M, Frankel S, Nanchahal K, Coast J and Donovan J (1992b), *Total Knee Replacement*, Bristol: Health Care Evaluation Unit.

Wilson WA and Hughes GRV (1979), Rheumatic diseases in Jamaica, *Annals of the Rheumatic Disorders*, 38: 320–5.

Winner SJ, Morgan CA and Evans JG (1989), Perimenopausal risk of falling and incidence of distal forearm fracture, *British Medical Journal* 298: 1486–8.

Wood PHN (1978), Special meeting on nomenclature and classification of arthritis in children, in *The Care of the Rheumatic Child* (ed. Munthe E), EULAR Monograph Series No 3, pp. 47–50: Basle.

Chapter 24 Accidents: trends in mortality and morbidity

Boyce WJ and Vessey MP (1985), Rising incidence of fracture of the proximal femur, *Lancet*, i: 150–151.

Breeze E, Trevor G and Wilmont A (1991), *General Household Survey 1989*, OPCS series GHS no. 20, London: HMSO.

Broughton J and Stark DC (1987), *The Effect of the 1983 Changes to the Law relating to Drink/Driving*, Research Report 106, Road Safety Division, Crowthorne: Transport and Road Research Laboratory (TRRL).

Broughton J (1987), *The Effect on Motorcycling of the 1981 Transport Act*, Research Report 106, Road Safety Division, Crowthorne: Transport and Road Research Laboratory (TRRL).

Chinn BP (1991), Motorcycle safety, in *Conference Proceedings, Safety 91*, Crowthorne: Transport and Road Research Laboratory (TRRL).

Christian MS and Bullimore DW (1989), Reduction in accident: severity in rear seat passengers using restraints, *Injury*, 20: 262–4.

Department of Health (1993 (i)), *The Health of the Nation, Key area handbook, Accidents*, Department of Health, London: HMSO.

Department of Health (1993 (ii)), *Hospital Episode Statistics, vol. 1, Finished consultant episodes by diagnosis, operation and specialty: England, financial year 1989–90, 1990–91, 1991–92, 1992–93*, London: DoH.

Department of Trade and Industry (1987), *Home Accident Surveillance System, Tenth Annual Report: 1986 data*, London: DTI.

Department of Trade and Industry (1993), *Consumer Safety Unit, Report on 1993 Accident data on safety research*, London: Home Accident Surveillance System.

Department of Transport (1975–94), *Road Accidents Great Britain 1974–93*, London: HMSO.

Department of Employment and Productivity (1971), *British Labour Statistics Historical Abstract 1886–1968*, London: HMSO.

Dewis M (1995), *Tolley's Health and Safety at Work Handbook, 1995, A comprehensive practical guide to health and safety law and practice*, British Safety Council, London: RoSPA.

DHSS and OPCS (1973), *Report on Hospital In-patient Enquiry for the year 1972, Preliminary Tables*, London: HMSO.

DHSS, OPCS, and Welsh Office (1982), *Hospital In-patient Enquiry, 1981, Summary Tables*, OPCS series MB4 no. 17, London: HMSO.

DHSS and OPCS (1983), *Hospital In-patient Enquiry, Summary Tables*, OPCS series MB4 no. 17, London: HMSO.

DoE and HSE (1989), Health and safety statistics 1986–87, *Employment Gazette*, Occasional Supplement no. 1: 97: (2) February.

DoE and HSE (1992), Health and safety statistics 1990–1, *Employment Gazette*, Occasional Supplement no. 3: 100: (9) September.

Drownings in the UK (1993), RoSPA.

Harvey AC and Durbin J (1986), The effects of seat belt legislation on British road casualties: A case study in structural time series modelling, *Journal of the Royal Statistical Society (A)*, 149: 187–227.

Health and Safety Commission (1995), *Annual Report 1994–5*, London: HMSO.

Health and Safety Commission (1993), *Annual Report Statistical Supplement 1992/3*, London: HMSO.

Health and Safety Executive (1988), *Health and Safety Statistics 1985–86*, London: HMSO.

McCormick A, Fleming D and Charlton J (1995), *Morbidity Statistics from General Practice 1991/2: Fourth National Study*, OPCS series MB5 no. 3, London: HMSO.

Nicholl JP, Coleman P and Williams BT (1993), *Injuries in Sport and Exercise: Main report*, London: The Sports Council of England.

OPCS (1985–1993), *Fatal Accidents occurring during Sporting and Leisure Activities*, OPCS Monitor, series DH4.

RCGP, OPCS and DHSS (1974), *Morbidity Statistics from General Practice 1971–2: Second National Study*, Studies in Medical and Population Subjects no. 36, London: HMSO.

RCGP, OPCS and DHSS (1984), *Morbidity Statistics from General Practice 1981–2: Third National Study*, OPCS series MB5 no. 1, London: HMSO.

Sabey BE (1995), Engineering safety on the road, *Injury Prevention*, 1(3): 182–186.

Sabey BE (1980), *Road Safety and Value for Money, Supplementary Report 581*, Accident Investigation Safety Division, Crowthorne: Transport and Road Research Laboratory.

Sheffield Health Authority (1995), Information Directorate personal communication.

Spector TD, Cooper C and Fenton-Lewis A (1990), Trends in admission for hip fracture in England and Wales 1968–1985, *British Medical Journal*, 300: 1173–4.

Stevens G (1992), Workplace Injuries: a view from HSE's Trailer to the 1990 Labour Force Survey, *Employment Gazette*, 100(1) December.

Watson GS, Zadar PL and Wilks A (1981), Helmet use, helmet use laws and motorcycle fatalities, *American Journal of Public Health*, 71(3): 297–300.

Wood T and Milne P (1988), Head injuries to the pedal cyclists and the promotion of helmet use in Victoria, *Accident Analysis and Prevention*, 1988: 20(3): 177–85.

Zadar PL and Ciccone MA (1993), Automobile driver fatalities in fatal impact: air bags compared with manual belts, *American Journal of Public Health*, 83: 661–6.

Chapter 25   Are we healthier?

Bennett N, Dodd T, Flatley J, Freeth S and Bolling K (1995), *Health Survey for England 1993*, Series K HS no 3, London: HMSO.

Bone M, Bebbington AC, Jagger C, Morgan K and Nicolaas G (1995), *Health Expectancy and its Uses*, London: HMSO.

Botting B (ed.), *The Health of our Children 1995*, London: HMSO.

Chief Medical Officer (1993), *On the State of the Public Health 1992*, London: HMSO.

Colhoun H and Prescott-Clark P (eds) (1996), *Health Survey for England 1994*, Series HS no.4, London: HMSO.

Department of Health (1995), *Fit for the Future, Second Progress Report on the Health of the Nation*, London: Department of Health.

Dunnell K (1991), Deaths among 15–44-year-olds, *Population Trends* 64, London: HMSO.

General Household Survey reports (annual), London: HMSO.

OPCS (1995), *GHS report for 1993*, London: HMSO.

OPCS (1996), *Living in Britain, report for 1994*, London: HMSO.

Martin J, Meltzer H and Elliot D (1988), *Prevalence of Disability among Adults*, London: HMSO.

Meltzer H, Gill B, Petticrew M and Hinds K (1995), *The Prevalence of Psychiatric Morbidity among Adults living in Private Households*, London: HMSO.

OPCS (1994), *Mortality Statistics – General, 1992*, Series DH1 no. 27, London: HMSO.

Todd JE and Lader D (1991), *Adult Dental Health 1988*, London: HMSO.

Chapter 26   The health and health care of older adults in England and Wales, 1841–1994

Abel-Smith B (1964), *The Hospitals 1800–1948*, London: Heinemann.

Abrams M (1951), *Social Surveys and Social Action*, London: Heinemann.

Adelstein A and Ashley J (1980), Recent trends in mortality and morbidity in England and Wales, in *Demographic Patterns in Developed Societies* (ed. Hiorns), London: Taylor & Francis Ltd.

Alderson MR and Ashwood F (1985), Projection of mortality rates for the elderly, *Population Trends*, 42: 22–9.

Alter G and Riley JC (1989), Frailty, sickness and death: models of morbidity and mortality in historical populations, *Population Studies*, 43: 25–46.

Aniansson A and Gustafsson E (1981), Physical training in elderly men with special reference to quadriceps muscle strength and morphology, *Clinical Physiology*, 1: 87–98.

Anonymous (1985), Geriatrics for all?, *Lancet*, i: 674–5.

Arie T and Isaacs AD (1978), The development of psychiatric services for the elderly in Britain, in *Studies in Geriatric Psychiatry* (eds Isaacs AD and Post F), Chichester: John Wiley & Sons, pp. 241–61.

Barker DJP (1992) (ed), *Fetal and Infant Origins of Adult Disease*, London: British Medical Journal.

Barker W (1987), *Adding Life to Years, Organized Geriatric Services in Great Britain and Implications for the United States*, Baltimore: John Hopkins University Press.

Barrett JC (1985), The mortality of centenarians, *Archives of Gerontology & Geriatric Medicine*, 4: 211–18.

Barrett JC (1986), The mortality of centenarians: a correction, *Archives of Gerontology & Geriatric Medicine*, 5: 81.

Bebbington AC and Darton RA (1996), *Healthy Life Expectancy in England and Wales: recent evidence*, Personal Social Services Research Unit, University of Kent, Discussion Paper 1205, Canterbury: University of Kent.

Benjamin B (1987), The demographic outlook, in *Pensions, the problems of today and tomorrow* (eds Benjamin B, Haberman S, Helowicz G, Kaye G and Wilkie D), London: Allen & Unwin.

Benjamin B and Overton E (1981), Prospects for mortality decline in England and Wales, *Population Trends*, 23: 22–8.

Birmingham Research Unit of the Royal College of General Practitioners (BRU, 1976), *Trends in National Morbidity*, London: Royal College of General Practitioners.

Blessed G and Wilson I (1982), The contemporary natural history of mental disorder in old age, *British Journal of Psychiatry*, 141: 59–67.

Bone M, Gregory J, Gill B and Lader D (1992), *Retirement and Retirement Plans*, London: HMSO.

Bone M, Bebbington A, Jagger C, Morgan K, and Nicholaas G (1996), *Health Expectancy and Its Uses*, London: HMSO. Chapter on: Calculations of trends in health expectancies 1976–1992.

Booth C (1894), *The Aged Poor in England and Wales*, London: Macmillan.

Bosanquet N and Gray A (1989), *Will you still love me? New Opportunities for Health Services for Elderly People in the 1990s and Beyond*, Birmingham: National Association of Health Authorities.

Boshuizen HC and van de Water HPA (1994), *An International Comparison of Health Expectancies*, TNO Report 94.06. Leiden: TNO.

Bourdelais P (1993), Review of 'Population âgées et révolution grise', *Population Studies*, 47: 177–8.

Bourgeois-Pichat J (1979), La transition démographique: vieillissement de la population, in *Population Science in the Service of Mankind*, Liége: IUSSP.

Bowling A (1991), *Measuring Health, a Review of Quality of Life Measurement Scales*, Milton Keynes: Open University Press.

Bowling A, Farquhar M, Grundy E and Formby J (1992), Psychiatric morbidity among people aged 85+ in 1987: A follow-up study at two and a half years: associations with changes in psychiatric morbidity, *International Journal of Geriatric Psychiatry*, 7: 307–21.

Branch LG and Jette AM (1982), A prospective study of long-term care institutionalization among the aged, *American Journal of Public Health*, 72: 1373–9.

Bury M (1992), The future of aging – changing perceptions and realities, in *Textbook of Geriatric Medicine and Gerontology*, 4th edn (eds Brocklehurst JC, Tallis RC and Fillitt HM), Edinburgh: Churchill Livingstone, pp.21–5.

Campbell J, Diep C, Reinken J, and McCosh L (1985), Factors predicting mortality in a total population sample of the elderly, *Journal of Epidemiology and Community Health*, 39: 337–42.

Carnegie Inquiry into the Third Age (1993), *Life, Work and Livelihood in the Third Age*, Dunfermline: Carnegie UK Trust.

Carrier N (1962), Demographic aspects of the aging of the population, in *Society, Problems and Methods of Study* (eds Welford AT, Argyle M, Glass DV and Morris JW), London: Routledge & Kegan Paul.

Christie A (1983), Changing patterns in mental illness in the elderly, *British Journal of Psychiatry*, 140: 154–9.

Colvez A and Blanchet M (1981), Disability trends in the United States population 1966–76: analysis of reported causes, *American Journal of Public Health*, 71: 464–71.

Cooper B (1991), The epidemiology of dementia, in *Psychiatry in the Elderly* (eds Jacoby R and Oppenheimer C), Oxford: Oxford University Press.

Crimmins E, Saito Y and Ingegneri D (1989), Changes in life expectancy and disability-free life expectancy in the United States, *Population and Development Review*, 15: 235–67.

DHSS (1989), *Caring for People, community care in the next decade and beyond*, London: HMSO.

Donaldson LJ (1992), Health and health care of elderly people, in *The Health of Elderly People, an Epidemiological Overview*, vol. II, Companion papers, Central Health Monitoring Unit, London: HMSO.

Elo IT and Preston SH (1992), Effects of early life conditions on adult mortality: a review, *Population Index*, 58: 186–212.

Evans JG (1985), Epidemiology of aging, in *Practical Geriatric Medicine* (eds Exton-Smith AN and Weksler ME), Edinburgh: Churchill Livingstone.

Evans JG, Goldacre MJ, Hodkinson HM, Lamb S and Savory S (1992), *Health and Abilities in the Third Age*, London: Carnegie UK Trust.

Finsen V (1988), Improvements in general health among the elderly: a factor in the rising incidence of hip fractures?, *Journal of Epidemiology and Community Health*, 42: 200–3.

Forsdahl A (1977), Are poor living conditions in childhood and adolescence an important risk factor for arteriosclerotic heart disease?, *British Journal of Preventive Social Medicine*, 31: 91–5.

Forsdahl A (1978), Living conditions in childhood and subsequent development of risk factors for arteriosclerotic heart disease, *Journal of Epidemiology and Community Health*, 32: 34–7.

Fries J (1980), Aging, natural death and the compression of morbidity, *New England Journal of Medicine*, 303: 130–5.

Gage TB (1993), The decline in mortality in England and Wales 1861–1964, *Population Studies*, 47: 47–66.

Gavrilov LA and Gavrilova NS (1991), *The Biology of Life Span: a quantitative approach*, London: Harwood Academic Publishers.

Gilleard L, Pattie A and Dearnan G (1980), Behavioural disabilities in psychogeriatric patients and residents of old people's homes, *Journal of Epidemiological and Community Health*, 34: 196–210.

Gonnot JP (1992), Changes in life expectancy and their impact on age distribution, in *Demographic Causes and Economic Consequences of Population Aging* (ed. Stolnitz GJ), New York: United Nations.

GRO (1958), *Morbidity Statistics from General Practice, 1955–56* (vols I–III), Studies on Medical and Population Subjects no. 14, London: HMSO.

Gruenberg EM (1977), The failures of success, *Millbank Memorial Fund Quarterly*, 55: 3–24.

Gruenberg HM and Hagnell O (1987), The rising prevalence of chronic brain syndrome in the elderly, in *Society, Stress and Disease* (ed. Levi L), vol.5 'Old Age', Oxford: Oxford University Press.

Grundy E (1987), Future patterns of morbidity in old age, in *Advanced Geriatric Medicine 6* (eds Caird, FI and Evans JG), Bristol: Wright.

Grundy E (1992a), The epidemiology of aging, in *Textbook of Geriatric Medicine and Gerontology*, 4th edn, (eds Brocklehurst, JL Tallis RC and Fillit HM), Edinburgh: Churchill Livingstone, pp.1–20.

Grundy E (1992b), Socio-demographic variations in rates of movement into institutions among elderly people in England and Wales: an analysis of linked census and mortality data 1971–1985, *Population Studies*, 46: 65–84.

Grundy E (1992c), The living arrangements of elderly people, *Reviews in Clinical Gerontology*, 2: 353–61.

Grundy E (1993), Moves into supported domestic environments among elderly people in England and Wales, *Environment and Planning A*, 25: 1467–79.

Harris A (1968), *Social Welfare for the Elderly*, London: HMSO.

Harris A (1971), *Handicapped and Impaired in Great Britain*, Part 1. London: HMSO.

Harris C (1987), Social ageing in the Macmillan era, *Continuity and Change* 2: 477–96.

Heikkenen E, Jokela J and Jylhn M (1996), Disability and functional status among elderly people: cross national comparisons, in Caselli Gard Lopez AD, *Health and Mortality among Elderly Populations*, Oxford: Clarendon press, pp.202-20.

Helowicz G (1987), A look at the past, in *Pensions: the Problems of Today and Tomorrow* (eds Benjamin B, Haberman S, Helowicz G, Kaye G and Wilkie D), London: Allen & Unwin.

Henretta JC (1994), Recent trends in retirement, *Reviews in Clinical Gerontology*, 4: 71–81.

Honigsbaum F (1979), *The Division in British Medicine*, London: Kogan Page.

Horrocks P (1982), The case for geriatric medicine as an age defined speciality, in *Recent Advances in Geriatric Medicine, II* (ed. Isaacs B), Edinburgh: Churchill Livingstone, pp.259–78.

Humphreys NA (1885) (ed.), William Farr, Vital Statistics, *A Memorial Volume of Selections from the Reports and Writings of William Farr*, London: Edward Stanford.

Hunt A (1978), *The Elderly at Home*, London: HMSO.

Johnson P (1989), The structured dependency of the elderly: a critical note, in *Growing Old in the Twentieth Century* (ed. Jeffreys M), London: Routledge, pp.62–72.

Katz S, Branch LG, Branson MH, Papsidero JA, Beck JC, Greer DS (1983), Active life expectancy, *New England Journal of Medicine*, 309: 1218–24.

Kay DWK, Beamish P and Roth M (1964), Old age mental disorders in Newcastle-upon-Tyne, I: A study of prevalence, *British Journal of Psychiatry*, 110: 146–58.

Kirkwood TBL (1988), The nature and causes of aging, in *Research and the Aging Population* (eds Evered D and Whelan J), CIBA Foundation Symposium 134, Chichester: John Wiley.

Kogevinas E (1990), *Socio-demographic Influences in Cancer Survival*, OPCS series LS no. 5, London: HMSO.

Kramer M (1984), The rising pandemic of mental disorders and associated chronic diseases and disabilities, *Acta Psychiatricus Scandinavica*, 62: suppl.285.

Laing W and Buisson (1991), *Care of elderly people market survey 1990–1991*.

Laslett P (1989), *A Fresh Map of Life: The Emergence of the Third Age*, London: Weidenfeld & Nicolson.

Lee R and Lam D (1983), Age distribution adjustments for English censuses 1821 to 1931, *Population Studies*, 37: 455–64.

Lin T (1953), A study of the incidence of mental disorder in Chinese and other cultures, *Psychiatry*, 16: 313–36.

Logan WPD and Brooke EM (1957), *The Survey of Sickness 1943–1952*, London: HMSO.

Logan WPD and Cushion AA (1958), *Morbidity Statistics from General Practice*, London: HMSO.

Manton KG (1982), Changing concepts of morbidity and mortality in the elderly population, *Millbank Memorial Fund Quarterly*, 60: 133–224.

Manton KG and Stallard E (1984), *Recent Trends in Mortality Analysis*, New York: Academic Press.

Martin J, Meltzer H and Elliot D (1988), *OPCS Surveys of Disability in Great Britain*, Report 1, London: HMSO.

McCormick A, Fleming D, Charlton J (1995), *Morbidity Statistics from General Practice: Fourth National Study, 1992–92*, OPCS series MB5 no. 3, London: HMSO.

McCormick A and Rosenbaum M (1990), *Mortality Statistics from General Practice. Third National Study: Socio-economic Analyses*, OPCS series MB5 no. 2, London: HMSO.

McPherson K and Coleman D (1988), Health, in *British Social Trends since 1900* (ed. Halsey AH), 2nd edn, Basingstoke: Macmillan.

Murphy MJ and Grundy E (1993), Co-residence of the elderly and household structure in Britain: aspects of change in the 1980s, in *Solidarity of Generations, Demographic, Economic and Social Change and its Consequences* (eds HA Becker and PLJ Hemken), Amsterdam: Thesis Publishers.

Notestein F (1954), Some demographic aspects of aging, *Proceedings of the American Philosophical Society*, 98: 229–33.

Olshansky SJ and Carnes BA (1996), Prospect for extended survival: a critical review of the biological evidence, in Caselli Gard Lopez AD, *Health and mortality among elderly populations*, Oxford: Clarendon Press, pp.202–20.

OPCS (1973 to 1993), *The General Household Survey*, Introductory Report and reports for subsequent years 1972–1991, London: HMSO.

OPCS (1981), *Trends in Respiratory Mortality 1951–1975*, OPCS series DHI no. 7, London: HMSO.

OPCS (1985), *Mortality Statistics: Cause*, OPCS series DH2 no. 11, Introduction – 'Rule 3', London: HMSO.

OPCS (1986), *Mortality Statistics*, OPCS series DH1 no. 16, Introduction – 'Rule 3', London: HMSO.

OPCS (1987), *Birth Statistics 1837–1983*, OPCS series FM1 no. 13, London: HMSO.

OPCS (1990), *Adult Dental Health 1988*, OPCS Monitor SS90/1, London: OPCS.

OPCS (1993), *Census Newsletter* no.27, London: OPCS.

Parker S (1980), *Older Workers and Retirement*, London: HMSO.

Phillipson C (1982), *Capitalism and the Construction of Old Age*, London: Macmillan.

Pinker R (1966), *English Hospital Statistics 1861–1938*, London: Heinemann.

Preston SH (1976), *Mortality Patterns in National Populations*, New York: Academic Press.

Quadagno J (1982), *Aging in Early Industrial Society: Work, Family and Social Policy in Nineteenth Century England*, London: Academic Press.

Ratcliffe H (1850), *Observations on the Rate of Mortality and Sickness Existing Among Friendly Societies, Particularized for Various Trades, Occupations and Localities*, Manchester: Manchester Unity of the Independent Order of Odd Fellows.

RCGP, OPCS and DH (1974), *Morbidity Statistics from General Practice: Second National Study, 1970–71*, OPCS Studies on Medical and Population Subjects 26, London: HMSO.

RCGP, OPCS and DH (1979), *Morbidity Statistics from General Practice: Second National Study, 1971–72*, OPCS Studies on Medical and Population Subjects 36, London: HMSO.

RCGP, OPCS and DH (1982), *Morbidity Statistics from General Practice, 1970–71: Socio-economic Analysis*, OPCS Studies on Medical and Population Subjects 46, London: HMSO.

RCGP, OPCS and DH (1986), *Morbidity Statistics from General Practice: Third National Study, 1981–82*, OPCS series MB5 no. 1, London: HMSO.

RCGP, OPCS and DH (1990), *Morbidity Statistics from General Practice, Third Morbidity Study: Socioeconomic Analysis 1981–82*, OPCS series MB5 no. 2, London: HMSO.

Richardson IM (1964), *Age and Need: a study of older people in North East Scotland*, Edinburgh: E and S Livingstone Ltd.

Riley J (1990), The risk of being sick: morbidity trends in four countries, *Population and Development Review*, 16: 403–32.

Robine JM, Blanchet M and Dowd JE (eds) (1992), *Health Expectancy. First Workshop of the International Healthy Life Expectancy Network (Reves)*, OPCS Studies on Medical and Population Subjects 54, London: HMSO.

Rothenberg R, Lentzner H and Parker R (1991), Population aging patterns: the expansion of morality, *Journal of Gerontology*, 46: S66–70.

Royal Commission on the Aged Deserving Poor (1895), *Report*, vol. 1, London: HMSO.

Royal Commission on National Health Insurance (1926), Appendix A: *Reports of the Departmental Actuarial Committee*, London: HMSO.

Ruzicka L and Kane P (1990), Health transition: the course of morbidity and mortality, in *What We Know About Health Transition: the cultural, social and behavioural determinants of health* (eds Caldwell J *et al*), vol. 1, Canberra: Health Transition Centre, Australian National University.

Ruigomez A, Alonso J, Anto JM (1993), Functional capacity and five year mortality in a sample of urban community elderly, *European Journal of Public Health*, 3: 165–71.

Sheldon JH (1948), *The Social Medicine of Old Age*, Oxford: Oxford University Press.

Shock NW (1983), Aging and physiological systems, *Journal of Chronic Diseases*, 36: 137–42.

Siegel JS (1992), *A Generation of Change: A Profile of America's Older Population*, New York: Russell Sage Foundation.

Smith FB (1979), *The People's Health*, London: Croom Helm.

Smith RM (1991), Introduction, in *Life, Death and the Elderly: historical perspectives* (eds Pelling M and Smith RM), London: Routledge.

Stocks P (1949), *Sickness in the Population of England and Wales 1944–1947*, Studies on Medical and Population Subjects 2, London: HMSO.

Strawbridge WJ, Kaphu GA, Camacho T and Cohen RD (1992), The dynamics of disability and functional change in an elderly cohort: results from the Alameda County study, *Journal of the American Geriatrics Society*, 40: 799–806.

Svanborg A (1988), The health of the elderly population: results from longitudinal studies with age-cohort comparisons, in *Research and the Aging Population* (eds Evered D and Whelan J), CIBA Foundation Symposium 134, Chichester: John Wiley.

Thatcher AR (1981), Centenarians in England and Wales, *Population Trends*, 25: 11–14.

Thomson D (1984), The decline of social welfare: falling state support for the elderly since early Victorian times, *Ageing and Society*, 4: 451–82.

Tinker A (1992), *Elderly People in Modern Society*, 3rd edn, London: Longman.

Tout K (1989), *Ageing in Developing Countries*, Oxford: Oxford University Press.

Townsend P (1962), *The Last Refuge: A survey of residential institutions and homes for the aged in England and Wales*, London: Routledge.

Townsend P (1981), Future policy trends: problems of implementation and their resolution, in *The Provision of Care for the Elderly* (eds Kinnaird J, Brotherston J and Williamson J), Edinburgh: Churchill Livingstone.

Townsend P and Wedderburn D (1965), *The Aged in the Welfare State*, London: G. Bell.

US Bureau of the Census (1992), Current Population Reports, Series P95/92–2, *Population and Health Transitions*, Washington DC: US Government Printing Office.

Vaupel JW, Manton KL and Stallard E (1979), The impact of heterogeneity in individual frailty on the dynamics of mortality, *Demography*, 16: 439–54.

Verbrugge L (1984), Longer life but worsening health? Trends in health and mortality in middle-aged and older persons, *Millbank Memorial Fund Quarterly*, 62: 475–19.

Victor CR (1989), Inequalities in health in later life, *Age and Ageing*, 18: 387–91.

Waldron I (1986), What do we know about sex differences in mortality? *Population Bulletin*, no. 18. New York: United Nations.

Walker A (1980), The social creation of poverty and dependency in old age, *Journal of Social Policy*, 9:49–75.

Warren MW (1946), Care of chronic aged sick, *Lancet*, 1: 841–3.

Warren MW (1948), The evolution of a geriatric unit, *Geriatrics*, 3: 47–50.

Warren MD and Knight R (1985), Mortality in relation to the functional capacities of people with disabilities living at home, *Journal of Epidemiology and Community Health*, 36: 220–3.

Weiner JM, Hanley RJ, Clark R and van Nostrand JF (1990), Measuring the activities of daily living: comparisons across national surveys, *Journal of Gerontology*, 45: S229–37.

Werner B (1987), Fertility statistics from birth registrations in England and Wales 1837–1987, *Population Trends*, 48: 4–10.

Wilkin D, Mashian T and Jolley D (1978), Changes in the behavioural characteristics of elderly populations of local authority homes and long-stay hospital wards 1976–77, *British Medical Journal*, ii: 1274–6.

Williamson J, Stokoe IH, Gray S, Fisher M, Smith A, McGhee A and Stephenson E (1964), Old people at home – their unreported needs, *Lancet*, i: 1117–20.

Wilmoth JR, Curtsinger JW and Horiuchi S (1995), *Rectangularisation Revisited: Survival Curves for Humans and Fruit Flies*, Paper presented at the annual meeting of the Population Association of America, San Francisco, 6–8 April 1995.

Winter J (1985), *The Great War and the British People*, London: Macmillan.

Wood E, Whitfield E and Christie A (1991), Changes in survival in demented hospital inpatients 1957–1987, *International Journal of Geriatric Psychiatry*, 6: 523–8.

Chapter 27   Trends and prospects at very high ages

Craig J (1983), The growth of the elderly population, *Population Trends*, 32: 28–33.

Fries JF (1980), Ageing, natural death and the compression of morbidity, *New England Journal of Medicine*, 303: 130–5.

Grundy E (1984), Mortality and morbidity amongst the old, *British Medical Journal*, 288: 663–4.

OPCS (1993), *National population projections 1991–based*, London: HMSO.

Perls TT (1995), The oldest old, *Scientific America*, January, 50–5.

Thatcher AR (1981), Centenarians, *Population Trends*, 25: 11–14.

Thatcher AR (1992), Trends in numbers and mortality at high ages in England and Wales, *Population Studies*, 46: 411–16.

Index

Printed in the United Kingdom
for The Stationery Office
4/97   N0008463